Cognitive impairment and dementia in Parkinson's disease

Errata

Cognitive Impairment and Dementia in Parkinson's Disease
Murat Emre, 9780199681648

pp. 9–12: *for citations* 30–94 *read* 29–93
pp. 81–85: *for citations* 18–36 *read* 17–35; *for citations* 41–66 *read* 36–61

Cognitive impairment and dementia in Parkinson's disease

SECOND EDITION

Edited by

Murat Emre

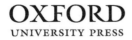

OXFORD

UNIVERSITY PRESS

OXFORD
UNIVERSITY PRESS

Great Clarendon Street, Oxford, OX2 6DP,
United Kingdom

Oxford University Press is a department of the University of Oxford.
It furthers the University's objective of excellence in research, scholarship,
and education by publishing worldwide. Oxford is a registered trade mark of
Oxford University Press in the UK and in certain other countries

© Oxford University Press 2015

The moral rights of the author have been asserted

First Edition published in 2010
Second Edition published in 2015

Impression: 1

Published in the United States of America by Oxford University Press
198 Madison Avenue, New York, NY 10016, United States of America

British Library Cataloguing in Publication Data

Data available

Library of Congress Control Number: 2014946888

ISBN 978-0-19-968164-8

Printed and bound by
CPI Group (UK) Ltd, Croydon, CR0 4YY

Preface to the second edition

The first edition of *Cognitive impairment and dementia in Parkinson's disease* was published 5 years ago. The book was well received by the scientific community, confirming that it filled a gap and satisfied an unmet need.

The first publication of the book proved to be timely. Since then, the topic of cognitive impairment and dementia in Parkinson's disease has become increasingly popular, and there have been a number of developments in the field, including new data on the natural course, clinical features, pathological correlates, neuroimaging, and treatment of this condition. Hence, we decided to work on a new edition of the book which would include these recent developments. All the authors of the original chapters kindly agreed to revise their contributions to reflect the new findings; I am very grateful to them. In the meantime, mild cognitive impairment in Parkinson's disease has been better recognized, criteria for its diagnosis have been published, and there has also been increasing interest in biomarkers of cognitive dysfunction and dementia. We decided to include several new chapters covering these topics.

We hope that the new edition of the book will be as useful for the scientific community as the previous one and that it will continue to serve as a major reference source for cognitive impairment and dementia in Parkinson's disease.

Murat Emre
İstanbul, December 2014

Contents

Contributors

Dag Aarsland
Karolinska Institutet, Department
of Neurobiology, Care Sciences and Society,
Alzheimer's Disease Research Center,
Stockholm, Sweden

Guido Alves
Norwegian Centre for Movement Disorders,
Stavanger University Hospital, Stavanger,
Norway

Clive Ballard
Wolfson Centre for Age-Related Diseases,
King's College London,
London, UK

Roger A. Barker
Department of Neurology and Cambridge
Centre for Brain Repair,
Addenbrooke's NHS Trust,
Cambridge, UK

Paolo Barone
University of Salerno, Department
of Medicine, Fisciano, Salerno, Italy

Alexandra Bernadotte
Karolinska Institutet, Department
of Neurobiology, Care Sciences and Society,
Alzheimer's Disease Research Center,
Stockholm, Sweden

Kolbjørn Brønnick
Norwegian Centre for Movement Disorders,
Stavanger University Hospital, Stavanger,
Norway

David J. Burn
Institute for Ageing and Health, Newcastle
University, Newcastle upon Tyne, UK

Elise Caccappolo
Department of Neurology, Columbia
University Medical Center, New York,
New York, USA

Gordon W. Duncan
Clinical Ageing Research Unit,
Newcastle University, Campus for Ageing
and Vitality, Newcastle upon
Tyne, UK

Murat Emre
İstanbul Faculty of Medicine, Department
of Neurology, Behavioral Neurology
and Movement Disorders Unit, İstanbul
University, İstanbul, Turkey

Michael J. Firbank
Institute for Ageing and Health, Wolfson
Research Centre, Newcastle General Hospital,
Newcastle upon Tyne, UK

Paul T. Francis
Wolfson Centre for Age-Related Diseases,
King's College London, London, UK

Sara Garcia-Ptacek
Department of Neurobiology, Care Sciences
and Society (NVS), Karolinska Institutet,
Stockholm, Sweden

Nir Giladi
Department of Neurology and Sagol School
of Neuroscience, Tel Aviv University and
Department of Neurology, Tel Aviv Sourasky
Medical Center, Tel-Aviv, Israel

Rita Guerreiro
Department of Molecular Neuroscience,
Institute of Neurology, University College
London, London, UK

John Hardy
Reta Lila Weston Institute, UCL Institute
of Neurology, London, UK

Alex Iranzo
Neurology Service, Institute of Neurosciences,
Hospital Clinic and University of Barcelona,
Barcelona, Spain

Jeffrey M. Hausdorff
Department of Physical Therapy and Sagol
School of Neuroscience, Tel Aviv University
and Department of Neurology, Tel Aviv
Sourasky Medical Center,
Tel Aviv, Israel

Jaime Kulisevsky
Sant Pau Hospital Universitat Autònoma
de Barcelona; CIBERNED (Centro de
Investigación Biomédica en Red sobre
Enfermedades Neurodegenerativas), Instituto
de Salud Carlos III, Madrid; and Universitat
Oberta de Catalunya, Barcelona, Spain

Guttalu K. Kumaraswamy
Medical University of South Carolina,
Department of Neurosciences, Movement
Disorders Program, Charleston, South
Carolina, USA

Jan Petter Larsen
Norwegian Centre for Movement Disorders,
Stavanger University Hospital, Stavanger,
Norway

Carol F. Lippa
Memory Disorders Program, Drexel
University College of Medicine, Philadelphia,
Pennsylvania, USA

Eugenia Mamikonyan
University of Pennsylvania, Department
of Geriatric Psychiatry, Philadelphia,
Pennsylvania, USA

Karen Marder
Columbia University, College of Physicians
and Surgeons, New York, New York, USA

Ian McKeith
Institute for Ageing and Health, Newcastle
University, Wolfson Research Centre, Campus
for Ageing and Vitality,
Newcastle upon Tyne, UK

Anat Mirelman
Department of Neurology, Tel Aviv Sourasky
Medical Center, Tel Aviv, Israel

Yoshikuni Mizuno
Juntendo University School of Medicine,
Tokyo, Japan

Judith Navarro-Otano
Neurology Service, Institute of Neurosciences,
Hospital Clinic and University of Barcelona,
Barcelona, Spain

John T. O'Brien
Institute for Ageing and Health, Wolfson
Research Centre, Newcastle General Hospital,
Newcastle upon Tyne, UK

Yasuyuki Okuma
Department of Neurology, Juntendo
University Shizuoka Hospital, Izunokuni,
Japan

Javier Pagonabarraga
Sant Pau Hospital Universitat Autònoma
de Barcelona and CIBERNED (Centro
de Investigación Biomédica en Red sobre
Enfermedades Neurodegenerativas), Instituto
de Salud Carlos III, Madrid, Spain

Kenn Freddy Pedersen
Norwegian Centre for Movement Disorders,
Stavanger University Hospital, Stavanger,
Norway

Elaine K. Perry
Institute for Ageing and Health, Newcastle
University, Campus for Ageing and Vitality,
Newcastle upon Tyne, UK

Margaret Ann Piggott
Institute for Ageing and Health, Newcastle
University, Campus for Ageing and Vitality,
Newcastle upon Tyne, UK

Gonzalo J. Revuelta
Medical University of South Carolina,
Department of Neurosciences, Movement
Disorders Program, Charleston,
South Carolina, USA

Gabriella Santangelo
Department of Neurological Sciences,
University of Napoli Federico II, Napoli,
Italy

Andrew Singleton
Molecular Genetics Section
and Laboratory of Neurogenetics,
National Institutes of Health, Bethesda,
Maryland, USA

Inger van Steenoven
Section of Geriatric Psychiatry, Rogaland
Psychiatric Hospital, Stavanger, Norway

Eduardo Tolosa
Neurology Service, Institute of Neurosciences,
Hospital Clinic and University of Barcelona,
Barcelona, Spain

Daniel Weintraub
University of Pennsylvania, Department
of Psychiatry and Neurology, Philadelphia,
Pennsylvania, USA

David Whitfield
Wolfson Centre for Age-Related Diseases,
King's College London, London, UK

Caroline H. Williams-Gray
Department of Neurology and Cambridge
Centre for Brain Repair, Addenbrooke's NHS
Trust, Cambridge, UK

Sophie E. Winder-Rhodes
Department of Neurology and Cambridge
Centre for Brain Repair, Addenbrooke's NHS
Trust, Cambridge, UK

Alison J. Yarnall
Institute for Ageing and Health, Newcastle
University, Newcastle upon Tyne, UK

Jenny Zitser
Department of Neurology, Tel Aviv Sourasky
Medical Center, Tel Aviv, Israel

Chapter 1

Introduction

Murat Emre

James Parkinson was more than a physician. One of his biographers records that 'Like many of his contemporaries he had absorbing and overwhelming interests which ranged successively, and successfully, through politics, the church, medicine and geology' and that 'James was a careful, perhaps obsessional, man' [1]. He had many intellectual skills, but above all he was a sharp and succinct observer, which enabled him to find associations no one had described before, resulting in discoveries and descriptions in medicine, geology, and palaeontology which still bear his name. Yet Parkinson's *An essay on the shaking palsy*, which otherwise so succinctly described the features of the disease that was later named after him, almost completely dismissed its mental aspects. He described the characteristic features of the disease as 'Involuntary tremulous motion with lessened muscular power, in parts not in action and even when supported, with a propensity to bend the trunk forwards and to pass from a walking to a running pace: the senses and intellects being uninjured' [2]. This statement, 'senses and intellects being uninjured', was probably one of the main reasons why mental dysfunction in Parkinson's disease (PD) was ignored for a long time to come, although his general description of the final stages of the disease ends with the statement that 'The urine and faeces are passed involuntarily; and at the last, constant sleepiness, with slight delirium, and other marks of extreme exhaustion, announce the wished-for release'. This brief statement on likely mental dysfunction attracted little attention as it was rather equivocal. Parkinson was honest about the potential shortcomings of his descriptions, as he admits in the opening remarks in his Preface: 'it therefore is necessary, that some conciliatory explanation should be offered for the present publication: in which, it is acknowledged, that mere conjecture takes the place of experiment; and, that analogy is the substitute for anatomical examination, the only sure foundation for pathological knowledge'. He realized that early and late stage symptoms may be different, stating that:

> The disease is of long duration: to connect, therefore, the symptoms, which occur in its later stages with those which mark its commencement, requires a continuance of observation of the same case, or at least a correct history of its symptoms, even for several years. Of both these advantages the writer has had the opportunities of availing himself; and has hence been led particularly to observe several other cases in which the disease existed in different stages of its progress.

Parkinson was a modest and unassuming man; true to form, he ended his opening remarks as follows: 'Should the necessary information be thus obtained, the writer will repine at no censure which the precipitate publication of mere conjectural suggestions may incur; but shall think himself fully rewarded by having excited the attention of those, who may point out the most appropriate means of relieving a tedious and most distressing malady'. He did excite attention for decades to come, for which he received well-deserved credit and recognition. His concluding remarks were exemplary and constitute a timely reminder for all contemprorary clinical scientists: 'Before concluding these pages, it may be proper to observe once more, that an important object proposed to be obtained by them is, the leading of the attention of those who humanely employ anatomical examination in detecting the causes and nature of diseases, particularly to this malady. By their benevolent labors its real nature may be ascertained and appropriate modes of relief, or even cure, pointed out'.

Why would such an excellent observer miss or ignore the mental aspects of the disease? The reasons are probably rather simple: James Parkinson did not observe a large number of patients—his essay was based on the study of only six. Two of them were 'casually met with in the street' (one aged 62 and the other about 65), questioned and observed once, while for a third case 'the particulars of which could not be obtained, and the gentleman, the lamented subject of which was only seen at a distance'. He personally attended to the other three patients, two of them in their 50s, and the third was examined at the age of 72, with a disease duration ranging from about 5–12 years. One of these patients was lost to follow-up after the first examination, and probably only one was followed to his terminal stages. Of particular note is that five of his six cases were seen at a relatively young age. We now know that age is the most important risk factor for dementia and that it rarely occurs in patients below the age of 60 years.

In fact, the occurrence of cognitive dysfunction and dementia in some patients with what came to be known as PD was recognized shortly after the description by Parkinson himself. Charcot, who in his *Lectures on diseases of the nervous system* (1877) called the disease 'maladie de Parkinson', stated that 'at a given point, the mind becomes clouded and the memory is lost'. Together with Vulpian, Charcot had already referred to these aspects of the disease during 1861–2: 'in general, psychic faculties are definitely impaired'. Nevertheless these statements attracted little attention, and for many years PD was perceived to be a pure motor disorder.

As patients with PD survived for substantially longer with modern dopaminergic treatment, cognitive dysfunction and dementia became more apparent. Descriptions from the 1960s onwards pointed out that dementia may accompany PD. Even then, it was assumed that dementia in PD (PD-D) may be a consequence of the ageing process, as ageing was recognized to be the main risk factor for PD-D. The observation that PD-D is frequently accompanied by Alzheimer's disease (AD)-type pathology, in particular plaques, subsequently led to the contention that PD-D simply represents coincident AD. This perception delayed the recognition of PD-D as a separate entity. Subsequently, however, prospective epidemiological studies clearly demonstrated that both the prevalence and incidence of dementia in PD are substantially increased compared with age-matched controls, indicating that dementia was related to the disease pathology itself. With the refinement of neuropsychological methods and an understanding of the circuits subserving discrete mental processes, the clinical profile of PD-D was better worked out in comparative studies, demonstrating the differences between PD-D and AD. In parallel, comprehensive clinico-pathological studies were conducted, which gained particular momentum after the discovery that α-synuclein is the main component of Lewy bodies (LB). The development of immunohisto-chemistry using antibodies against this protein, which turned out to be more sensitive in detecting LB-type pathology than the conventional ubiquitin staining, was crucial in dissecting out the underlying pathology. All these developments were instrumental in the recognition of PD-D as a separate entity and dementia as an integral part of the disease spectrum of PD.

The consequences of considering dementia as part of the pathological substrate of PD are not only academic. As PD patients survive for longer due to more efficient treatment for their motor symptoms, cognitive deficits and dementia occur more often and constitute one of the main reasons for severe disability in the later stages of the disease. These deficits are not responsive to dopaminergic substitution and often worsen under such treatment. Hence, understanding and managing all aspects of PD-D are of practical relevance for patients and their families. Full recognition of its clinical features would allow accurate diagnosis as well as development of assessment measures to evaluate the natural course of the disease and the potential benefits of future treatments. Understanding the associated biochemical deficits, pathophysiology, and pathology would allow such potential treatments to be developed.

Much has already been achieved. Major epidemiological studies have produced valuable data about the point prevalence, cumulative incidence, and risk factors associated with PD-D. A number of clinical studies have been able to discern the profile of cognitive deficits and the frequency as well as the spectrum of accompanying behavioural symptoms. Comprehensive clinico-pathological correlation studies have successfully described the type and topography of the underlying pathology, and genetic findings have provided data supporting the role of α-synuclein. Finally, specific clinical diagnostic criteria have been published and the first specific treatment has become available.

The purpose of this book is to compile in one volume the data that have accumulated over the course of the last few decades. Physicians treating patients with PD will be able to find information on all aspects of the disease without the need for time-consuming searches. It is also hoped that this book could lead to more interest in PD-D, giving rise to new ideas and research initiatives. It would be appropriate to echo James Parkinson's concluding remarks: the editor and the authors of this book would feel fulfilled and satisfied if this latter purpose is served.

References

1. **Gardner-Thorpe C.** *James Parkinson, 1755–1824.* Exeter: A Wheaton & Co. Ltd, 1988.
2. **Parkinson J.** *An essay on the shaking palsy.* London: Whittingham & Rowland, 1817.

Chapter 2

Epidemiology of dementia associated with Parkinson's disease

Dag Aarsland and Alexandra Bernadotte

Introduction

Studies of the frequency of dementia in Parkinson's disease (PD) have used a variety of methods and designs, and this may affect the outcome. Important methodological features include tests to assess cognition, definitions of dementia, and the criteria for selecting patients. For example, results vary according to whether attempts were made to identify all patients in a defined region or whether the study was based on convenience samples from hospital clinics. The optimal method for case identification is a door-to-door survey, but few studies have used this method to report the prevalence or incidence of PD with dementia (PD-D) in the general population. Most studies have been cross-sectional, providing an estimate of the proportion of PD patients who have dementia (point prevalence). For several reasons, including the higher mortality rate in people with PD-D versus PD patients without dementia [1], more accurate information regarding the true frequency of PD-D can be drawn from longitudinal studies. Such studies provide information on the incidence of PD-D. Furthermore, if a healthy control group is included, such studies can also deduce the relative increase in the risk of developing dementia related to PD pathology. In addition, by combining prevalence, incidence, and mortality rates, period prevalence, i.e. the proportion of people with dementia in a PD cohort during a specified time, provides important information concerning the total proportion of PD patients who will eventually develop dementia.

Point prevalence

In a 1988 review of 27 studies representing 4336 patients with PD, Cummings [2] found a mean prevalence of dementia of 40%. Although the studies were critically considered, most were based on patients who had been referred to neurology clinics and might therefore not be representative of unselected PD populations. Also, at that time studies did not include the identification and exclusion of patients with dementia with Lewy bodies (DLB).

In 2005, a systematic review was conducted employing strict methodological inclusion and exclusion criteria; it included 13 studies with a total of 1767 patients [3]. Of these, 554 were diagnosed with dementia, yielding a prevalence of 31.3% (95% confidence interval 29.2–33.6). This review also included 24 studies that explored the prevalence of dementia in the general population and included patients with PD. In this analysis 3–4% of patients with dementia in the general population had PD-D. The estimated prevalence of PD-D in the general population aged 65 years and over was found to be 0.3–0.5% [3]. The results of studies published after this review are in line with these findings, reporting rates of dementia in PD of 48% [4], 35% [5], 23% [6], and 22% [7]. In a recent German study of 886 people with PD, 28% were found to suffer from dementia, increasing from 13.8% in those under 65 years to 40.2% in those aged over 76 [8].

Incidence

Most studies on the incidence of PD-D have been based on longitudinal studies of community-based cohorts. These studies have reported incidence rates per 1000 PD patients per year of 54.7 [9] in the UK, 95.3 [10] in Norway, and 112.5 [11] in the United States, indicating that about 10% of people with PD will develop dementia per year.

The relative risk for developing dementia in PD patients compared with people without PD has been reported to be 1.7 [11], 2.6 [9], 4.7 [7], 5.1 [4], and 5.9 [10]. There are several reasons for this variation, including case selection procedures, definitions of dementia, and the use of different estimates of risk.

Whereas most incidence studies have explored the probability of developing dementia in defined PD populations, the frequency of dementia in PD patients as part of a large, prospective, population-based cohort study of the general population has been recently reported in some studies. In the MRC Cognitive Function and Ageing Study [12], all subjects aged 65 years and over living in defined geographical regions of the UK were invited to participate, and more than 13 000 participants had a screening interview. Participants were assessed at baseline and in two follow-up waves. The proportion of PD patients among those with dementia was 2% at 2 years and 3% at 6 years after baseline, compared with 1% in those without dementia, and the total adjusted odds ratio for PD-D compared with non-PD dementia was 3.5 (1.3–9.3).

The Rotterdam study was based on a door-to-door survey of nearly 8000 people aged 55 years and above at baseline in 1990–3 [7]. Two follow-up visits were performed, and patients were diagnosed with prevalent PD at baseline ($n = 99$) and incident PD during follow-up ($n = 67$). The mean follow-up time was 6.9 years (4.3 years in the incident PD group). During follow-up, 15% of the prevalent PD group developed dementia compared with 4.9% of the control group, with a hazard ratio of 2.80 (1.79–4.38). In the incident cohort, the hazard ratio was 4.74 (2.49–9.02). The association of PD with dementia was more pronounced in those with at least one *APOE* ε4 allele, compared with ε3 carriers.

The majority of 'incidence' studies of PD-D have been longitudinal studies of prevalence cohorts, meaning that patients with a variety of disease durations have been followed. Since the risk for developing dementia depends on the duration of disease, variations among cohorts in the duration of PD will affect the incidence of dementia. Thus, following patients from the onset of their disease provides a more accurate and representative estimate of the incidence of PD-D. In the first study of PD-D based on an incident PD cohort, the CamPaIGN (Cambridgeshire Parkinson's Incidence from GP to Neurologist) study, 180 PD patients were re-examined 3 and 5 years after baseline. The annual incidence of dementia was 30 (16–53) per 1000 person-years [13]. In addition to the shorter duration of disease, the lower incidence of dementia may also be related to the younger age at baseline in this cohort compared with most prevalence studies (Table 2.1). In a subsequent analysis of the CamPaIGN cohort after 10 years, the incidence of dementia in the PD cohort was 54.7 per 1000 person-years, which was 2.6 times higher than the estimated incidence of dementia in the general Cambridgeshire population aged over 65 years [9]. In a prospective population-based incidence study of 182 cases in Norway, the ParkWest study, the overall incidence of PD-D was 20.5 per 1000 person-years [14].

In an incidence study over 15 years in Olmsted, MN, United States, 542 incident cases of PD were identified, and the incidence of PD-D in the population was 2.5 per 100 000 person-years. The incidence of PD-D was similar in men and women, but increased with age and was 47.0 in people aged 80–99 years [15].

Table 2.1 Studies of the incidence and relative risk for dementia in patients with PD

Study	Population	No. of PD patients	Age at baseline (years)	Duration of PD at baseline assessment (years)	Rate/1000 per year	Relative risk of dementia in PD (95% CI)	Country
Mayeux, 1990 [16]	Incident[a]	249	71.4	4.75	69		USA, New York
Marder, 1995 [17]	Community[a]	140	71	7	113	1.7 (1.1–2.7)	USA, New York
Hughes, 2000 [18]	Hospital	83	64	4	43	–	UK
Aarsland, 2001 [10]	Community[a]	130	70	8.5	95	5.9 (3.9–9.1)	Norway
Hobson, 2005 [19]	Community[a]	86	74	7	107	5.1 (2.1–12.5)	North Wales
De Lau, 2005 [7]	Incident[b]	67	–	–	–	4.7 (2.5–9.0)	Netherlands
Hely, 2005 [21], 2008 [20]	Incident[a]	136	71.6	10.9	44	2.3	Australia
Buter, 2008 [22]	Incident	233	75	8	82	5.9	Norway
Williams-Gray, 2013 [9]	Incident[a]	121	70.2		54.7	2.5	UK
Savica, 2013 [15]	Community[a]	542[c]	80+		47		USA, Minnesota
Pedersen, 2013 [14]	Incident[a]	182	67.5	2.3	20.5		Norway
Perez, 2012 [23]	Community[a]	44	82.4	6.8	74	2.5 (1.55–3.95)	France

[a] Aged 65+.

[b] Door-to-door survey of whole population.

[c] Cases of parkinsonism, including DLB and PD-D.

Period (cumulative) prevalence

Since the mortality is higher among PD-D patients than PD patients without dementia [1], point prevalence is an underestimate of the true frequency of PD-D. Accordingly, reporting the cumulative proportion of PD patients who develop dementia with time provides a more accurate estimate of the frequency of PD-D. Some, but not all, longitudinal studies have controlled for the selected attrition due to death. Thus, merely adding up the number of patients who develop dementia before they die will underestimate the true proportion with dementia. Another potential bias is the interval between assessments, since attrition due to death increases with the duration of the interval.

The Sydney study [24] prospectively followed newly diagnosed PD patients to assess the frequency of dementia over more than 10 years. In that study, 149 patients with carefully diagnosed PD were recruited from neurologists for inclusion in a clinical trial. Patients were assessed at baseline with a comprehensive neuropsychological assessment, and 17% were classified as having dementia, defined as impairment of memory and two additional cognitive domains [24] (these patients would thus have been classified today as having DLB). After 3 and 5 years, 26 and 28%, respectively, had dementia [24]. After 15 years, 48% of the evaluated patients had dementia and a further 36% had evidence of cognitive impairment; only 15% had no evidence of cognitive impairment [21]. Recently, data from a 20-year follow-up were presented [20], reporting that 83% of the 30 survivors had dementia after 20 years, and altogether 75% had developed dementia prior to death. No attempt to control for selective attrition due to death was made.

The Stavanger Parkinson study [25] was based on a prevalence cohort of people with PD in south-western Norway, after a careful extensive search in the community. At baseline, the average duration of PD was 9 years, and 28% of the cohort had dementia. After 8 years, after adjustment for mortality, the cumulative prevalence of dementia was found to be 78% [25]. Based on the 12-year follow-up period, Markov analysis was performed to enable a more precise estimate of the risk of developing dementia for an individual patient based on age, gender, and duration of PD [22]. Without correcting for attrition due to death the proportion who developed dementia was stable at about 60%, but the cumulative prevalence steadily increased to 80–90% by the age of 90.

More specifically, at the age of 70 a man with PD but no dementia has a life expectancy of 8 years, of which 3 years would be expected to be with dementia. At any age, the life expectancy after onset of dementia was substantially reduced. At 12-year follow-up [22], only 10% of the population were alive and without dementia after having suffered from PD for an average of 19 years. In the CamPaIGN study, the cumulative probability of dementia after 10 years was 46% [9].

Time to dementia in PD

The majority of studies report that the mean duration from onset of PD to the development of dementia is about 10 years [11, 18, 21]. There are, however, wide variations. In a study with two large community-based cohorts of patients with PD, a linear relationship was found between time from onset of PD to the diagnosis of dementia. Whereas some patients develop cognitive impairment and subsequent dementia within a few years of disease onset, others remain free from dementia for 20 or more years [11, 26]. The time from onset of PD to dementia is related to clinical risk factors and the type and extent of brain pathology [27]. As well as demonstrating a high risk for the development of PD-D, the Sydney and Stavanger studies also convincingly demonstrated that even after decades with PD there are some people who remain free of dementia. Thus, in addition to identifying the risk factors for developing PD-D, a key research question is to identify factors which protect against dementia in long-standing PD. Similarly, since the vast majority of PD patients will eventually develop dementia, another important question is to identify factors that are associated with the time to develop dementia.

Risk factors for dementia in PD

Many demographic and clinical features have been assessed as potential risk factors for dementia in PD. The most consistent risk factors in longitudinal studies are more severe parkinsonism, in particular non-tremor dominant parkinsonism, higher age, olfactory dysfunction, and mild cognitive impairment (MCI) at baseline, visual hallucinations (VH), and rapid eye movement sleep behaviour disorder (RBD) (Table 2.2).

Table 2.2 Risk factors for dementia in patients with PD

Risk factor	Risk rate
Parkinsonism	Increased risk [1]
Age	Nine-fold increased risk in group over 80 years compared with group aged 50–59 years [15]. Four- to six-fold increased risk in group over 76 years of age compared with those <65 years [8, 28]
Mild cognitive impairment	Risk increased 3–3.9-fold [14, 30]
Olfactory dysfunction	Twenty-fold higher [31]
Visual hallucinations	Four-fold increased risk [31]
Rapid eye movement sleep behaviour disorder	Two-fold increased risk [32]
Gender	1.7-fold increased risk for men [15]
Genetics	Increased cumulative risk
Cerebrovascular factors	Increased risk [33–36]

Parkinsonism

Patients with severe parkinsonism have increased risk for dementia, but there is evidence that the risk of dementia differs among different parkinsonian symptoms. In one study, speech and axial impairment, thought to be predominantly due to non-dopaminergic deficits, was found to predict incident dementia, whereas dopaminergic symptoms, such as rigidity and bradykinesia, were not [1].

The motor profile may vary with time, the most common change being transition from tremor dominance to the postural instability and gait disturbance (PIGD) type, and in nearly all dementia cases dementia is preceded by PIGD-dominant disease, or by transition from tremor-dominant to PIGD type [1, 37, 38]. In the CamPaIGN study, the severity of non-tremor type PD (i.e. mixed or PIGD type) was associated with a higher risk for dementia, independent of age [13]. A meta-analysis confirmed that patients with non-tremor pre-dominant symptoms had more severe cognitive decline than those with tremor-dominant symptoms [39].

Age

The majority of studies have found that age and age at onset are both associated with a higher risk of dementia. This is not surprising, given that age is the most prominent risk factor for dementia in the general population. Interestingly, age and the severity of motor symptoms seem to have a combined rather than an additive effect on the risk of dementia [1]. Age, disease duration, and age at onset are highly correlated in PD cohorts, and thus it can be difficult to disentangle their relative importance, i.e. whether it is age, disease duration, or age of onset of PD that is driving the age-associated risk for dementia. Some studies suggest that age, but not age at onset or duration of disease, is the key risk factor for PD-D. The incidence of PD-D increases consistently with age [15], and ageing seems to play a substantial role in the pathogenesis through an interaction with the disease process in non-dopaminergic structures.

Mild cognitive impairment

Many PD patients have MCI which does not significantly influence daily functioning, and thus the criteria for dementia are not fulfilled. In 2012, a Movement Disorders Society Task Force proposed criteria for PD-MCI [40]. There is good evidence that approximately 25% of PD patients without dementia have MCI [41], and that 15–20% of PD patients have MCI even at the time of diagnosis and before dopaminergic treatment [42–45].

Longitudinal studies suggest that MCI represents an early stage on the trajectory to dementia, at least in some patients. In a cohort of patients with advanced PD, more than 60% of PD patients with cognitive impairment had developed dementia compared with only 20% of those with normal cognition [30]. Similarly, in the CamPaIGN study, those with evidence of cognitive impairment at disease onset had a higher risk of dementia [13].

In the ParkWest incident PD study, 27% of those with MCI converted to dementia within 3 years of follow-up, compared with <1% of patients without MCI [14]. Of note, some patients with MCI reverted to normal cognition. In a 5-year study, the proportion with MCI increased, and all patients who developed dementia had MCI at an earlier assessment [46].

The overall pattern of cognitive impairment in PD differs from that in Alzheimer's disease (AD) [47], but there is considerable cognitive heterogeneity even within PD. Some patients exhibit a typical executive–visuospatial impairment, whereas others show a more memory-dominant impairment. We found numerical evidence of some difference in the risk for dementia among patients with PD and different cognitive profiles [30]. This was also found in the CamPaIGN study, where patients with impairment in tests with a more posterior cortical basis, including semantic memory, had a higher risk for developing dementia than those with impairment in tests depending on frontal functions [13, 48].

Visual hallucinations

VH are among the most characteristic neuropsychiatric features of PD, and may even aid in the differentiation of PD from other parkinsonian disorders [49]. VH are associated with both a higher rate of cognitive decline [50] and a higher risk for development of dementia [25, 31]. The association of VH with dementia is probably related to VH being associated with both Lewy body pathology in the temporal lobe, particularly in the amygdala [51], and cholinergic deficits [52]. Patients who develop VH soon after the initiation of dopaminergic treatment are also at higher risk of developing dementia [53].

Rapid eye movement sleep behaviour disorder

RBD is another common and characteristic symptom of PD. Rates of MCI are about six to seven times higher in PD patients with RBD compared with PD patients without RBD [54], and RBD in PD is a marker for earlier onset of PD-D compared with PD patients without RBD [32, 55]. RBD is associated with a lower Braak neurofibrillary tangle stage and much lower neuritic plaque scores [56, 57]. Of note, it may be more difficult to diagnose RBD in PD patients than in those without PD [56, 58, 59].

Olfactory dysfunction

The risk of dementia is higher in PD patients with severe hyposmia than in those who do not exhibit olfactory dysfunction. Furthermore, severe hyposmia is correlated with profound cerebral atrophy which can be observed before the onset of dementia. It has been shown that hyposmia and visuoperceptual impairment should be considered as independent risk factors for future PD-D [31].

Cerebrovascular risk factors

Cerebrovascular disease is common in the elderly and is associated with cognitive decline; it may thus contribute to PD-D as well. There is, however, inconsistent evidence regarding the role of cerebrovascular disease in PD-D. Some studies have shown that cerebrovascular risk factors are not associated with PD-D [33–36], whereas others suggest that chronic cerebral hypoperfusion with large and small vessel disease negatively affects cognition in PD [34, 60, 61].

Genetics

The genetics of PD has received much attention during the last decade, but few studies have systematically explored the potential relationship between genetics and PD-D. There is some evidence of an association between genes and the risk of PD-D [63]. In a recent large historical cohort study, a higher risk for cognitive impairment and dementia was found in relatives of PD patients compared with relatives of control subjects, particularly for patients with an early age of onset of PD [64].

The gene dosage of *SNCA*, the gene encoding α-synuclein, has been found to be a cause of autosomal dominant PD, late-onset PD, disease progression, and the development of dementia [65–70]. Compared with duplication, triplication of the *SNCA* gene is associated with a higher risk of PD-D. Mutations in the glucocerebrosidase gene (*GBA*) represent the most prevalent genetic risk factor for the development of cognitive decline in PD patients [71–73]. The autosomal recessive genes *PARK2*, *PINK1* (formerly *PARK6*), and *PARK7* correlate with an early onset of PD and seem to have a good prognosis regarding cognitive impairment and dementia [67, 74]. Mutation in the leucine-rich repeat kinase 2 gene (*LRRK2*) is the most frequent autosomal dominant genetic cause of PD. In some studies carriers of the G2019S mutation in the *LRRK2* gene demonstrated poorer performance in executive functions on a computerized cognitive battery [75]. Other studies have found small differences between carriers and non-carriers of G2019S [76], and polymorphisms in the dual specificity tyrosine-phosphorylation-regulated kinase 1A (*DYRK1A*) gene have been associated with PD-D [77] (DYRK1A phosphorylates α-synuclein and amyloid precursor protein).

A Val66Met polymorphism in brain-derived neurotrophic factor (BDNF) is also significantly correlated with cognitive impairment in PD [78]. The apolipoprotein (*APOE*) ε4 allele is associated with a higher risk of AD and an earlier onset, and several studies have explored the role of *APOE* in PD, with inconsistent results. An autopsy study suggested that the ε4 allele was associated with PD-D [79], and a similar conclusion was reached in a meta-analysis [80]. However, no association between PD-D and *APOE* ε4 could be seen when PD-D was more carefully defined [81]. The H1/H1 haplotype of the microtubule-associated protein tau (*MAPT*) gene shows a positive association with PD and increased risk for PD-D [82, 83].

Smoking

There is convincing evidence of an association between smoking and reduced risk for PD, possibly mediated by an effect on nicotinic receptors. Nicotinic receptors are involved in learning and memory, and smoking may therefore theoretically protect against cognitive decline and dementia in PD. However, smoking also increases inflammation and oxidative stress and is associated with cardiovascular disease. Longitudinal studies have supported the hypothesis that smoking may reduce the risk for dementia and cognitive decline [84] in PD. However, another longitudinal study did not find an association between smoking and cognitive impairment [37].

Medications and cholinergic deficits

Patients with cholinergic deficits have a higher risk of developing dementia. It has been shown that cholinergic dysfunction in the cerebral cortex was significantly higher in PD-D patients than in a PD cohort without cognitive dysfunction [62, 67, 85–89]. Thus it is not surprising that anticholinergic drugs, which are traditionally used in PD, are associated with cognitive decline [90]. Autopsy studies in PD patients who were treated with anticholinergic medications for a long time revealed that amyloid plaque densities were more than 2.5 times higher than in PD patients who had no or limited anticholinergic treatment [88, 91]. Another drug used in PD, amantadine, was found to decrease the risk of dementia in a retrospective, naturalistic longitudinal study [92]; this finding, however, needs confirmation. Dopaminergic antiparkinsonian drugs may affect cognition in a complex way, but a significant association with risk for dementia has not been convincingly demonstrated.

Gender

The incidence of PD-D has been shown to be higher in men than in women, particularly in elderly patients [15].

Other factors

Risk factors common for AD and vascular dementia, such as high cholesterol [81], head trauma, diabetes mellitus, and hypertension, were not associated with risk for PD-D [1, 33]. There is also conflicting evidence regarding the association of hyperhomocysteinaemia, a well-known risk factor for cognitive decline in the general population, with the risk for PD-D. Some [93], but not all [94], studies have found such an association.

Conclusions

The point prevalence of PD-D is close to 30% and the incidence rate is increased four to six times compared with people without PD. In addition, MCI occurs in 20–25% of PD patients without dementia. The cumulative prevalence is very high—at least 75% of PD patients who survive for more than 10 years will develop dementia. The time from onset of PD to dementia varies considerably. The most established risk factors are old age, severity of motor symptoms, in particular PIGD, and the presence of MCI, VH, and RBD.

References

1. Levy G, Tang MX, Louis ED, et al. The association of incident dementia with mortality in PD. Neurology 2002; **59**: 1708–13.
2. Cummings JL. Intellectual impairment in Parkinson's disease: clinical, pathologic, and biochemical correlates. J Geriatr Psychiatry Neurol 1988; **1**: 24–36.
3. Aarsland D, Zaccai J, Brayne C. A systematic review of prevalence studies of dementia in Parkinson's disease. Mov Disord 2005; **20**: 1255–63.
4. Hobson P, Meara J. Risk and incidence of dementia in a cohort of older subjects with Parkinson's disease in the United Kingdom. Mov Disord 2004; **19**: 1043–9.
5. Mekawichai CL. The prevalence and the associated factors of dementia in patients with Parkinson's disease at Maharat Nakhon Ratchasima hospital. J Med Assoc Thai 2013; **96**: 440–5.
6. Athey RJ, Porter RW, Walker RW. Cognitive assessment of a representative community population with Parkinson's disease (PD) using the Cambridge Cognitive Assessment-Revised (CAMCOG-R). Age Ageing 2005; **34**: 268–73.
7. De Lau LM, Schipper CM, Hofman A, et al. Prognosis of Parkinson disease: risk of dementia and mortality: the Rotterdam Study. Arch Neurol 2005; **62**: 1265–9.

8. **Riedel O, Schneider C, Klotsche J, et al**. The prevalence of Parkinson's disease, associated dementia, and depression in Dresden. Fortschr Neurol Psychiatry 2013; **81**: 81–7.
9. **Williams-Gray CH, Mason SL, Evans JR, et al**. The CamPaIGN study of Parkinson's disease: 10-year outlook in an incident population-based cohort. J Neurol Neurosurg Psychiatry 2013; **84**: 1258–64.
10. **Aarsland D, Andersen K, Larsen J, et al**. Risk of dementia in Parkinson's disease: a community-based, prospective study. Neurology 2001; **56**: 730–6.
11. **Marder K, Tang MX, Alfaro B, et al**. Risk of Alzheimer's disease in relatives of Parkinson's disease patients with and without dementia. Neurology 1999; **52**: 719–24.
12. **Yip AG, Brayne C, Matthews FE**. Risk factors for incident dementia in England and Wales: the Medical Research Council Cognitive Function and Ageing Study. A population-based nested case–control study. Age Ageing 2006; **35**: 154–60.
13. **Williams-Gray CH, Foltynie T, Brayne C, et al**. Evolution of cognitive dysfunction in an incident Parkinson's disease cohort. Brain 2007; **130**: 1787–98.
14. **Pedersen KF, Larsen JP, Tysnes OB, et al**. Prognosis of mild cognitive impairment in early Parkinson disease: the Norwegian ParkWest study. J Am Med Assoc Neurol 2013; **70**: 580–6.
15. **Savica R, Grossardt BR, Bower JH, et al**. Incidence of dementia with Lewy bodies and Parkinson disease dementia. J Am Med Assoc Neurol 2013; **70**: 1396–402.
16. **Mayeux R, Chen J, Mirabello E, et al**. An estimate of the incidence of dementia in idiopathic Parkinson's disease. Neurology 1990; **40**: 1513–17.
17. **Marder K, Tang MX, Cote L, Stern Y, Mayeux R**. The frequency and associated risk factors for dementia in patients with Parkinson's disease. Arch Neurol 1995; **52**: 695–701.
18. **Hughes TA, Ross HF, Musa S, et al**. A 10-year study of the incidence of and factors predicting dementia in Parkinson's disease. Neurology 2000; **54**: 1596–602.
19. **Hobson P, Gallacher J, Meara J**. Cross-sectional survey of Parkinson's disease and parkinsonism in a rural area of the United Kingdom. Mov Disord 2005; **20**: 995–8.
20. **Hely MA, Reid WGJ, Adena MA, et al**. The Sydney multicenter study of Parkinson's disease: the inevitability of dementia at 20 years. Mov Disord 2008; **23**: 837–44.
21. **Hely MA, Morris JGL, Reid WGJ, et al**. Sydney Multicenter Study of Parkinson's disease: non-L-dopa-responsive problems dominate at 15 years. Mov Disord 2005; **20**: 190–9.
22. **Buter TC, Van Den Hout A, Matthews FE, et al**. Dementia and survival in Parkinson disease: a 12-year population study. Neurology 2008; **70**: 1017–22.
23. **Perez F, Helmer C, Foubert-Samier A, et al**. Risk of dementia in an elderly population of Parkinson's disease patients: a 15-year population-based study. Alzheimers Dement 2012; **8**: 463–9.
24. **Reid WGJ, Hely MA, Morris JG, et al**. A longitudinal of Parkinson's disease: clinical and neuropsychological correlates of dementia. J Clin Neurosci 1996; **3**: 327–33.
25. **Aarsland D, Andersen K, Larsen JP, et al**. Prevalence and characteristics of dementia in Parkinson disease: an 8-year prospective study. Arch Neurol 2003; **60**: 387–92.
26. **Aarsland D, Kvaløy JT, Andersen K, et al**. The effect of age of onset of PD on risk of dementia. J Neurol 2007; **254**: 38–45.
27. **Halliday G, Hely M, Reid WGJ, et al**. The progression of pathology in longitudinally followed patients with Parkinson's disease. Acta Neuropathol 2008; **115**: 409–15.
28. **Wada K, Nakashima K**. Mild cognitive impairment in Parkinson's disease. Brain Nerve 2012; **64**: 1365–75.
29. **Janvin CC, Larsen JP, Aarsland D, et al**. Subtypes of mild cognitive impairment in Parkinson's disease: progression to dementia. Mov Disord 2006; **21**: 1343–9.
30. **Baba T, Kikuchi A, Hirayama K, et al**. Severe olfactory dysfunction is a prodromal symptom of dementia associated with Parkinson's disease: a 3 year longitudinal study. Brain 2012; **135**: 161–9.

31. **Marion MH, Qurashi M, Marshall G, et al.** Is REM sleep behaviour disorder (RBD) a risk factor of dementia in idiopathic Parkinson's disease? J. Neurol 2008; **255**: 192–6.

32. **Haugarvoll K, Aarsland D, Wentzel-Larsen T, et al.** The influence of cerebrovascular risk factors on incident dementia in patients with Parkinson's disease. Acta Neurol Scand 2005; **112**: 386–90.

33. **Rektor I, Goldemund D, Sheardová K, et al.** Vascular pathology in patients with idiopathic Parkinson's disease. Parkinsonism Relat Disord 2009; **15**: 24–9.

34. **Rodriguez-Oroz MC, Lage PM, Sanchez-Mut J, et al.** Homocysteine and cognitive impairment in Parkinson's disease: a biochemical, neuroimaging, and genetic study. Mov Disord 2009; **24**: 1437–44.

35. **Slawek J, Wieczorek D, Derejko M, et al.** The influence of vascular risk factors and white matter hyperintensities on the degree of cognitive impairment in Parkinson's disease. Mov Disord 2008; **42**: 505–12.

36. **Alves G, Larsen JP, Emre M, et al.** Changes in motor subtype and risk for incident dementia in Parkinson's disease. Mov Disord 2006; **21**: 1123–30.

37. **Burn DJ, Rowan EN, Allan LM, et al.** Motor subtype and cognitive decline in Parkinson's disease, Parkinson's disease with dementia, and dementia with Lewy bodies. J Neurol Neurosurg Psychiatry 2006; **77**: 585–9.

38. **Tremblay C, Achim AM, Macoir J, et al.** The heterogeneity of cognitive symptoms in Parkinson's disease: a meta-analysis. J Neurol Neurosurg Psychiatry 2013; **84**: 1265–72.

39. **Litvan I, Goldman JG, Tröster AI, et al.** Diagnostic criteria for mild cognitive impairment in Parkinson's disease: Movement Disorder Society Task Force guidelines. Mov Disord 2012; **27**: 349–56.

40. **Aarsland D, Bronnick K, Williams-Gray C, et al.** Mild cognitive impairment in Parkinson disease: a multicenter pooled analysis. Neurology 2010; **75**: 1062–9.

41. **Aarsland D, Brønnick K, Larsen JP, et al.** Cognitive impairment in incident, untreated Parkinson disease: the Norwegian ParkWest study. Neurology 2009; **72**: 1121–6.

42. **Elgh E, Domellöf M, Linder J, et al.** Cognitive function in early Parkinson's disease: a population-based study. Eur J Neurol 2009; **16**: 1278–84.

43. **Foltynie T, Brayne CEG, Robbins TW, et al.** The cognitive ability of an incident cohort of Parkinson's patients in the UK. The CamPaIGN study. Brain 2004; **127**: 550–60.

44. **Muslimovic D, Post B, Speelman JD, et al.** Cognitive profile of patients with newly diagnosed Parkinson disease. Neurology 2005; **65**: 1239–45.

45. **Broeders M, de Bie RM, Velseboer DC, et al.** Evolution of mild cognitive impairment in Parkinson disease. Neurology 2013; **81**: 346–52.

46. **Bronnick K, Emre M, Lane R, et al.** Profile of cognitive impairment in dementia associated with Parkinson's disease compared with Alzheimer's disease. J Neurol Neurosurg Psychiatry 2007; **78**: 1064–8.

47. **Williams-Gray CH, Evans JR, Goris A, et al.** The distinct cognitive syndromes of Parkinson's disease: 5 year follow-up of the CamPaIGN cohort. Brain 2009; **132**: 2958–69.

48. **Williams DR, Warren JD, Lees AJ.** Using the presence of visual hallucinations to differentiate Parkinson's disease from atypical parkinsonism. J Neurol Neurosurg Psychiatry 2008; **79**: 652–5.

49. **Aarsland D, Andersen K, Larsen JP, et al.** The rate of cognitive decline in Parkinson disease. Arch Neurol 2004; **61**: 1906–11.

50. **Harding AJ, Broe GA, Halliday GM.** Visual hallucinations in Lewy body disease relate to Lewy bodies in the temporal lobe. Brain 2002; **125**: 391–403.

51. **Perry AF, Kerwin EK, Perry J, et al.** Visual hallucinations and the cholinergic system in dementia. J Neurol Neurosurg Psychiatry 1990; **53**: 88.

52. **Factor SA, Feustel PJ, Friedman JH, et al.** Longitudinal outcome of Parkinson's disease patients with psychosis. Neurology 2003; **60**: 1756–61.

53. **Gagnon JF, Vendette M, Postuma RB, et al.** Mild cognitive impairment in rapid eye movement sleep behavior disorder and Parkinson's disease. Ann Neurol 2009; **66**: 39–47.

54. **Vendette M, Gagnon JF, Décary A, et al**. REM sleep behavior disorder predicts cognitive impairment in Parkinson disease without dementia. Neurology 2007; **69**: 1843–9.

55. **Yoritaka A, Ohizumi H, Tanaka S, et al**. Parkinson's disease with and without REM sleep behaviour disorder: are there any clinical differences? Eur Neurol 2009; **61**: 164–70.

56. **Dugger BN, Boeve BF, Murray ME, et al**. Rapid eye movement sleep behavior disorder and subtypes in autopsy-confirmed dementia with Lewy bodies. Mov Disord 2012; **27**: 72–8.

57. **Eisensehr I, Lindeiner H, Jäger M, et al**. REM sleep behavior disorder in sleep-disordered patients with versus without Parkinson's disease: is there a need for polysomnography? J Neurol Sci 2001; **186**: 7–11.

58. **Scaglione C, Vignatelli L, Plazzi G, et al**. REM sleep behaviour disorder in Parkinson's disease: a questionnaire-based study. Neurol Sci 2005; **25**: 316–21.

59. **Derejko M, Sławek J, Wieczorek D, et al**. Regional cerebral blood flow in Parkinson's disease as an indicator of cognitive impairment. Neurol Neurochir Pol 2008; **24**: 505–12.

60. **Mehanna R, Jankovic J**. Movement disorders in cerebrovascular disease. Lancet Neurol 2013; **12**: 597–608.

61. **Shin J, Choi S, Lee JE, et al**. Subcortical white matter hyperintensities within the cholinergic pathways of Parkinson's disease patients according to cognitive status. J Neurol Neurosurg Psychiatry 2012; **83**: 315–21.

62. **Kurz MW, Schlitter AM, Larsen JP, et al**. Familial occurrence of dementia and parkinsonism: a systematic review. Dement Geriatr Cogn Disord 2006; **22**: 288–95.

63. **Rocca WA, Bower JH, Ahlskog JE, et al**. Risk of cognitive impairment or dementia in relatives of patients with Parkinson disease. Arch Neurol 2007; **64**: 1458–64.

64. **Fuchs J, Nilsson C, Kachergus J, et al**. Phenotypic variation in a large Swedish pedigree due to SNCA duplication and triplication. Neurology 2007; **68**: 916–22.

65. **Ross OA, Braithwaite AT, Skipper LM, et al**. Genomic investigation of alpha-synuclein multiplication and parkinsonism. Ann Neurol 2008; **63**: 743–50.

66. **Johansen KK, White LR, Sando SB, et al**. Biomarkers: Parkinson disease with dementia and dementia with Lewy bodies. Parkinsonism Relat Disord 2010; **16**: 307–15.

67. **Chartier-Harlin MC, Kachergus J, Roumier C, et al**. Alpha-synuclein locus duplication as a cause of familial Parkinson's disease. Lancet 2004; **364**: 1167–9.

68. **Farrer M, Kachergus J, Forno L, et al**. Comparison of kindreds with parkinsonism and alpha-synuclein genomic multiplications. Ann Neurol 2004; **55**: 174–9.

69. **Krüger R, Kuhn W, Müller T, et al**. Ala30Pro mutation in the gene encoding alpha-synuclein in Parkinson's disease. Nature Genet 1998; **18**: 106–8.

70. **Clark LN, Kartsaklis LA, Wolf Gilbert R, et al**. Association of glucocerebrosidase mutations with dementia with Lewy bodies. Arch Neurol 2009; **66**: 578–83.

71. **Neumann J, Bras J, Deas E, et al**. Glucocerebrosidase mutations in clinical and pathologically proven Parkinson's disease. Brain 2009; **132**: 1783–94.

72. **Sidransky E, Nalls MA, Aasly JO, et al**. Multicenter analysis of glucocerebrosidase mutations in Parkinson's disease. N Engl J Med 2009; **361**: 1651–61.

73. **Ahlskog JE**. Parkin and PINK1 parkinsonism may represent nigral mitochondrial cytopathies distinct from Lewy body Parkinson's disease. Parkinsonism Relat Disord 2009; **15**: 721–7.

74. **Thaler A, Mirelman A, Gurevich T, et al**. Lower cognitive performance in healthy G2019S LRRK2 mutation carriers. Neurology 2012; **79**: 1027–32.

75. **Hentati E, Nabli F, Trabelsi M, et al**. Cognitive dysfunction in Tunisian LRRK2 associated Parkinson's disease. Parkinsonism Relat Disord 2012; **18**: 243–6.

76. **Jones EL, Aarsland D, Londos E, et al**. A pilot study examining associations between DYRK1A and α-synuclein dementias. Neurodegener Dis 2012; **10**: 229–31.

77. **Białecka M, Kurzawski M, Roszmann A, et al.** BDNF G196A (Val66Met) polymorphism associated with cognitive impairment in Parkinson's disease. Neurosci Lett 2014; **561:** 86–90.

78. **Papapetropoulos S, Farrer MJ, Stone JT, et al.** Phenotypic associations of tau and ApoE in Parkinson's disease. Neurosci Lett 2007; **414:** 141–4.

79. **Huang X, Chen P, Kaufer DI, et al.** Apolipoprotein E and dementia in Parkinson disease: a meta-analysis. Arch Neurol 2006; **63:** 189–93.

80. **Jasinska-Myga B, Opala G, Goetz CG, et al.** Apolipoprotein E gene polymorphism, total plasma cholesterol level, and Parkinson disease dementia. Arch Neurol 2007; **64:** 261–5.

81. **Goris A, Williams-Gray CH, Clark GR, et al.** Tau and alpha-synuclein in susceptibility to, and dementia in, Parkinson's disease. Ann Neurol 2007; **62:** 145–53.

82. **Healy DG, Abou-Sleiman PM, Lees AJ, et al.** Tau gene and Parkinson's disease: a case–control study and meta-analysis. J Neurol Neurosurg Psychiatry 2004; **75:** 962–5.

83. **Weisskopf MG, Grodstein F, Ascherio A.** Smoking and cognitive function in Parkinson's disease. Mov Disord 2007; **22:** 660–5.

84. **Bohnen NI, Kaufer DI, Hendrickson R, et al.** Cortical cholinergic denervation is associated with depressive symptoms in Parkinson's disease and parkinsonian dementia. J Neurol Neurosurg Psychiatry 2007; **78:** 641–3.

85. **Shimada H, Hirano S, Shinotoh H, et al.** Mapping of brain acetylcholinesterase alterations in Lewy body disease by PET. Neurology 2009; **73:** 273–8.

86. **Mattila PM, Röyttä M, Lönnberg P, et al.** Choline acetyltransferase activity and striatal dopamine receptors in Parkinson's disease in relation to cognitive impairment. Acta Neuropathol 2001; **102:** 160–6.

87. **Grujic Z.** Cognitive disturbances in Parkinson's disease. Dis Mon 2007; **53:** 302–8.

88. **Braak H, Del Tredici K, Rüb U, et al.** Staging of brain pathology related to sporadic Parkinson's disease. Neurobiol Aging 2003; **24:** 197–211.

89. **Ehrt U, Broich K, Larsen JP, et al.** Use of drugs with anticholinergic effect and impact on cognition in Parkinson's disease: a cohort study. J Neurol Neurosurg Psychiatry 2010; **81:** 160–5.

90. **Perry EK, Kilford L, Lees AJ, et al.** Increased Alzheimer pathology in Parkinson's disease related to antimuscarinic drugs. Ann Neurol 2003; **54:** 235–8.

91. **Inzelberg R, Bonuccelli U, Schechtman E, et al.** Association between amantadine and the onset of dementia in Parkinson's disease. Mov Disord 2006; **21:** 1375–9.

92. **Religa D, Czyzewski K, Styczynska M, et al.** Hyperhomocysteinemia and methylenetetrahydrofolate reductase polymorphism in patients with Parkinson's disease. Neurosci Lett 2006; **404:** 56–60.

93. **O'Suilleabhain PE, Sung V, Hernandez C, et al.** Elevated plasma homocysteine level in patients with Parkinson disease: motor, affective, and cognitive associations. Arch Neurol 2004; **61:** 865–8.

Chapter 3

General features, mode of onset, and course of dementia in Parkinson's disease

Murat Emre

Introduction

Dementia associated with Parkinson's disease (PD-D) demonstrates characteristic features, making it a clinically recognizable entity that is frequently associated with typical pathological changes. These features include its mode of onset, the chronology and course of the symptoms, the profile of cognitive deficits and behavioural symptoms, the associated motor phenotype, and other accompanying features. The characteristic symptoms and signs in each of these domains are described in detail in subsequent chapters. The objective of this chapter is to describe the general features of PD-D including its mode of onset, its course, and its prognosis.

General features of PD-D

The prototypical form of PD-D can be described as a dysexecutive syndrome commonly associated with behavioural symptoms and a postural instability and gait disturbance (PIGD)-dominant motor phenotype [1]. The defining neuropsychological deficits, described in detail in Chapter 4, include prominent and fluctuating impairment in attention, deficits in most aspects of executive function, early and prominent visuospatial deficits (often disproportionate to the overall severity of dementia), relatively mild and usually of retrieval type memory impairment, and largely preserved core language functions except for difficulties with word finding and impaired fluency. Behavioural symptoms include depression, hallucinations, apathy, delusions, and anxiety [2]. Tremor is less frequent and a PIGD phenotype prevails; autonomic dysfunction, especially incontinence, is common. The cognitive, behavioural, and motor features of PD-D are similar to dementia with Lewy bodies (DLB) and different from those seen in Alzheimer's disease (AD) [3].

Unlike the majority of patients with AD, who often deny that anything is wrong with their memory, insight into their mental deficits is usually preserved in people with PD-D; they tend to either complain themselves or admit when asked the presence of mental problems. Another defining feature is that patients who have initiation problems or frequent pauses during the performance of a task perform better if provided with guidance, or if external cues are given when they pause. In other words, internally driven performance is worse than that driven by external cues or help. This is similar to the ability of PD patients to walk better when visual guidance is provided. In this sense, cognitive deficits and dementia in PD (at least before the deficits become more advanced and severe) are more characterized by difficulties in the modulation of cognitive functions than losses in their contents.

Dysexecutive syndrome is the prototypical form of dementia seen in patients with PD. There are, however, some patients in whom deviations from this pattern are observed. For example, in the majority of patients the pattern of memory impairment is retrieval-type, with storage of new information being relatively spared, but some may develop a limbic-type amnesia where the new information is not stored, which is more typical of AD [4]. Likewise some patients may show a more AD-like 'cortical' pattern of deficits [5]. The extent and topography of Lewy body (LB)-type degeneration as well as the magnitude of the coexisting AD-type pathology are likely to determine the profile, severity, and time course of cognitive and behavioural symptoms. In a clinico-pathological study, patients with a pure LB pathology had a more dysexecutive syndrome, those with pure AD pathology an amnestic syndrome, and those with both pathologies a more mixed cognitive profile [6].

Mode and age of onset

Mode of onset

The mode of onset of PD-D is insidious; it is often difficult for the patient and family members to remember when the first signs of mental dysfunction became apparent. It is not uncommon for mental dysfunction to emerge or be visible following a minor trauma, surgery, infection, or dehydration; the symptoms may then not be fully reversible although the triggering insult has vanished. This in fact represents an incipient dementia becoming overt; such constellations may mislead caregivers to conclude that the onset of mental dysfunction was acute. Conversely, acute confusion (delirium) due to systemic diseases or adverse effects of drugs may be mistaken for dementia. Therefore, an acute onset or acute worsening of mental dysfunction should always be suspicious for exogenous factors and necessitates a careful history, detailed clinical examination, and appropriate laboratory investigations.

Age at onset of dementia and time from disease onset to dementia

Although marked cognitive dysfunction can be found in de novo populations or at the time of diagnosis [8% of newly diagnosed patients were found to have marked cognitive impairment defined as a Mini-Mental State Examination (MMSE) score <24] [7], dementia at the time of diagnosis of PD is rare. By current definitions, such cases would qualify for a diagnosis of DLB. A diagnosis of PD-D requires the preceding diagnosis of PD, followed by dementia developing on the background of established PD.

In the majority of patients cognitive dysfunctions are usually subtle at the time of disease onset and develop during the later stages. In a cohort of patients with newly diagnosed PD, 10% developed dementia at a mean of 3.5 years from diagnosis; the annual incidence of dementia was calculated to be 30 per 1000 person-years [8] (see Chapter 2). In the prospectively followed Sydney cohort the prevalence of dementia was 16% at baseline [9], whereas 84% of patients developed cognitive dysfunction, 48% severe enough to justify the diagnosis of dementia 15 years after the diagnosis of PD [10]. In the same cohort, dementia was present in 83% of all surviving patients 20 years after the diagnosis [11]. In another prospective study, old age and longer disease duration were found to be strong determinants of dementia [12]. The reason for the delay to the onset of dementia may be the relatively late involvement of brain structures subserving mental functions in typical PD patients. This is suggested by the staging of disease pathology described by Braak et al. [13]. According to this hypothesis, LB pathology in PD has its onset in certain susceptible nuclei of the brainstem, subsequently ascending to the upper brainstem, limbic structures, and finally to the cerebral cortex, heteromodal association cortices succumbing first, followed by homomodal association and primary sensory-motor cortices. However, there also seem to be patients with a greater burden of cortical pathology who have a more malignant disease course and a shorter time before the emergence of dementia [14].

The average time to the onset of PD-D was found to be about 9 years in one cohort [15]. An important determinant of time to occurrence of dementia is current age; the older the patient the more likely is a shorter time to the onset of dementia. Estimates of age-specific incidence of cognitive impairment suggest that it is 2.7% per year at ages 55–64 increasing to 13.7% at 70–79 years [16–18]. Similar effects of age were observed in the Sydney cohort: the prevalence of dementia at baseline was 5% in those aged <60, 14% at 60–69, and 35% in patients aged ≥70 years [9]. The effect of age at disease onset is, however, debated: whereas several studies have reported that a younger age of onset is associated with a lower risk of dementia, a recent analysis suggested that it is age per se rather than age of onset which determines the risk [19].

Predictors and early signs

Several clinical and demographic features are associated with increased risk for dementia. These are described in detail in the chapter 2; the most important ones will be mentioned here. Among many reported associations three can be singled out: one demographic (age), one related to motor phenotype (PIGD type), and the other cognitive performance at the time of assessment.

Predictors of dementia

As repeatedly confirmed in a number of studies, advanced age and severe motor symptoms are the most significant risk factors for dementia [18, 20, 21]. In a population-based cross-sectional study, dementia was not present in any of the patients aged under 50, whereas 69% of all those aged over 80 had dementia [22]. The combination of old age and severe motor symptoms seems to indicate a particularly bleak prognosis, increasing the risk by almost ten-fold compared with patients who are young and have mild disease [23]. There are certain constellations and clinical vignettes which, when present, render patients more susceptible to developing dementia. One such feature is the motor phenotype. Patients with more symmetrical signs, higher disability and bradykinesia scores, and more impairment of gait and balance are more likely to develop dementia [9]. In contrast, patients with the tremor-predominant subtype are less likely to develop dementia than those who suffer from a PIGD subtype [8]. In a group of patients who were prospectively followed up, those who suffered from a tremor-dominant subtype at baseline had converted to a PIGD-predominant subtype by the time they developed dementia [24].

Performance in neuropsychological tests also provides clues as to the risk of developing dementia. Patients with low overall cognitive scores, mild deficits in executive functions, word-finding difficulties, mild impairment of memory, poor attentional function, reduced verbal fluency, and impairments in picture completion tests are more likely to develop dementia than those patients with normal cognitive performance [18, 21, 25–27]. Letter and especially semantic fluency tests seem to be particularly sensitive measures, as well as copying a figure of intersecting pentagons [8, 25]. The appearance of visual hallucinations or confusion soon after initiation of dopaminergic medication may also be a harbinger of incipient dementia [28]. The reverse is also true: the main risk factor for appearance of hallucinations in treated PD patients is cognitive impairment [29]. Patients with a diagnosis of mild cognitive impairment (MCI) at the time of examination have a higher risk of developing dementia than those without. In a prospective study, 62% of patients with MCI at baseline converted to dementia as opposed to 20% of those who were cognitively intact. Single-domain non-memory MCI and multiple-domain slightly impaired MCI were associated with a high risk of developing dementia, whereas the amnestic MCI subtype was not; however, the numbers in this latter group were small [30]. In the 10-year follow-up of the CamPaIGN study, which has been designed to prospectively track disease evolution from diagnosis in an unselected population, 46% of patients had developed dementia. Baseline predictors of dementia were age, motor impairment, 'posterior-cortical' cognitive deficits, and *MAPT* genotype [31]. In the Norwegian ParkWest study, 182 patients with incident PD were monitored for 3 years; they were classified as having MCI and received a diagnosis of dementia according to published consensus criteria. Significantly more patients with MCI than without MCI at baseline (27.0 versus 0.7%) progressed to dementia during follow-up. Of those with MCI at baseline, 21.6% had reverted to normal cognition during follow-up. MCI at the 1-year visit was associated with a similar progression rate to dementia and reversion rate to normal cognition. However, among the 22 patients with persistent MCI at baseline and the 1-year visit, 45.5% developed dementia and only two had reverted to normal cognition by the end of study. The authors concluded that MCI at PD diagnosis predicts a highly increased risk for early dementia [32].

Early symptoms of incipient dementia

Before overt signs of dementia become visible to friends and family, many patients develop subtle symptoms (Box 3.1). One such symptom is disturbance of the sleep–wake cycle. Caregivers notice that patients develop an increasing amount of daytime sleepiness, they often fall asleep when seated, reading a newspaper, or watching television. Although excessive daytime sleepiness (EDS) can also be seen in PD patients without dementia, or sleep attacks may occur as a result of dopaminergic treatment, EDS is more frequent in patients with dementia [33] and is often an early sign. On awakening, patients may have a brief confused episode, not realizing for a moment where they are, or have continuation of the dream they were just having by asking or searching for non-existent people or animals.

Another sleep-related phenomenon is rapid eye movement sleep behaviour disorder (RBD), designating dream-enacting such as speaking, shouting, or moving during sleep. Although it may also occur in patients without dementia and may precede the onset of the disease by many years,

Box 3.1 Early signs and symptoms preceding dementia in Parkinson's disease

- Disturbances of the sleep–wake cycle
- Excessive daytime sleepiness
- Brief confusion on awakening
- Feelings of presence, occasional hallucinations
- Disturbances of visual orientation
- Increasing forgetfulness
- Impaired attentiveness and concentration
- Apathy

it is significantly more frequent in PD-D patients [34]. RBD has been found to predict cognitive decline in PD patients without dementia [35], especially if it is combined with hallucinations [36]. Thus, de novo emergence of RBD in a patient with PD may signal the onset of cognitive dysfunction.

Psychotic phenomena such as feelings of presence (the feeling that there is somebody in the room or in the house, although the patient does not actually see this person), the feeling that somebody is standing behind the patient, the sensation of passage of a shadow or of an animal, or isolated brief episodes of visual hallucinations usually occurring at nighttime or on awakening can also precede the other signs of dementia. Hallucinations may develop on relatively low doses of dopamine agonists or levodopa, which the patient may have tolerated well previously.

Due to deterioration of attention, patients become more and more inattentive; they seem not to understand what they are being told and their reactions become delayed. They become with-drawn and apathetic; they lose their spontaneity, doing less and less on their own. Visuospatial deficits are one of the earliest cognitive impairments in PD-D. Accordingly, having orientation problems in a new environment can be an early symptom of mental dysfunction, worsening as the disease progresses—patients can have navigational problems in familiar places, mixing up rooms and not finding the direction to the toilet in their own home.

Course of dementia and rate of progression

The course of dementia in PD is relentlessly progressive over years—a reversible course has not been observed [37]. At times patients may seem to have been stabilized for months; they may, however, also show episodes of rapid worsening for no obvious reason. Fluctuations during the day and from day to day, as occur in DLB, are also frequent in patients with PD-D. When asked, family members would admit that the patient is clearly better on certain days or at certain times of the day, usually in the morning, and tending to perform worse after a bad night's sleep. As dementia progresses patients become increasingly more confused, living in almost a continu-ous confusional state, with prolonged blank stares and signs of visual hallucinations, although these may not be verbalized. Speech and postural problems often worsen in parallel and patients become more and more dependent.

Rate of progression

There have been two studies in which the rate of progression was evaluated prospectively in patients with PD-D, using MMSE as the cognitive measure. In one of these studies patients with PD-D were compared with those with AD and with healthy controls. Over a 4-year period the annualized decline was a mean score of 2.3 in the PD-D group compared with 2.6 in patients with AD; the change in the PD group without dementia was small and similar to that for healthy controls [38]. The annualized decline in the PD-D group was variable across the patients and ranged from 1 (18%) to >4 (16%) points. In the other study, cognitive decline was compared in patients with PD-D, DLB, and controls. Over a 2-year period cognitive decline was a mean score of 4.5 in the PD-D group, 3.9 in the DLB group, 0.2 in the PD group and 0.3 in the controls [39], thus yielding annual rates of decline very similar to those in the previous study. Although these studies provide useful information, they may not reflect the true progression of the dis-ease because MMSE is rather insensitive for the assessment of executive dysfunction, which is one of the core features of PD-D. Indirect evidence as to the rate of progression using other parameters, albeit over a shorter period, can also be deduced from placebo-controlled clinical trials. One such trial, performed in a large PD-D population with mild to moderate dementia, included a sizeable placebo arm. All cognitive and functional measures worsened in the placebo group; the decrease in the MMSE score over a period of 6 months was 0.2 (out of 20 at baseline), Alzheimer's Disease Assessment Scale–cognitive subscale (ADAS-cog) score decreased by 0.7 (out of 24 at baseline), and the Alzheimer Disease Consortium Study activities of daily living (ADL) score decreased by 3.6 (out of 41 at baseline) [40]. These decreases were smaller than those observed in AD patients receiving placebo in clinical studies with a comparable design and duration, suggesting a slower rate of progression in PD-D. Such comparisons, however, have limited value as they are indirect.

Determinants of progression rate

Patients with atypical neurological features such as early occurrence of autonomic failure, symmetrical disease presentation, and limited response to dopaminergic therapy tend to have more severe dementia [41]. In a prospective study spanning 2 years there was an association between PIGD subtype and increased rate of cognitive decline [39]. Likewise the presence of major depression, visual hallucinations, or of moderate-to-severe EDS predicts significantly greater or faster cognitive decline [33, 38, 42]. The amount of attentional deficit may also determine the severity of functional impairment. In a multiple regression analysis performed on the baseline data of a large patient population which participated in a clinical trial, the attention factor was the single strongest cognitive predictor of ADL score, matching the strength of the effects of motor functions on ADL score [43]. Disease prognosis is likely to be poorer and progression faster in patients who have mixed LB- and AD-type pathologies [6].

Survival

In a prospective study with follow-up of approximately 4 years, among those who died 49% had developed dementia compared with 23% of those who remained alive. Incident dementia had an independent effect on mortality when controlling for the severity of extrapyramidal symptoms; the development of dementia was associated with a two-fold increased mortality risk [44]. In another prospective 12-year study the cumulative incidence of dementia steadily increased with age and duration of PD, increasing to 80–90% by the age of 90 years conditional on survival. Women with PD lived longer than men and spent more years with dementia. At the age of 70, a man with PD without dementia was predicted to have a life expectancy of 8 years, of which 5 years would be expected to be dementia free followed by 3 years with dementia. In a 70-year-old PD-D patient the life expectancy is substantially reduced to 4.2 years for men and 5.7 years for women [12]. In a prospective study of autonomic dysfunction, patients with persistent orthostatic hypotension had a significantly shorter survival than those with no or non-persistent orthostatic hypotension; patients with constipation and/or urinary incontinence in addition to persistent orthostatic hypotension had a poorer prognosis than those with isolated persistent orthostatic hypotension or no orthostatic hypotension [45].

Pathological determinants of dementia in PD

An important question is why some patients with PD develop dementia relatively early whereas others do so late in the disease course, or not at all. It may simply be a matter of time, as the vast majority of surviving patients in the Sydney cohort did develop dementia 20 years into the diagnosis. This may be determined by how fast the disease pathology progresses to involve relevant brain structures. The predominance of the PIGD phenotype in PD-D patients, and conversion of initially tremor-dominant patients to the PIGD phenotype by the time they developed dementia, indicate that the involvement of certain brain structures subserving both postural–gait functions and cognition may be necessary for the development of dementia.

The amount and topography of the α-synuclein pathology, the main component of LBs, may be an important determinant. Dementia is not a common feature in families with a duplication of the α-synuclein gene locus, whereas those carrying a triplication mutation frequently develop dementia (see Chapter 13). This indicates that total α-synuclein burden may be an important factor in determining which patients will develop dementia. It is, however, unlikely to be the only factor: in an autopsy study, subjects with 'reasonable' burden of α-synuclein pathology in both brainstem and cortical areas had not developed motor or mental dysfunction during their lifetime. The distribution or load of α-synuclein pathology did not permit a dependable post-mortem diagnosis of extrapyramidal symptoms or cognitive impairment [46]. The same group recently reported that around 55% of subjects with widespread α-synuclein pathology (Braak PD stages 5–6) lacked clinical signs of dementia or extrapyramidal signs ante mortem [47]. Another clinico-pathological correlation study demonstrated that the presence of limbic or cortical LBs may not always be associated with dementia in PD: nine out of 17 patients with a clinical diagnosis of PD and no history of cognitive impairment showed a neuropathological picture consistent with limbic LBs and eight of them a pathology consistent with neocortical DLB [48]. It is unclear why some individuals appear to 'tolerate' high levels of synuclein deposition without developing symptoms. The specific pattern of LB distribution may be important for dementia to develop; in a multivariate analysis of various pathologies in the brains of patients with PD-D, only LB densities in the entorhinal and anterior cingulate cortex were significantly associated with cognitive scores [49]. The contribution of non-LB pathologies may be an additional factor, modifying or enhancing the impact of synuclein pathology. In an autopsy study, patients carrying both LB- and AD-type pathologies had a worse ante-mortem prognosis than patients with predominantly one type of pathology [6]. In a review of studies conducted at the Queen Square Brain Bank, cortical Lewy- and Alzheimer-type pathologies were associated with milestones of poorer prognosis and with non-tremor predominance, which in turn are linked to dementia. A combination of these pathologies was found to be the most robust neuropathological substrate of PD-D, with cortical amyloid-β burden determining a faster progression to dementia [50].

The severity and topography of cortical involvement seems to be another factor. Widespread areas of cortical atrophy, in both temporal and frontal lobes as well as in the left parietal lobe, were found in patients with PD-D compared with normal controls. Compared with PD patients with MCI but no dementia, grey matter reductions were found in the frontal, parietal, limbic, and temporal lobes of patients with PD-D [51]. In a comparative study of PD patients who developed dementia early versus late in the disease course, those with early dementia had more atrophy in certain brain areas while the late dementia group had symmetrical reduction in grey matter in the insula bilaterally. The authors suggested that the early development of PD-D is associated with more severe degeneration of cortical and subcortical structures [52]. In another study, in which correlation between time to dementia and different types of cortical pathological findings was analysed, there was an association between longer duration of parkinsonism prior to dementia and less severe cortical α-synuclein pathology and lower plaque scores. There was an unexpected correlation between more pronounced cortical cholinergic deficits and longer duration of parkinsonism prior to dementia, implying a greater loss of ascending cholinergic projections in this population before the onset of dementia [15]. By contrast, a more 'top-down' pathological process has also been described, with a greater burden of cortical pathology in patients with a more malignant disease course and a shorter time before dementia supervenes [14].

Conclusion

The typical profile of PD-D is characterized by a dysexecutive syndrome with prominent impairment of attention, visuospatial function, memory, and frequent behavioural symptoms. Dementia in PD has an insidious onset and slow progression, and overt symptoms are usually preceded by more subtle changes. The annual rate of decline is similar to or somewhat less than that seen in AD. Old age, longer duration of disease, and a PIGD subtype are associated with higher risk and faster progression. The severity and topography of LB-type degeneration, as well as the presence and amount of coexisting pathologies, may determine the risk of developing dementia, time to onset, and the rate of progression.

References

1. **Emre M, Aarsland D, Brown R, et al**. Clinical diagnostic criteria for dementia associated with Parkinson's disease. Mov Disord 2007; **22**: 1689–707.

2. **Aarsland D, Brønnick K, Ehrt U, et al**. Neuropsychiatric symptoms in patients with Parkinson's disease and dementia: frequency, profile and associated care giver stress. J Neurol Neurosurg Psychiatry 2007; **78**: 36–42.

3. **Metzler-Baddeley C**. A review of cognitive impairments in dementia with Lewy bodies relative to Alzheimer's disease and Parkinson's disease with dementia. Cortex 2007; **43**: 583–600.

4. **Weintraub D, Moberg PJ, Culbertson WC, et al**. Evidence for impaired encoding and retrieval memory profiles in Parkinson disease. Cogn Behav Neurol 2004; **17**: 195–200.

5. **Aarsland D, Litvan I, Salmon D, et al**. Performance on the dementia rating scale in Parkinson's disease with dementia and dementia with Lewy bodies: comparison with progressive supranuclear palsy and Alzheimer's disease. J Neurol Neurosurg Psychiatry 2003; **74**: 1215–20.

6. **Kraybill ML, Larson EB, Tsuang DW, et al**. Cognitive differences in dementia patients with autopsy-verified AD, Lewy body pathology, or both. Neurology 2005; **64**: 2069–73.

7. **Foltynie T, Brayne CEG, Robbins TW, et al**. The cognitive ability of an incident cohort of Parkinson's patients in the UK. The CamPaIGN study. Brain 2004; **127**: 1–11.

8. **Williams-Gray CH, Foltynie T, Brayne CE, et al**. Evolution of cognitive dysfunction in an incident Parkinson's disease cohort. Brain 2007; **130**: 1787–98.

9. **Reid WG, Hely MA, Morris JG, et al**. A longitudinal study of Parkinson's disease: clinical and neuropsychological correlates of dementia. J Clin Neurosci 1996; **3**: 327–33.

10. **Hely MA, Morris JG, Reid WG, et al**. Sydney Multicenter Study of Parkinson's disease: non-dopa responsive problems dominate at 15 years. Mov Disord 2005; **20**: 190–9.

11. **Hely MA, Reid WG, Adena MA, et al**. The Sydney multicenter study of Parkinson's disease: the inevitability of dementia at 20 years. Mov Disord 2008; **23**: 837–44.

12. **Buter TC, Van Den Hout A, Matthews FE, et al**. Dementia and survival in Parkinson disease. Neurology 2008; **70**: 1017–22.

13. **Braak H, Del Tredici K Rub U, et al**. Staging of brain pathology related to sporadic Parkinson's disease. Neurobiol Aging 2003; **24**: 197–211.

14. **Halliday G, Hely M, Reid W, et al**. The progression of pathology in longitudinally followed patients with Parkinson's disease. Acta Neuropathol 2008; **115**: 409–15.

15. **Ballard C, Ziabreva I, Perry R, et al**. Differences in neuropathologic characteristics across the Lewy body dementia spectrum. Neurology 2006; **67**: 1931–4.

16. **Mayeaux R, Chen J, Mirabello E, et al**. An estimate of the incidence of dementia in idiopathic Parkinson's disease. Neurology 1990; **40**: 1513–17.

17. **Biggins CA, Boyd JL, Harrop FM et al**. A controlled, longitudinal-study of dementia in Parkinson's disease. J Neurol Neurosurg Psychiatry 1992; **55**: 566–71.

18. **Aarsland D, Andersen K, Larsen JP, et al.** Risk of dementia in Parkinson's disease: a community-based, prospective study. Neurology 2001; **56**: 730–6.

19. **Aarsland D, Kvaloy JT, Andersen K, et al.** The effect of age of onset of PD on risk of dementia. J Neurol 2007; **254**: 38–45.

20. **Hughes TA, Ross HF, Musa S, et al.** A 10-year study of the incidence of and factors predicting dementia in Parkinson's disease. Neurology 2000; **54**: 1596–602.

21. **Hobson P, Meara J.** Risk and incidence of dementia in a cohort of older subjects with Parkinson's disease in the United Kingdom. Mov Disord 2004; **19**: 1043–9.

22. **Mayeux R, Denaro J, Hemenegildo N, et al.** A population-based investigation of Parkinson's disease with and without dementia. Relationship to age and gender. Arch Neurol 1992; **49**: 492–7.

23. **Levy G, Schupf N, Tang MX, et al.** Combined effect of age and severity on the risk of dementia in Parkinson's disease. Ann Neurol 2002; **51**: 722–9.

24. **Alves G, Larsen JP, Emre M, et al.** Changes in motor subtype and risk for incident dementia in Parkinson's disease. Mov Disord 2006; **21**: 1123–30.

25. **Jacobs DM, Marder K, Cote LJ, et al.** Neuropsychological characteristics of preclinical dementia in Parkinson's disease. Neurology 1995; **45**: 1691–6.

26. **Mahieux F, Fenelon G, Flahault A, et al.** Neuropsychological prediction of dementia in Parkinson's disease J Neurol Neurosurg Psychiatry 1998; **65**: 804–5.

27. **Taylor JP, Rowan EN, Lett D, et al.** Poor attentional function predicts cognitive decline in patients with non-demented Parkinson's disease independent of motor phenotype. J Neurol Neurosurg Psychiatry 2008; **79**: 1318–23.

28. **Stern Y, Marder K, Tang MX, et al.** Antecedent clinical features associated with dementia in Parkinson's disease. Neurology 1993; **43**: 1690–2.

29. **Fenelon G, Mahieux F, Huon R, et al.** Hallucinations in Parkinson's disease: prevalence, phenomenology and risk factors. Brain 2000; **123**: 733–45.

30. **Janvin CC, Larsen JP, Aarsland D, et al.** Subtypes of mild cognitive impairment in Parkinson's disease: progression to dementia. Mov Disord 2006; **21**: 1343–9.

31. **Williams-Gray CH, Mason SL, Evans JR, et al.** The CamPaIGN study of Parkinson's disease: 10-year outlook in an incident population-based cohort. J Neurol Neurosurg Psychiatry 2013; **84**: 1258–64.

32. **Pedersen KF, Larsen JP, Tysnes OB, et al.** Prognosis of mild cognitive impairment in early Parkinson disease: the Norwegian ParkWest study. J Am Med Assoc Neurol 2013; **70**: 580–6.

33. **Gjerstad MD, Aarsland D, Larsen JP.** Development of daytime somnolence over time in Parkinson's disease. Neurology 2002; **85**: 1544–6.

34. **Marion MH, Qurashi M, Marshall G, et al.** Is REM sleep behaviour disorder (RBD) a risk factor of dementia in idiopathic Parkinson's disease? J Neurol 2008; **255**: 192–6.

35. **Vendette M, Gagnon JF, Decary A et al.** REM sleep behavior disorder predicts cognitive impairment in Parkinson disease without dementia. Neurology 2007; **69**: 1843–9.

36. **Sinforiani E, Pacchetti C, Zangaglia R, et al.** REM behaviour disorder, hallucinations and cognitive impairment in Parkinson's disease: a two-year follow up. Mov Disord 2008; **23**: 1441–5.

37. **Aarsland D, Andersen K, Larsen JP, et al.** Prevalence and characteristics of dementia in Parkinson disease: an 8-year prospective study. Arch Neurol 2003; **60**: 387–92.

38. **Aarsland D, Andersen K, Larsen JP.** The rate of cognitive decline in Parkinson's disease. Arch Neurol 2004; **61**: 1906–11.

39. **Burn DJ, Rowan EN, Allan LM, et al.** Motor subtype and cognitive decline in Parkinson's disease, Parkinson's disease with dementia, and dementia with Lewy body disease. J Neurol Neurosurg Psychiatry 2006; **77**: 585–9.

40. **Emre M, Aarsland D, Albanese A, et al.** Rivastigmine for dementia associated with Parkinson's disease. N Engl J Med 2004; **351**: 2509–18.

41. **Aarsland D, Tandberg E, Larsen JP, et al.** Frequency of dementia in Parkinson disease. Arch Neurol 1996; **53**: 538–42.

42. **Starkstein SE, Mayberg HS, Leiguarda R, et al.** A prospective longitudinal study of depression, cognitive decline, and physical impairments in patients with Parkinson's disease. J Neurol Neurosurg Psychiatry 1992; **55**: 377–82.

43. **Bronnick K, Ehrt U, Emre M, et al.** Attentional deficits affect activities of daily living in dementia-associated with Parkinson's disease. J Neurol Neurosurg Psychiatry 2006; **77**: 1136–42.

44. **Levy G, Tang MX Louis ED, et al.** The association of incident dementia with mortality in PD. Neurology 2002; **59**: 1708–13.

45. **Parkkinen L, Kauppinen T, Pirttila T, et al.** Alpha-synuclein pathology does not predict extrapyramidal symptoms or dementia. Ann Neurol 2005; **57**: 82–91.

46. **Stubendorff K, Aarsland D, Minthon L, et al.** The impact of autonomic dysfunction on survival in patients with dementia with Lewy bodies and Parkinson's disease with dementia. PLoS ONE 2012; **7**: e45451, doi: 10.1371/journal.pone.0045451.

47. **Parkkinen L, Pirttilä T, Alafuzoff I.** Applicability of current staging/categorization of alpha-synuclein pathology and their clinical relevance. Acta Neuropathol 2008; **115**: 399–407.

48. **Colosimo C, Hughes AJ, Kilford L, et al.** Lewy body cortical involvement may not always predict dementia in Parkinson's disease. J Neurol Neurosurg Psychiatry 2003; **74**: 852–6.

49. **Kovari, Gold G, Herrmann FR, et al.** Lewy body densities in the entorhinal and anterior cingulate cortex predict cognitive deficits in Parkinson's disease. Acta Neuropathol 2003; **106**: 83–8.

50. **Compta Y, Parkkinen L, Kempster P, et al.** The significance of α-synuclein, amyloid-β and tau pathologies in Parkinson's disease progression and related dementia. Neurodegener Dis 2014; **13**: 154–6.

51. **Beyer MK, Janvin CC, Larsen JP, et al.** A magnetic resonance imaging study of patients with Parkinson's disease with mild cognitive impairment and dementia using voxel-based morphometry. J Neurol Neurosurg Psychiatry 2007; **78**: 254–9.

52. **Beyer MK, Aarsland D.** Grey matter atrophy in early versus late dementia in Parkinson's disease. Parkinsonism Relat Disord 2008; **14**: 620–5.

Chapter 4

Cognitive profile in Parkinson's disease dementia

Kolbjørn Brønnick

Introduction

The focus of research in Parkinson's disease (PD) and Parkinson's disease dementia (PD-D) has shifted somewhat since the first edition of this book in 2010. There is increased emphasis on mild cognitive impairment (MCI) and how it affects the risk of dementia, and the new criteria for MCI in PD [1] have facilitated research in this area. Further, the work of Kehagia and colleagues regarding the 'dual syndrome' hypothesis [2] is central to the discussion of the dementia syndrome in PD and new purely descriptive studies of cognition in PD-D are not as relevant as in the past.

Nevertheless, studying and describing the cognitive profile of patients with PD-D is still of fundamental importance. If PD-D is characterized as having a specific cognitive impairment profile, cognitive assessment may be a useful tool in the diagnostic workup of individual patients. Further, the pattern of cognitive deficits can contribute to knowledge about relationships between brain function, brain structure, and cognitive processes in PD-D in relation to other neurodegenerative dementias. Finally, the cognitive profile in PD-D provides in itself a valuable insight regarding the phenomenology of PD-D. Thus, the aim of the present chapter is to describe the relative cognitive profile of patients with PD-D compared with other forms of dementia, as well as with healthy individuals.

While there is a large literature on the cognitive features of PD in general [3], research on cognition in PD-D is still relatively scarce. In several older studies in particular the diagnostic status of the PD patients regarding dementia was not reported according to explicit criteria. Further, studies preceding the first consensus criteria for dementia with Lewy bodies (DLB) proposed in 1996 [4] did not employ the 1-year rule concerning the interval between onset of parkinsonism and onset of cognitive dysfunction. In the literature review presented in the article outlining the criteria for PD-D [5] this problem was solved by restricting the reviewed papers to those investigating patients with PD and dementia according to clearly operationalized criteria. The same approach will be adopted in this chapter.

Cognitive domains and their assessment

When describing the cognitive profile in PD-D there are at least two implicit assumptions that should be elaborated: (1) the existence of distinct cognitive functions or domains, and (2) that cognitive functions may be quantified and compared between groups of individuals. Assumption (1) has been extensively discussed in the cognitive neuropsychology literature. Although most researchers would probably agree that cognitive domains are separable, there is still some disagreement about the interrelationship between them, and the terminology may be inconsistent and confusing between studies.

For instance, 'executive functions' is a term for processes that regulate all goal-directed behaviour [6]. This implies that these 'executive functions' should exert a global effect on tests that were designed to assess other cognitive domains if those tests require goal-directed behaviour, such as planning, monitoring, effort, and flexibility. This is problematic, however, considering that the 'double dissociation' method has often been used in order to analytically identify independent cognitive functions [7]. According to this method, it should be demonstrated that the hypothetical cognitive function A could be impaired in some patients while cognitive function B could be intact, and there should be patients in whom function B is impaired while function A is intact. However, as executive and attentional deficits, by definition, should have modulatory effects on a wide range of cognitive functions, the 'double dissociation' method does not always apply. Rather, it has been demonstrated that brain pathology in fronto-subcortical areas leads to a global deficit in all types of tests that require controlled attention. This is of particular relevance to PD-D, as it has been proposed that cognitive deficits in PD, in general, are caused by disruption of fronto-subcortical loops [3]. In the dual -syndrome hypothesis of Kehagia and colleagues [2], it is proposed that such a fronto-striatal dysfunction mediates a dysexecutive syndrome seen in PD without dementia, while PD-D is characterized by more widespread memory and visuospatial deficits.

Another important issue concerns phenomena such as alertness and arousal. In DLB and PD-D, attentional 'fluctuation' is a feature of the cognitive profile. Such fluctuation could possibly be related to changes in arousal or alertness, this could exert a global effect on other cognitive and behavioural functions [8]. Thus, when interpreting patterns of cognitive dysfunction in PD-D one should be mindful of the possible influence of executive dysfunction and of reduced arousal/alertness. I will return to this issue later and discuss the term 'bradyphrenia' as related to deficits in arousal and alertness.

Assumption (2) (i.e. that it is possible to quantify and compare cognitive functions across groups) is more straightforward. Cognitive measures are constructed according to statistical psychometric principles and can be subjected to relative comparisons between groups. The fundamental 'gold standard' for describing a cognitive profile in a patient group is comparison with a healthy control group matching the patients on background variables that are known to affect cognition, such as age, gender, and education. Further, cognitive comparisons can be carried between patient groups.

Average effect size: a meta-analytic approach

The simplest way of comparing cognitive functions between different groups is to simply arrange them ordinally (e.g. group A are worse than group B), as in qualitative reviews. This strategy was employed in two reviews on cognitive functions in PD-D and DLB [9, 10]. The problem with this is that it is very difficult to draw an overall conclusion regarding the literature as a whole. Another method is to compare standardized effect sizes to identify differences in standardized group mean values (Cohen's *d*), a strategy used in quantitative meta-analysis. In this strategy, the differences of the means are divided by the pooled standard deviations of the groups, enabling a comparison of the magnitude of differences in various cognitive domains, in this case between PD-D and the comparison groups. In the present review this will be done for studies on cognition in PD-D that reported means, standard deviations, and group sizes. Other studies will be described in a qualitative manner. The cognitive profile of patients with PD-D as compared with healthy control subjects (HC) will be described, representing the cognitive deficits in PD-D relative to healthy ageing. Further, the cognitive profile of PD-D compared with other neurodegenerative dementias, i.e. PD-D versus Alzheimer's disease (AD), and PD-D versus DLB, will be presented. A fixed-effects meta-analysis of the average standardized difference between DLB and PD-D on attention and executive functions, memory, and visuospatial functions will also be presented, as the distinction between DLB and PD-D remains contested.

Deficits in individual cognitive domains in PD-D

Attention and executive functions

The term 'executive functions' refers to a set of cognitive functions that are responsible for the planning, initiation, sequencing, and monitoring of complex goal-directed behaviour [6]. Historically, 'executive functions' has been used in at least two different ways. The older use of the term referred to 'higher'/'frontal' functions such as insight, will, abstraction, and judgement. In the recent literature, the term usually means cybernetic 'control' functions [6] and is used more or less synonymously with concepts such as 'top-down' cognitive control or attentional control functions [11].

Thus, attentional control refers to the same phenomena as the cybernetic executive control functions. However, the term attention may also refer to 'bottom-up' phenomena such as orienting to stimulus novelty and startle, as well as to basic alertness or vigilance. Alertness and vigilance may be defined as readiness to detect and respond to stimuli, related to cortical arousal. Further, the term 'selective attention' refers to the ability to filter out task-irrelevant stimuli and to facilitate the processing of task-relevant stimuli [11]. Alertness and vigilance are basic requisites for behaviour involving the processing of external events and have a global impact on behaviour and cognition [8]. Focus on the importance of alertness and vigilance has increased as the concept of 'fluctuating attention' has become a 'core feature' in the diagnostic criteria for DLB [12], since such fluctuations could be viewed as a form of alertness deficit.

A problem in measuring executive functions and attention is that there are no pure tests of such functions. These functions are cognitive component-processes of both goal-directed behaviour and bottom-up driven processing of external stimuli. This may pose a problem if, for instance, one only uses visual test-paradigms for measuring attention in a patient group with severe visuospatial impairment. However, different tasks have different requirements for attention and executive functions, and executive and attentional deficits may be inferred if patients tend to perform worse on such tasks than on less demanding ones.

An overview of studies in which PD-D was diagnosed according to explicit criteria is shown in Table 4.1. In the columns of the table, effect sizes, measured with Cohen's d [13], defined as the difference of the means divided by the pooled standard deviations, are given for the comparisons of PD-D with different patients groups (DLB, AD, and PD patients without dementia) and healthy controls (HC). The pooled standard deviation of the compared groups was calculated as recommended by Hedges and Olkin [14]. An effect size of 0.2 to 0.3 is considered small, 0.5 medium, and ≥ 0.8 a 'large' effect [13]. A positive number indicates that the group represented in the column performed better than the PD-D group, while a negative number indicates worse performance than the PD-D group.

Attention and executive functions are somewhat more severely affected in PD-D than in AD, with a medium average effect size of 0.14. It appears that attention and executive functions are

Table 4.1 Executive functions and attention

Test	HC	DLB	AD	PD
CAMCOG: attention [15]	1.71	−0.04	0.49	1.46
Verbal fluency:				
Letter [16]		−0.13	0.52	
Letter [17]		0		
Letter [18]	1.91		0.43	
Letter [19]			0.23	
Letter [20]		−0.70	−0.22	
Letter [21]	1.94		−0.01	
Category [16]		0.26	0.38	
Category [17]		−0.33		
Category [18]	1.65		−0.19	
Category (supermarket) [20]		−0.18	−0.61	
Category (animals) [20]		−0.71	−0.65	
Category [21]	1.21		−0.05	
Category and letter [22]	0.65		−0.14	0.33
Trail making test:				
Part A [17]		−1.36[a]		
Part A [22]	1.48		0.05[a]	0.66
Part B [17]		−0.13[a]		
Part A (ZVT version) [21]	1.46		−0.34[a]	
Dementia Rating Scale:				
Initiation and perseveration [18]	2.04		0	
Attention [23]			0.03	
Initiation and perseveration [23]			0.30	
Wisconsin card sorting test:				
Criteria [17]		−0.29		
Categories [18]	1.66		0.54	
Categories [19]			−0.04	
Cancellation				
Shape time [16]		−0.04[a]	1.06[a]	
TMX time [16]		−0.41	0.83	
Stroop test:				
Interference [17]		−0.41		
Interference [20]		−0.24	0.55	
Frontal assessment battery [17]		0		

Table 4.1 (continued) Executive functions and attention

Test	HC	DLB	AD	PD
Digit span:				
WAIS total [17]		0		
Forward [19]			−0.09	
Forward [20]		0.18	0.06	
Forward [21]	1.67		−0.33	
Forward [22]	0		−0.40	0.32
Backward [19]			−0.10	
Backward [20]		−0.66	0.08	
Backward [21]	2.72		0.17	
Backward [22]	0.40		−0.23	0.44
RBANS: attention [24]			0.72	1.46
Mental control (WMS) [22]	0.38		−0.43	0.41
Digit symbol (WAIS) [22]	1.72		0	0.92
Choice reaction time [25][b]	1.60[a]	0.04[a]	0.86[a]	1.20[a]
Simple reaction time [25][b]	1.39	0.34[1]	0.74	1.21
Serial 7s [26]			0.72	
Average effect size	1.42	−0.21, −0.11[c]	0.14	0.84

Numbers represent Cohen's *d* relative to PD-D.

CAMCOG, Cambridge Cognitive Examination [27]; ZVT, Zahlen-Verbindungs-Test; RBANS, Repeatable Battery for the Assessment of Neuropsychological Status [28]; TMX, Consonant Trigram Cancellation; WAIS, Wechsler Adult Intelligence Scale; WMS, Wechsler Memory Scale.

[a] Reaction time data reversed.

[b] This study had large MMSE and age differences.

[c] Weighted meta-analytic average effect size, according to sample size; *p* = 0.106.

more severely affected in DLB than in PD-D, with a small average effect size of −0.21, but a fixed-effects meta-analysis revealed a weighted average mean difference of −0.11 (*p* = 0.106). Hence, there is no proven statistical difference between DLB and PD-D with regard to attention and executive functions. Fig. 4.1 gives a graphical depiction.

This meta-analytic review should be interpreted with caution as there are several results that come from the same sample, just with different tests, and hence sample characteristics specific to these studies may exert too much weight in the results.

There were a few studies that could not be included in Table 4.1 as the required statistics were not reported. In a study by Aarsland et al. [29], 60 patients with DLB, 35 with PD-D, 49 with progressive supranuclear palsy (PSP), and 29 with AD were compared using subscores from the Mattis Dementia Rating Scale (DRS) [30]. The groups were not matched for age, education, and severity of dementia, but statistical correction was used. Further, results were presented separately for mild to moderate versus severe dementia. The main findings showed that patients with DLB and PD-D suffering from severe dementia had a similar cognitive profile. For mild to moderate dementia, the PD-D group had a higher conceptualization score than the DLB group. This subscale measures semantic language abilities and abstraction. No other differences were found.

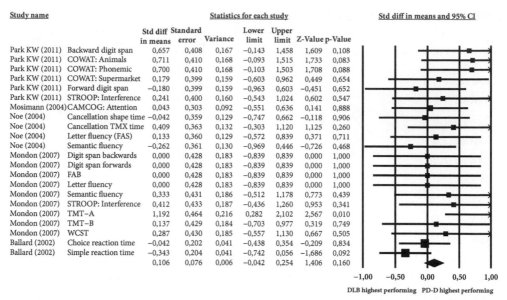

Study name		Statistics for each study							Std diff in means and 95% CI
		Std diff in means	Standard error	Variance	Lower limit	Upper limit	Z-Value	p-Value	
Park KW (2011)	Backward digit span	0,657	0,408	0,167	−0,143	1,458	1,609	0,108	
Park KW (2011)	COWAT: Animals	0,711	0,410	0,168	−0,093	1,515	1,733	0,083	
Park KW (2011)	COWAT: Phonemic	0,700	0,410	0,168	−0,103	1,503	1,708	0,088	
Park KW (2011)	COWAT: Supermarket	0,179	0,399	0,159	−0,603	0,962	0,449	0,654	
Park KW (2011)	Forward digit span	−0,180	0,399	0,159	−0,963	0,603	−0,451	0,652	
Park KW (2011)	STROOP: Interference	0,241	0,400	0,160	−0,543	1,024	0,602	0,547	
Mosimann (2004)	CAMCOG: Attention	0,043	0,303	0,092	−0,551	0,636	0,141	0,888	
Noe (2004)	Cancellation shape time	−0,042	0,359	0,129	−0,747	0,662	−0,118	0,906	
Noe (2004)	Cancellation TMX time	0,409	0,363	0,132	−0,303	1,120	1,125	0,260	
Noe (2004)	Letter fluency (FAS)	0,133	0,360	0,129	−0,572	0,839	0,371	0,711	
Noe (2004)	Semantic fluency	−0,262	0,361	0,130	−0,969	0,446	−0,726	0,468	
Mondon (2007)	Digit span backwards	0,000	0,428	0,183	−0,839	0,839	0,000	1,000	
Mondon (2007)	Digit span forwards	0,000	0,428	0,183	−0,839	0,839	0,000	1,000	
Mondon (2007)	FAB	0,000	0,428	0,183	−0,839	0,839	0,000	1,000	
Mondon (2007)	Letter fluency	0,000	0,428	0,183	−0,839	0,839	0,000	1,000	
Mondon (2007)	Semantic fluency	0,333	0,431	0,186	−0,512	1,178	0,773	0,439	
Mondon (2007)	STROOP: Interference	0,412	0,433	0,187	−0,436	1,260	0,953	0,341	
Mondon (2007)	TMT−A	1,192	0,464	0,216	0,282	2,102	2,567	0,010	
Mondon (2007)	TMT−B	0,137	0,429	0,184	−0,703	0,977	0,319	0,749	
Mondon (2007)	WCST	0,287	0,430	0,185	−0,557	1,130	0,667	0,505	
Ballard (2002)	Choice reaction time	−0,042	0,202	0,041	−0,438	0,354	−0,209	0,834	
Ballard (2002)	Simple reaction time	−0,343	0,204	0,041	−0,742	0,056	−1,686	0,092	
		0,106	0,076	0,006	−0,042	0,254	1,406	0,160	

−1,00   −0,50   0,00   0,50   1,00

DLB highest performing   PD-D highest performing

Fig. 4.1 Fixed-effects meta-analysis: DLB versus PD-D, attention and executive functions. Studies cited in the figure are Park et al. [20], Mosimann et al. [15], Noe et al. [16], Mondon et al. [17], and Ballard et al. [25].

PD-D patients with mild to moderate dementia performed worse than AD patients on 'initiation and perseveration', a measure of executive functions. However, this subscale contains several complex motor tasks, possibly confounding the results.

There are two studies analysing components of attentional processes in PD-D using event-related potentials (ERPs). Perriol and colleagues [73] investigated a sensory filtering mechanism, pre-pulse inhibition (PPI), in PD-D, DLB, AD, and HC (10 subjects in each group). PPI is calculated as the amplitude of N1/P2 ERPs to a startle stimulus after a preceding (about 120 ms in this case) non-startling stimulus. The authors found reduced PPI in DLB and PD-D compared with the HC, and the DLB group also showed reduced PPI when compared with the AD group. Thus, the authors concluded that sensory filtering was most severely affected in DLB, followed by PD-D, while the AD patients did not differ significantly from the HC.

Brønnick and colleagues [31] investigated an auditory automatic stimulus change-detection mechanism by measuring the mismatch negativity (MMN) ERP [32] in PD-D, DLB, AD, PD, and HC subjects. The amplitude of the MMN for the PD-D group was significantly attenuated compared with DLB, PD, and HC. Further, as compared with PD, DLB, AD, and HC, the PD-D group significantly regularly missed target stimuli in an auditory 'oddball-distracter' task which significantly correlated with MMN amplitude. Thus, the authors concluded that the PD-D patients had a more severe auditory attention deficit than DLB and AD, related to automatic (bottom-up driven) detection of stimulus deviance. A notable finding was that the MMN of the PD group was equal to that of the HC group, there was not even a tendency towards amplitude-attenuation. Hence, there appears to be a qualitative difference in automatic stimulus detection in PD-D versus PD that may be associated with the development of dementia in PD. The more severe deficit in PD-D compared with DLB was also surprising. A possible explanation could be that the attentional deficit in DLB is more pronounced in visual modality, as most of the research on attentional deficits in DLB and PD-D has used visual tests. Clearly, it should not be concluded that attention in general is impaired based on tests in a single sensory modality.

The finding that executive impairment is marked in PD-D is not surprising, given that cognitive impairment in PD without dementia is also frequently characterized by a dysexecutive syndrome [3, 33, 34]. However, it is not clear how the cognitive deficits in PD progress to PD-D, i.e. if this process is one of gradual change or of qualitative differences. While in earlier studies progression of dopaminergic deficits was held responsible for cognitive impairment in PD-D, the role of other neural systems and neurotransmitters, including noradrenergic, serotonergic, and cholinergic systems, was subsequently emphasized [35]. This view has been most clearly put forward by Kehagia et al. [2], who argue that PD-D is first and foremost associated with a severe cholinergic deficit that sets this condition apart from PD with dysexecutive features. Kehagia calls this 'the dual-syndrome hypothesis'.

The deficits of attention and executive functions in PD-D have a special significance, as it has been shown that attentional deficits in PD-D are the most important cognitive predictor of ability to perform activities of daily living (ADL) in a very large sample of PD-D patients [36]. Further, it has been shown that attention [37] and executive functions [38] appear to be the cognitive functions that are most closely associated with visual hallucinations in PD. There is a possibility that such attentional–executive deficits may partly underlie impairments in other cognitive domains, especially visuospatial dysfunction [39] (later in this chapter we shall see that this may not be the whole story, as DLB appears to be associated with more severe visuospatial deficits).

Attention and bradyphrenia

In 1922, the neurologist F. Naville introduced the concept of bradyphrenia, a condition characterized by slow cognition, apathy, and impaired concentration [40]. The term originated in the context of an epidemic of encephalitis lethargica in the 1920s which resulted in parkinsonism and the psychiatric syndrome that became to be known as bradyphrenia. The term 'bradyphrenia' is frequently used in the older literature on cognitive deficits in PD. However, even initially there were conflicting results regarding the relationship between parkinsonism and bradyphrenia. In 1924, Worster-Drought and Hardcastle found that reduced psychomotor speed, but not an increase in 'cerebration time' ('thinking time'), was associated with parkinsonism [40]. Authors such as Mayeux have suggested that slowed cognition is a cause of, or at least closely related to, deficits of alertness in PD [41].

In PD-D, there is consistent ERP-based evidence of slowed cognition. In a study investigating both auditory and visual ERPs in HC, PD-D, AD, and PD, auditory P300 and flash visual-evoked potential latency measures were significantly increased in the PD-D group compared with controls [42]. Increased ERP-latencies in PD-D have also been found in other studies [43]. Two studies have directly compared P300 latency in both PD-D and PD relative to HC. In both studies P300 latencies were normal in the PD groups but increased in the PD-D groups [44, 45].

Pate and Margolin [46], who used two reaction time tasks, concluded that motor, as well cognitive, slowing was present in both PD and PD-D, and that such slowing was disproportionate to the level of general cognitive impairment compared with a group of AD patients. However, Goldman et al. [47] compared 22 patients with mild PD-D with 58 non-impaired PD patients and 48 HC. They found slow movement time, but no increase in cognitive reaction time in either PD or mild PD-D. Nevertheless, the study of Ballard et al. [25] showed that cognitive reaction time was slower in PD-D than in PD and AD, being comparable to that in DLB. The PD patients without dementia had slower choice reaction time than the HC but a similar variability of reaction time. Thus, this study indicates that slow cognition is associated with cognitive decline in PD, and its severity is disproportionately large in PD-D and DLB compared with AD.

The concept of bradyphrenia and 'slow cognition' may be problematic in relation to the attention construct and also to other cognitive functions. The study by Mayeux et al. [41] illustrates the problem. Poor performance on a vigilance task was deemed to be due to 'bradyphrenia'. What then is the relationship between 'bradyphrenia' and 'vigilance' or 'alertness'? A solution is offered in Timothy Salthouse's [48] processing speed theory of adult age differences in cognition. Salthouse proposes that slowed cognition (bradyphrenia) is a general mechanism underlying the age-related decline in cognitive performance. The assumption is that any complex mental task is executed by multiple cognitive component processes with associated neural underpinnings. If one or more of these processes runs more slowly because of pathology affecting the associated neural substrate(s), the mental task will either be solved more slowly or not solved successfully at all (if it depends on a timing restraint). This is the case in perceptual detection tasks, where the presentation of external stimuli cannot be slowed down by the perceiver. In this case, slowed cognition may, for instance, lead to missed target stimuli. Salthouse calls this phenomenon a 'limited time' mechanism. Slow component cognitive processes can also lead to deficits when the product of early processing stages is no longer available for use in a later processing stage. Salthouse calls this the 'simultaneity mechanism' [48]. The latter may, for instance, be the case in working memory tasks where cognitive manipulation of working memory content is dependent upon active maintenance of this content. Thus, slow cognition and deficits in vigilance/alertness are phenomena on different analytical levels. Slow cognition is a neural and mental mechanism, while vigilance/alertness deficits are behavioural manifestations of this mechanism. The evidence overall indicates that not all PD patients experience cognitive slowing, but that cognitive slowing is associated with cognitive decline and dementia and that it may be closely related to the aetiology of the cognitive decline in PD to a larger degree than in AD.

In summary, the combined evidence shows that executive and attentional dysfunctions are cognitive hallmarks of PD-D compared with AD. When compared with DLB, the deficits overall appear to be somewhat less severe. However, the studies that have compared 'fluctuations', defined as variability of reaction time [25, 31], both showed that fluctuating attention was at least as severe in PD-D as in DLB.

Visuospatial functions

The term 'visuospatial functions' is used to describe a wide range of cognitive functions measured by several different tests. The unifying theme of the term is that these tests rely on visual perception, visual representation, or a visually guided response. The term can be misleading, as it lumps together very different cognitive processes, perhaps too broadly. Ungerleider and Mishkin [49] proposed two distinct cortical processing pathways of visual information, the occipito-temporal pathway (the 'what is it' pathway) and the occipito-parietal pathway (the 'where is it' pathway). It has since become clear that visual processing is performed in several widely distributed cortical areas [50, 51] and that spatial cognition is very different from the perception of visual form and object categorization [50]. In the clinical neuropsychology literature, many 'visuospatial tests' are tests of the ability to draw complex figures (visual construction). Unfortunately, the performance of such tasks demands attentional/executive control as well as fine-motor control. In addition, such tests do not usually assess spatial cognition well. These issues are problematic in the research on PD-D, as it has been difficult to interpret findings. An overview of studies on PD-D in which visuospatial functions were reported is given in Table 4.2.

Table 4.2 Visuospatial functions

Test	HC	DLB	AD	PD
Pentagon drawing [52]		−0.13	0.42	1.33
DRS construction [23]			0.53	
Rey–Osterrieth complex figure test:				
Copy [17]		−0.22		
Copy [20]		−0.08	0.41	
Poppelreuter test [17]		−0.61		
CERAD neuropsychological battery copy test [21]	1.17		0.09	
CAMCOG:				
Construction [15]	3.16	−0.12	0.84	2.32
Perception [15]	1.60	−0.55	0.59	1.32
BVRT: matching [16]		−0.14	0.88	
Rosen drawing test [16]		−0.94	0.08	
ADAScog: construction [26]			0.49	
RBANS: visuospatial [24]			0.51	1.23
Benton visual retention test (copy) [22]	0.98		0.10	0.52
Average effect-size	1.73	−0.35, −0.31[a]	0.44	1.34

Numbers represent Cohen's d, relative to PD-D.

[a]Weighted meta-analytic average effect size, according to sample size; $p = 0.009$.

CAMCOG, Cambridge Cognitive Examination [27]; DRS, Dementia Rating Scale; BVRT: Benton Visual Retention Test [53]; ADAScog, cognitive part of Alzheimer's Disease Assessment Scale [54]; RBANS, Repeatable Battery for the Assessment of Neuropsychological Status [28].

PD-D patients have more pronounced visuospatial dysfunctions than patients with AD, with a medium effect size (Cohen's $d = 0.44$). It is also evident that according to the fixed-effect meta-analysis, visuospatial functions are statistically significantly less severely affected in PD-D than in DLB, approaching a medium effect size ($d = -0.35$, average weighted fixed effect = -0.21, $p = 0.009$) (see Fig. 4.2 for a graphical depiction).

Some of the studies used perception tasks that required no eye–hand coordination or motor control, and less executive control; for instance there was a larger deficit in DLB compared with PD-D on the Cambridge Cognitive Examination (CAMCOG) perception task relative to the CAMCOG construction task [15]. Patients with PD-D also performed better than patients with DLB on other perception tasks [16, 17].

The study by Mosimann et al. [15] is probably the most comprehensive study published to date regarding visuospatial functions in PD-D compared with other patient groups. In addition to the CAMCOG results listed in Table 4.2, the study included tests of visual object-form perception, space-motion perception, and visual discrimination of various lengths and sizes. DLB, AD, PD, and HC groups were compared with PD-D, and separate analyses were conducted for patients with and without hallucinations. No statistically significant differences between DLB and PD-D patients were found on any tasks, and both these groups performed worse than patients with AD. Patients with visual hallucinations performed worse than non-hallucinators in both the DLB and

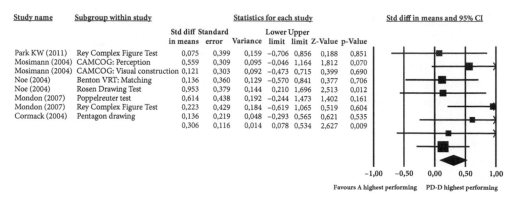

Study name	Subgroup within study	Statistics for each study							Std diff in means and 95% CI
		Std diff in means	Standard error	Variance	Lower limit	Upper limit	Z-Value	p-Value	
Park KW (2011)	Rey Complex Figure Test	0,075	0,399	0,159	−0,706	0,856	0,188	0,851	
Mosimann (2004)	CAMCOG: Perception	0,559	0,309	0,095	−0,046	1,164	1,812	0,070	
Mosimann (2004)	CAMCOG: Visual construction	0,121	0,303	0,092	−0,473	0,715	0,399	0,690	
Noe (2004)	Benton VRT: Matching	0,136	0,360	0,129	−0,570	0,841	0,377	0,706	
Noe (2004)	Rosen Drawing Test	0,953	0,379	0,144	0,210	1,696	2,513	0,012	
Mondon (2007)	Poppelreuter test	0,614	0,438	0,192	−0,244	1,473	1,402	0,161	
Mondon (2007)	Rey Complex Figure Test	0,223	0,429	0,184	−0,619	1,065	0,519	0,604	
Cormack (2004)	Pentagon drawing	0,136	0,219	0,048	−0,293	0,565	0,621	0,535	
		0,306	0,116	0,014	0,078	0,534	2,627	0,009	

−1,00 −0,50 0,00 0,50 1,00

Favours A highest performing   PD-D highest performing

Fig. 4.2 Fixed-effects meta-analysis: DLB versus PD-D, visuospatial functions. Studies as in Fig. 4.1 plus Cormack et al. [52].

PD-D group. While the authors concluded that the performance of the PD-D and DLB groups was worse in the object-form perception tasks than in the space-motion perception task, the very low error scores in the AD, PD, and HC groups indicate a probable floor-effect that is likely lead to underestimation of the real differences. Thus, it is difficult to draw conclusions regarding relative impairment in subdomains of visuospatial functioning in PD-D based on this study.

The previously mentioned study on PD-D, AD, DLB, and PSP by Aarsland et al. [29] also showed that in the groups with mild to moderate dementia the DLB patients performed worse than the PD-D group on the Mattis DRS construction (drawing) tasks. No difference was found in the severe dementia groups.

In conclusion, PD-D is associated with visuospatial dysfunctions that are more severe than in AD but very likely less severe than in DLB.

Memory

In several diagnostic manuals (DSM-IV, DSM-IIIR, ICD10), memory impairment is required for the diagnosis of dementia. This requirement is arbitrary and a historical relic related to the importance of AD in earlier dementia research and in the clinic. In AD, the earliest sign of impairment is usually observed in episodic memory, related to pathology affecting the medial temporal lobes, most notably the hippocampus and enthorinal cortex [55]. As AD is the most common cause of dementia, memory impairment has become a defining feature of dementia. The newly published DSM-V diagnostic manual has finally changed this rule, and in the consensus criteria for diagnosing DLB memory impairment is not essential [12]. Likewise, in the clinical criteria for PD-D memory impairment is not a prerequisite [5], impairment in 'free recall' is listed as one of the four core cognitive features, of which two are required to make a diagnosis of 'probable' PD-D.

Like executive and visuospatial functions, memory is a broad term that encompasses several different phenomena. However, the present discussion will be restricted to declarative, episodic memory, which is the form of memory that has been commonly investigated. The basic features of this kind of memory are that: (1) the memory content is consciously available for access and can be expressed verbally or by other means, such as drawing or by other behavioural means, and (2) the memory trace pertains to an experienced past event [56]. As mentioned, this type of memory depends on the integrity of the medial temporal lobes, and impairment of episodic memory is usually the first cognitive symptom of AD [55]. Table 4.3 presents the effect sizes for verbal

Table 4.3 Verbal memory

Test	HC	DLB	AD	PD
Buschke selective reminding test:				
Total recall [19]			−0.17	
Total recall [17]		−0.70		
Total recall [16]		−0.08	−0.26	
Delayed recall [16]		0.10	−1.26	
Total recall [57]	1.96		−0.08	1.12
Delayed recall [57]	1.74		−0.42	1.41
Total recall [58]	2.96		−0.08	
Delayed recall [58]	3.02		−0.15	
Delayed recognition [58]	1.99		−1.15	
ADAScog memory:				
Recall [26]			−0.37	
Recognition [26]			−0.23	
Grober–Buschke procedure:				
Total free immediate recall [59]			−2.05	
Long delay free recall [59]			−2.53	
Recognition correct [59]			−7.83[a]	
Recognition false positives [59]			−4.81[a]	
RBANS memory:				
Immediate recall [24]			−0.08	1.01
Delayed memory [24]			−1.17	0.75
Rey auditory verbal learning:				
Free recall list A [60]	1.86		−0.16	
Recognition discriminability [60]	0.83		−0.94	
Luria memory test:				
Immediate recall [58]	1.51		−0.32	
Delayed recall [58]	1.69		−0.82	
Story recall:				
Short delay [58]	1.46		−0.84	
Short delay [22]	0.95		−0.75	0.26
California verbal learning test:				
Short delay free recall [61]				1.75
Long delay free recall [61]				1.50
Short delay cued recall [61]				1.86
Long delay cued recall [61]				1.57

Table 4.3 (continued) Verbal memory

Test	HC	DLB	AD	PD
Recognition [61]				1.84
Immediate memory total [62]	1.80	−0.99		
Long delay free recall [62]	1.69	−0.91		
Seoul verbal learning test:				
Immediate recall [20]		−0.49	−0.22	
Delayed recall [20]		−0.98	−1.30	
CERAD neuropsychological battery:				
Word list learning [21]			−0.67	
Word list delayed recall [21]			−0.38	
Average effect size	1.80	−0.57	−0.68	1.30

Numbers represent Cohen's *d*, relative to PD-D.

ADAScog, cognitive part of Alzheimer's Disease Assessment Scale [54]; RBANS, Repeatable Battery for the Assessment of Neuropsychological Status [28].

[a]These figures are not normally distributed and are not included in the averages.

memory in PD-D. As visuospatial impairment in PD-D may affect the memory performance for visual material, findings in visual memory tests are presented separately in Table 4.4.

As seen from these results, verbal memory performance in PD-D is severely deficient when compared with healthy controls. The pooled data show that patients with PD-D clearly have better verbal memory functioning than patients with AD, with an average effect size of 0.68. A fixed-effects meta-analysis also showed that the standardized mean difference between verbal memory in PD-D and DLB was −0.57, a statistically significant difference ($p < 0.001$) (see Fig. 4.3).

In interpreting the findings in Table 4.4 it should be kept in mind that the average effect sizes are calculated from very few studies; thus the results may not be generalizable. Nevertheless, it is interesting to note that visual memory in PD-D is more deficient than in DLB, as confirmed by a fixed-effects meta-analysis of the results (weighted effect size −0.437, $p = 0.006$; see Fig. 4.4). These results mimic those of the verbal memory comparisons, indicating that memory in general is less affected in PD-D than in DLB.

There are four studies that compared AD with PD-D using composite memory scales [15, 18, 23, 59], including both verbal and visual tasks (see Table 4.5). The average effect size is very large (Cohen's $d = −1.30$), indicating that memory performance in AD overall is worse than in PD-D.

An important discussion concerning memory dysfunction in PD without dementia concerns whether there exists a genuine episodic memory deficit that affects learning (encoding) and the retention of learned material or if memory deficits are secondary consequences of executive/attentional deficits [63]. For instance, it has been claimed that patients with PD may show dysfunction on free recall measures of memory but be able to recognize the material when it is presented to them [33]. Thus, the deficit could be related to deficient retrieval of memory content, and this has been called 'the retrieval deficit hypothesis'. It is still not clear whether there exists a recognition memory deficit in PD without dementia. In a quantitative meta-analytic review [64], the authors divided studies on memory in PD into three groups: studies of (1) patients with

Table 4.4 Visual memory in PD-D compared with other diseases and healthy controls

Test	HC	DLB	AD	PD
Benton visual retention test:				
Visual recognition [19]			0.21	
Visual recognition [17]		−0.78		
Visual recognition [16]		−0.25	0.74	
Visual recognition [57]	1.64		0.56	2.07
WMS associate memory [22]	0.85		−0.56	0.47
Delayed matching to sample:				
Instant visual recognition [17]		−1.70		
Delayed visual recognition [17]		−1.50		
Rey–Osterrieth complex figure test:				
Short delay, visual construction [17]		−0.18		
Immediate [20]		0.20		
Delayed [20]		0.26		
CERAD neuropsychological battery: visuoconstructive delayed recall [21]	3.08		−0.31	
Average effect size	1.86	−0.56	0.13	1.27

Numbers represent Cohen's *d*, relative to PD-D.

WMS, Wechsler Memory Scale.

dementia, (2) patients without dementia, and (3) patients unselected according to cognitive status. A small effect size (Cohen's *d* = 0.16) for the patients without dementia suggested that there is a recognition memory deficit in PD but that the magnitude is small, requiring studies with large samples for it to be detected. In the unselected patients, the effect size was moderate (*d* = 0.52). The patients with PD-D had clear recognition memory deficits, as shown by a large effect size (*d* = 1.3) compared with the controls.

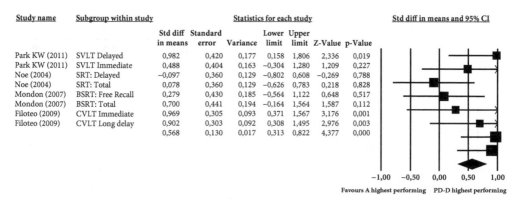

Fig. 4.3 Fixed-effects meta-analysis: DLB versus PD-D, verbal memory. Studies as in Fig. 4.1 plus Filoteo et al. [62].

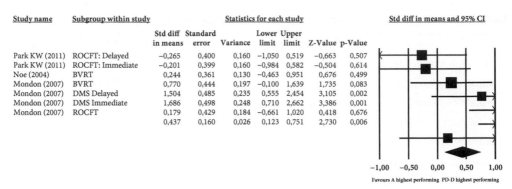

Study name	Subgroup within study	Std diff in means	Standard error	Variance	Lower limit	Upper limit	Z-Value	p-Value
Park KW (2011)	ROCFT: Delayed	−0,265	0,400	0,160	−1,050	0,519	−0,663	0,507
Park KW (2011)	ROCFT: Immediate	−0,201	0,399	0,160	−0,984	0,582	−0,504	0,614
Noe (2004)	BVRT	0,244	0,361	0,130	−0,463	0,951	0,676	0,499
Mondon (2007)	BVRT	0,770	0,444	0,197	−0,100	1,639	1,735	0,083
Mondon (2007)	DMS Delayed	1,504	0,485	0,235	0,555	2,454	3,105	0,002
Mondon (2007)	DMS Immediate	1,686	0,498	0,248	0,710	2,662	3,386	0,001
Mondon (2007)	ROCFT	0,179	0,429	0,184	−0,661	1,020	0,418	0,676
		0,437	0,160	0,026	0,123	0,751	2,730	0,006

Fig. 4.4 Fixed-effects meta-analysis: DLB versus PD-D, visual memory. Studies as in Fig. 4.1.

When averaging effect sizes from all studies on memory in PD-D, we find that PD-D patients perform better than patients with DLB (d = 0.63) and AD (d = 0.65), but show a severe memory dysfunction compared with HC (d = 2.05) and PD without dementia (d = 1.51). Thus, while memory deficits are less pronounced than in AD and DLB, they are severe compared with subjects without dementia. However, as the included studies employed diagnostic criteria for dementia that required memory impairment, this may be an artefact of these criteria. Future research using the proposed criteria for PD-D [5] should be useful for gaining more accurate knowledge about memory impairment in PD-D.

Language

As shown in Table 4.1, several studies have assessed executive functions through verbal fluency tests, which may also be viewed as tests of expressive language. Patients with PD-D are not able to produce as many words within a given time span as patients with AD, and they show a severe deficit when compared with HC. However, these deficits have been interpreted as being caused by a more general executive control deficit [65] and few studies have focused on core language functions in PD-D.

Table 4.5 Composite memory scales

Test	HC	DLB	AD	PD
Dementia Rating Scale:				
Memory [23]			−0.86	
Memory [18]	2.54		−1.51	
Wechsler Memory Scale [18] (composite scale)	2.90		−1.19	
CAMCOG memory [15] (composite scale)	2.11	−0.37	−1.44	1.71
Wechsler Memory Scale [59] (composite scale)			−1.48	
Average effect size	2.52	−0.37	−1.30	1.71

Numbers represent Cohen's d, relative to PD-D.

CAMCOG, Cambridge Cognitive Examination [27].

Cummings et al. [66] have published the most comprehensive study of language in PD-D to date. In this study, 16 patients with PD-D, 35 with PD, and 10 patients with AD were compared using a comprehensive language assessment battery derived from the Boston Diagnostic Aphasia Examination [67] and the Western Aphasia Battery [68]. Speech, writing, comprehension of spoken language, naming, verbal fluency, reading comprehension, reading aloud, and repetition were assessed. The PD-D and AD patients did not differ in age, Mini-Mental State Examination (MMSE) score, or disease duration. Several differences were found between AD and PD-D. The PD-D patients had more severe dysarthric speech deficits (loudness, pitch, articulation, rate, and intelligibility), shorter phrase length, poorer speech melody, reduced grammatical complexity, and poorer writing mechanics. Thus, the PD-D group mostly had deficits that could be attributed to the motor impairment. The PD-D patients showed fewer naming deficits (anomia), better word list generation, and had higher information content in spontaneous speech than the patients with AD.

Thus, the sparse research on language functions in PD-D indicates that language impairment is likely to be primarily due to executive/attentional deficits.

Conclusion: the overall cognitive profile in PD-D

Fig. 4.5 summarizes the data from Tables 4.1–4.5 and the cognitive profile of PD-D is shown graphically. Language functions are not shown as the literature does not warrant a quantitative comparison.

The bars represent average effect size (Cohen's d) of comparisons where PD-D represents the reference group for each comparison with HC, DLB, AD, and PD without dementia. A positive number represents that the indicated group performed better than PD-D patients, while negative numbers indicate worse performance than in PD-D.

Perhaps somewhat surprisingly, memory is most severely affected compared with HC, followed by visuospatial functions, and finally attention and executive functions. Further, as was also

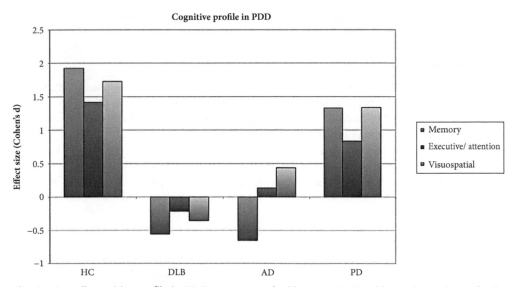

Fig. 4.5 Overall cognitive profile in PD-D as compared with AD, DLB, PD without dementia, and HC.

revealed by the meta-analyses shown graphically in Figs 4.1–4.4, PD-D patients performed better than DLB patients on visuospatial functions and on memory, while being very similar for attention and executive functions. This is important, as the distinction between DLB and PD-D is not clear, and these results indicate that there are differences that should be investigated further with regard to aetiology and pathophysiology.

Compared with AD, PD-D is clearly characterized with better memory functions but somewhat worse attention/executive functions, and clearly worse visuospatial functions. Finally, we see that PD patients without dementia have poorer performance on attention and executive functions than HC, using PD-D as the reference, and also performing worse overall on other functions.

Taken as a whole, there is some evidence that Kehagia's dual-syndrome hypothesis [2] is supported, as PD-D appears to be qualitatively quite different from PD with regard to cognitive profile, and the largest effect sizes are seen for visuospatial functions, as predicted by this hypothesis, but also for memory, while attention and executive functions are less different. Early cognitive impairments in PD without dementia should be driven by dopaminergically mediated frontostriatal executive impairments and PD-D should be associated with visuospatial deficits in which cholinergic deficits are prominent, and this is to some degree what is seen. However, there is still considerable research required in order to clarify how PD-D develops from PD and how the cognitive impairment seen in early PD [69] relates to PD-D, as there are very few studies which deal with these questions. A recent and methodologically sound study is the Norwegian ParkWest study, and in a recent article Pedersen et al. [70] reported that MCI was a strong predictor of PD-D and that verbal memory and executive inhibition as measured by the Stroop test were the strongest cognitive predictors.

The study by Janvin et al. [71] suggests that MCI in PD is associated with increased risk for developing dementia but that amnestic-type MCI is not associated with increased risk for dementia. Further, the same group have shown that there is heterogeneity in the cognitive profile of patients with PD-D; it was suggested that some patients show a 'cortical' profile while others demonstrate a 'subcortical' profile [72]. In the future, the impact of deficits in alertness and arousal should be systematically assessed, as such deficits could be important factors regarding the fluctuation of cognition in PD-D and the development of 'bradyphrenia'. The general impact of such deficits on other cognitive domains should also be more thoroughly assessed in future research.

References

1. **Litvan I, Goldman JG, Troster AI, et al.** Diagnostic criteria for mild cognitive impairment in Parkinson's disease: Movement Disorder Society Task Force guidelines. Mov Disord 2012; **27**: 349–56.
2. **Kehagia AA, Barker RA, Robbins TW.** Cognitive impairment in Parkinson's disease: the dual syndrome hypothesis. Neurodegener Dis 2013; **11**: 79–92.
3. **Zgaljardic DJ, Borod JC, Foldi NS, et al.** A review of the cognitive and behavioral sequelae of Parkinson's disease: relationship to frontostriatal circuitry. Cogn Behav Neurol 2003; **16**: 193–210.
4. **McKeith IG, Galasko D, Kosaka K, et al.** Consensus guidelines for the clinical and pathologic diagnosis of dementia with Lewy bodies (DLB): report of the consortium on DLB international workshop. Neurology 1996; **47**: 1113–24.
5. **Emre M, Aarsland D, Brown R, et al.** Clinical diagnostic criteria for dementia associated with Parkinson's disease. Mov Disord 2007; **22**: 1689–707.
6. **Royall DR, Lauterbach EC, Cummings JL, et al.** Executive control function: a review of its promise and challenges for clinical research. A report from the Committee on Research of the American Neuropsychiatric Association. J Neuropsychiatry Clin Neurosci 2002; **14**: 377–405.

7. **Van Orden GC, Pennington BF, Stone GO**. What do double dissociations prove? Cogn Sci 2001; **25**: 111–72.

8. **Mesulam MM**. A cortical network for directed attention and unilateral neglect. Ann Neurol 1981; **10**: 309–25.

9. **Troster AI**. Neuropsychological characteristics of dementia with Lewy bodies and Parkinson's disease with dementia: differentiation, early detection, and implications for 'mild cognitive impairment' and biomarkers. Neuropsychol Rev 2008; **18**: 103–19.

10. **Metzler-Baddeley C**. A review of cognitive impairments in dementia with Lewy bodies relative to Alzheimer's disease and Parkinson's disease with dementia. Cortex 2007; **43**: 583–600.

11. **Parasuraman R**. The attentive brain: issue and prospects. In: Parasuraman R (ed.) *The attentive brain*. Cambridge, MA: MIT Press, 1998; pp. 221–56.

12. **McKeith IG, Dickson DW, Lowe J, et al**. Diagnosis and management of dementia with Lewy bodies: third report of the DLB Consortium. Neurology 2005; **65**: 1863–72.

13. **Cohen J**. *Statistical power analysis for the behavioral sciences*. Hillsdale, NJ: Laurence Erlbaum, 1988.

14. **Hedges LV, Olkin I**. *Statistical methods for meta-analysis*. Orlando, FL: Academic Press, 1985.

15. **Mosimann UP, Mather G, Wesnes KA, et al**. Visual perception in Parkinson disease dementia and dementia with Lewy bodies. Neurology 2004; **63**: 2091–6.

16. **Noe E, Marder K, Bell KL, et al**. Comparison of dementia with Lewy bodies to Alzheimer's disease and Parkinson's disease with dementia. Mov Disord 2004; **19**: 60–7.

17. **Mondon K, Gochard A, Marque A, et al**. Visual recognition memory differentiates dementia with Lewy bodies and Parkinson's disease dementia. J Neurol Neurosurg Psychiatry 2007; **78**: 738–41.

18. **Litvan I, Mohr E, Williams J, et al**. Differential memory and executive functions in demented patients with Parkinson's and Alzheimer's disease. J Neurol Neurosurg Psychiatry 1991; **54**: 25–9.

19. **Starkstein SE, Sabe L, Petracca G, et al**. Neuropsychological and psychiatric differences between Alzheimer's disease and Parkinson's disease with dementia. J Neurol Neurosurg Psychiatry 1996; **61**: 381–7.

20. **Park KW, Kim HS, Cheon SM, et al**. Dementia with Lewy bodies versus Alzheimer's disease and Parkinson's disease dementia: a comparison of cognitive profiles. J Clin Neurol 2011; **7**: 19–24.

21. **Hildebrandt H, Fink F, Kastrup A, et al**. Cognitive profiles of patients with mild cognitive impairment or dementia in Alzheimer's or Parkinson's disease. Dement Geriatr Cogn Disord Extra 2013; **3**: 102–12.

22. **Johnson DK, Galvin JE**. Longitudinal changes in cognition in Parkinson's disease with and without dementia. Dement Geriatr Cogn Disord 2011; **31**: 98–108.

23. **Paolo AM, Troster AI, Glatt SL, et al**. Differentiation of the dementias of Alzheimer's and Parkinson's disease with the dementia rating scale. J Geriatr Psychiatry Neurol 1995; **8**: 184–8.

24. **Beatty WW, Ryder KA, Gontkovsky ST, et al**. Analyzing the subcortical dementia syndrome of Parkinson's disease using the RBANS. Arch Clin Neuropsychol 2003; **18**: 509–20.

25. **Ballard CG, Aarsland D, McKeith I, et al**. Fluctuations in attention: PD dementia vs DLB with parkinsonism. Neurology 2002; **59**: 1714–20.

26. **Bronnick K, Emre M, Lane R, et al**. Profile of cognitive impairment in dementia associated with Parkinson's disease compared with Alzheimer's disease. J Neurol Neurosurg Psychiatry 2007; **78**: 1064–8.

27. **Roth M, Tym E, Mountjoy CQ, et al**. CAMDEX. A standardized instrument for the diagnosis of mental disorder in the elderly with special reference to the early detection of dementia. Br J Psychiatry 1986; **149**: 698–709.

28. **Randolph C, Tierney MC, Mohr E, et al**. The repeatable battery for the assessment of neuropsychological status (RBANS): preliminary clinical validity. J Clin Exp Neuropsychol 1998; **20**: 310–19.

29. **Aarsland D, Litvan I, Salmon D, et al**. Performance on the dementia rating scale in Parkinson's disease with dementia and dementia with Lewy bodies: comparison with progressive supranuclear palsy and Alzheimer's disease. J Neurol Neurosurg Psychiatry 2003; **74**: 1215–20.

30. **Mattis S.** Dementia rating scale. In: Bellak L, Karasu TB (ed.) *Geriatric psychiatry. A handbook for psychiatrists and primary care physicians.* New York: Grune and Stratton, 1976; pp. 108–21.

31. **Brønnick KS, Nordby H, Larsen JP, et al.** Disturbance of automatic auditory change detection in dementia associated with Parkinson's disease: a mismatch negativity study. Neurobiol Aging 2010; **31**: 104–13.

32. **Naatanen R, Paavilainen P, Rinne T, et al.** The mismatch negativity (MMN) in basic research of central auditory processing: a review. Clin Neurophysiol 2007; **118**: 2544–90.

33. **Dubois B, Pillon B.** Cognitive deficits in Parkinson's disease. J Neurol 1997; **244**: 2–8.

34. **Zgaljardic DJ, Borod JC, Foldi NS, et al.** An examination of executive dysfunction associated with frontostriatal circuitry in Parkinson's disease. J Clin Exp Neuropsychol 2006; **28**: 1127–44.

35. **Braak H, Del Tredici K, Rub U, et al.** Staging of brain pathology related to sporadic Parkinson's disease. Neurobiol Aging 2003; **24**: 197–211.

36. **Brønnick K, Ehrt U, Emre M, et al.** Attentional deficits affect activities of daily living in dementia-associated with Parkinson's disease. J Neurol Neurosurg Psychiatry 2006; **77**: 1136–42.

37. **Meppelink AM, Koerts J, Borg M, et al.** Visual object recognition and attention in Parkinson's disease patients with visual hallucinations. Mov Disord 2008; **23**: 1906–12.

38. **Barnes J, Boubert L.** Executive functions are impaired in patients with Parkinson's disease with visual hallucinations. J Neurol Neurosurg Psychiatry 2008; **79**: 190–2.

39. **Miyake A, Friedman NP, Rettinger DA, et al.** How are visuospatial working memory, executive functioning, and spatial abilities related? A latent-variable analysis. J Exp Psychol Gen 2001; **130**: 621–40.

40. **Rogers D.** Bradyphrenia in parkinsonism: a historical review. Psychol Med 1986; **16**: 257–65.

41. **Mayeux R, Stern Y, Sano M, Cote L, et al.** Clinical and biochemical correlates of bradyphrenia in Parkinson's disease. Neurology 1987; **37**: 1130–4.

42. **O'Mahony D, Rowan M, Feely J, et al.** Parkinson's dementia and Alzheimer's dementia: an evoked potential comparison. Gerontology 1993; **39**: 228–40.

43. **Matsui H, Nishinaka K, Oda M, et al.** Auditory event-related potentials in Parkinson's disease: prominent correlation with attention. Parkinsonism Relat Disord 2007; **13**: 394–8.

44. **Tanaka H, Koenig T, Pascual-Marqui RD, et al.** Event-related potential and EEG measures in Parkinson's disease without and with dementia. Dement Geriatr Cogn Disord 2000; **11**: 39–45.

45. **Goodin DS, Aminoff MJ.** Electrophysiological differences between demented and nondemented patients with Parkinson's disease. Ann Neurol 1987; **21**: 90–4.

46. **Pate DS, Margolin DI.** Cognitive slowing in Parkinson's and Alzheimer's patients: distinguishing bradyphrenia from dementia. Neurology 1994; **44**: 669–74.

47. **Goldman WP, Baty JD, Buckles VD, et al.** Cognitive and motor functioning in Parkinson disease: subjects with and without questionable dementia. Arch Neurol 1998; **55**: 674–80.

48. **Salthouse TA.** The processing-speed theory of adult age differences in cognition. Psychol Rev 1996; **103**: 403–28.

49. **Ungerleider LG, Mishkin M.** Two cortical visual systems. In: Eagle DJ, Goodale MA, Mansfield RJ (ed.) *Analysis of visual behavior.* Cambridge, MA: MIT Press, 1982; pp. 549–86.

50. **Jeannerod M, Jacob P.** Visual cognition: a new look at the two-visual systems model. Neuropsychologia 2005; **43**: 301–12.

51. **Gattass R, Nascimento-Silva S, Soares JG, et al.** Cortical visual areas in monkeys: location, topography, connections, columns, plasticity and cortical dynamics. Phil Trans R Soc Lond B: Biol Sci 2005; **360**: 709–31.

52. **Cormack F, Aarsland D, Ballard C, et al.** Pentagon drawing and neuropsychological performance in dementia with Lewy bodies, Alzheimer's disease, Parkinson's disease and Parkinson's disease with dementia. Int J Geriatr Psychiatry 2004; **19**: 371–7.

53. **Benton AL.** A multiple choice type of the visual retention test. Am Med Assoc Arch Neurol Psychiatry 1950; **64**: 699–707.

54. **Rosen WG, Mohs RC, Davis KL**. A new rating scale for Alzheimer's disease. Am J Psychiatry 1984; **141**: 1356–64.

55. **Dubois B, Feldman HH, Jacova C, et al.** Research criteria for the diagnosis of Alzheimer's disease: revising the NINCDS-ADRDA criteria. Lancet Neurol 2007; **6**: 734–46.

56. **Baddeley AD**. The psychology of memory. In: Baddeley AD, Kopelman MD, Wilson BA (ed.) *Memory disorders.* Chichester: John Wiley, 2002; 3–15.

57. **Kuzis G, Sabe L, Tiberti C, et al.** Explicit and implicit learning in patients with Alzheimer disease and Parkinson disease with dementia. Neuropsychiatry Neuropsychol Behav Neurol 1999; **12**: 265–9.

58. **Helkala EL, Laulumaa V, Soininen H, et al.** Different error pattern of episodic and semantic memory in Alzheimer's disease and Parkinson's disease with dementia. Neuropsychologia 1989; **27**: 1241–8.

59. **Pillon B, Deweer B, Agid Y, et al.** Explicit memory in Alzheimer's, Huntington's, and Parkinson's diseases. Arch Neurol 1993; **50**: 374–9.

60. **Tierney MC, Nores A, Snow WG, et al.** Use of the Rey auditory verbal learning test in differentiating normal aging from Alzheimer's and Parkinson's dementia. Psychol Assess 1994; **6**: 129–34.

61. **Higginson CI, Wheelock VL, Carroll KE, et al.** Recognition memory in Parkinson's disease with and without dementia: evidence inconsistent with the retrieval deficit hypothesis. J Clin Exp Neuropsychol 2005; **27**: 516–28.

62. **Filoteo JV, Salmon DP, Schiehser DM, et al.** Verbal learning and memory in patients with dementia with Lewy bodies or Parkinson's disease with dementia. J Clin Exp Neuropsychol 2009; **31**: 823–34.

63. **Higginson CI, King DS, Levine D, et al.** The relationship between executive function and verbal memory in Parkinson's disease. Brain Cogn 2003; **52**: 343–52.

64. **Whittington CJ, Podd J, Kan MM**. Recognition memory impairment in Parkinson's disease: power and meta-analyses. Neuropsychology 2000; **14**: 233–46.

65. **Bayles KA**. Language and Parkinson disease. Alzheimer Dis Assoc Disord 1990; **4**: 171–80.

66. **Cummings JL, Darkins A, Mendez M, et al.** Alzheimer's disease and Parkinson's disease: comparison of speech and language alterations. Neurology 1988; **38**: 680–4.

67. **Goodglass H, Kaplan E**. *The assessment of aphasia and related disorders.* Philadelphia: Lea and Febiger, 1976.

68. **Kertesz A**. *Aphasia and associated disorders: taxonomy, localization and recovery.* New York: Grune and Stratton, 1979.

69. **Aarsland D, Brønnick K, Larsen JP, et al.** Cognitive impairment in incident, untreated Parkinson disease: the Norwegian ParkWest Study. Neurology 2009; **72**: 1121–6.

70. **Pedersen KF, Larsen JP, Tysnes OB, et al.** Prognosis of mild cognitive impairment in early Parkinson disease: the Norwegian ParkWest study. J Am Med Assoc Neurology 2013; **70**: 580–6.

71. **Janvin CC, Larsen JP, Aarsland D, et al.** Subtypes of mild cognitive impairment in Parkinson's disease: progression to dementia. Mov Disord 2006; **21**: 1343–9.

72. **Janvin CC, Larsen JP, Salmon DP, et al.** Cognitive profiles of individual patients with Parkinson's disease and dementia: comparison with dementia with Lewy bodies and Alzheimer's disease. Mov Disord 2006; **21**: 337–42.

73. **Perriol MP, Dujardin K, Derambure P, et al.** Disturbance of sensory filtering in dementia with Lewy bodies: comparison with Parkinson's disease dementia and Alzheimer's disease. J Neurol Neurosurg Psychiatry 2005; **76**(1): 106–8. doi:10.1136/jnnp.2003.035022

Chapter 5

Neuropsychiatric symptoms in Parkinson's disease dementia

Eugenia Mamikonyan and Daniel Weintraub

Introduction

Dementia affects approximately 30% of Parkinson's disease (PD) patients at any given time [1], with a long-term cumulative prevalence rate close to 80% [2]. In addition to clinically significant cognitive impairment that defines the disorder, dementia in PD (PD-D) is often accompanied by a range of neuropsychiatric symptoms (NPS), including psychosis, affective symptoms (e.g. depression and anxiety), apathy, and behavioural disturbances (e.g. aggression and agitation). This chapter provides an overview of the epidemiology and presentation, clinical impact, correlates and risk factors, neuropathophysiology, assessment, and clinical management of NPS in PD-D (see Table 5.1 for an overview).

Epidemiology

Prevalence of neuropsychiatric symptoms

The Neuropsychiatric Inventory (NPI) [3] is the most commonly used instrument to assess the range of NPS that can occur in neurodegenerative diseases. In a placebo-controlled clinical trial of rivastigmine for the treatment of PD-D, 537 patients were assessed with the NPI at baseline and serially during the course of the study [4]. Almost all (about 90%) experienced at least one NPS, and 77% had two or more. In that study five distinct NPI clusters were identified: one group with few and mild symptoms (52%); a mood cluster (11%; high depression, anxiety, and apathy scores); an apathy cluster (24%; high apathy score but low scores on other items); an agitation cluster (5%; high score on agitation and high total NPI score); and a psychosis cluster (8%; high scores on delusions and hallucinations). This study sample, however, may not be fully representative as PD-D patients with severe dementia were excluded.

Five NPI clusters were identified in a community-based study that used the NPI to identify NPS in 100 PD patients with (43%) and without dementia (57%) [5]. The clusters with the highest representation of PD-D patients were a group characterized primarily by hallucinations (79% PD-D) and a group with high scores on several NPI items (57% PD-D).

In a study that used factor analysis to determine patterns of NPI symptoms in PD patients with (36%) and without dementia (64%), the most common NPS in the sample overall (patients with and without dementia were not described separately) were depression (38%) and hallucinations (27%), and the least common were euphoria and disinhibition [6]. Factor analysis showed that hallucinations, delusions, and irritability clustered into one factor and apathy and anxiety constituted another factor.

A study utilizing the 12-item NPI to compare NPS in PD patients with normal cognition (NC), mild cognitive impairment (MCI), and PD-D found that apathy was reported in 50% of PD patients with MCI and PD-D. The presence of apathy was found to be the differentiating factor between PD patients with NC and MCI. Additionally, hallucinations and delusions (psychosis) were much more common in the PD-D group, with 48% of patients reporting symptoms; only 12.9% of PD patients with NC and 16.7% with MCI reported similar symptoms. Notably, evaluating the prevalence of psychosis in PD patients with MCI may prove beneficial in monitoring the conversion from PD-MCI to PD-D [7].

Comparison with other disease states

Several studies have also used the NPI to compare the frequency and patterns of NPS in PD-D with those in other neurodegenerative diseases. In one study, NPS overall were very common in both PD-D and Alzheimer's disease (AD), with hallucinations being more severe in PD-D and aberrant motor behaviour, agitation, disinhibition, irritability, euphoria, and apathy more common in AD [8]. In a comparative study of PD patients unselected with regard to their cognitive status and patients with progressive supranuclear palsy (PSP), PD patients had a higher frequency of hallucinations, delusions, and depression, but less apathy and disinhibition than PSP patients [9].

PD-D and dementia with Lewy bodies (DLB) overlap to a great extent in terms of neuropathophysiology and clinical presentation. Regarding NPS, a comparative study of PD-D and DLB found that delusions and hallucinations were more common in DLB, with little difference between the groups otherwise [10]. Another study found that cognitive fluctuations, visual and auditory hallucinations, depression, and sleep disturbances were equally common in both PD-D and DLB, and all these symptoms were more common in PD-D and DLB than in an AD comparison group [11].

Clinical presentation

Depression and anxiety

Depression is common in PD-D, occurring in 30–60% of patients [4, 6, 8]. In addition, depression in PD patients without dementia is a risk factor for cognitive decline and development of PD-D [12–14]. This may be due in part to shared risk factors for dementia and depression in PD, including increasing age and more severe disease [13, 15]. Although not specifically examined in PD-D patients, in PD there is high co-morbidity between depression and anxiety disorders [16].

Most PD-D patients are on chronic levodopa treatment, and many experience motor fluctuations (MF), which involve 'off' periods characterized by worsening parkinsonism along with 'on' periods with improved motor function. In addition to MF, non-motor fluctuations (NMF) also occur. Increasing anxiety and discrete anxiety attacks have been associated with MF, particularly with the onset of 'off' periods, although this relationship does not hold for all patients [17]. When it does occur, patients often describe a sensation of feeling 'trapped' as they become increasingly immobilized, with anxiety symptoms typically resolving only after improvement in motor symptoms. Other NMF include slowness of thinking, fatigue, and dysphoria. NMF can be more disabling than MF for a substantial percentage of PD patients [18]. Patients may rarely experience hypomanic symptoms during 'on' periods [19].

A large national study in Germany assessing the frequency of NPS in 1449 PD patients found that at least one symptom occurred in 71% of PD patients. Depression was present in 23.8% of all PD patients and anxiety was present in 19.6%. Additionally, the co-morbidity of depression and dementia was analysed: patients experiencing both depression and dementia were more likely to experience additional NPS [20].

Apathy

Apathy is another common co-morbid condition in PD-D [1], one that overlaps with some motor symptoms of PD, but is a distinct clinical syndrome characterized by diminished spontaneous activity, motivation, and affect. It is common in a range of neurodegenerative diseases, including frontotemporal dementia (FTD) [21], PSP [9], DLB [21], and AD [22]; its frequency and severity increase with disease progression [22].

Studies have examined the prevalence of apathy in PD-D and determined that it affects 15–50% of patients [4, 6, 8, 9, 23]. In a study comparing PD patients with a similarly disabled group (osteoarthritis patients) [24], apathy was significantly more common in the PD group and was associated with cognitive impairment, but was not associated with either depression or anxiety. Another study reported similar findings using the Lille Apathy Rating Scale [25, 26], with apathy being more common in PD-D patients than in PD patients without dementia. All PD patients showed a decrease in action initiation compared with healthy controls, but PD-D patients were significantly more impaired in this regard. Additionally, they exhibited lower emotional responses and decreased self-awareness compared with PD patients without dementia.

A recent study assessed the association between the presence of apathy and the course of cognitive decline or dementia in 40 PD patients without depression or dementia. The patients were assessed twice over an 18-month period; over this time the rate of cognitive decline as well as conversion to dementia was found to be significantly higher in PD patients with apathy [27].

Psychosis

While disorders of affect in PD-D are common and clinically significant, psychosis may be the most clinically significant NPS in PD, as it is associated with cognitive decline and the development of dementia, worsening of motor symptoms, caregiver burden, and institutionalization [4, 28, 29]. Psychosis is defined by the presence of either hallucinations (i.e. false sensory perception) or delusions (i.e. fixed false beliefs). While hallucinations are common in PD overall, affecting approximately 25–44% of patients, the prevalence in PD-D is markedly higher than in PD patients without dementia [30], ranging from 45 to 65% [4, 8, 10]. Hallucinations are generally visual, well formed, recurrent, and complex [10, 31–33]; however, auditory [31, 34], tactile [35], gustatory [32], and olfactory [36, 37] hallucinations may occur as well. Delusions are not as common as hallucinations, and typically co-occur with hallucinations. The most frequent forms are the 'phantom boarder' phenomenon (the belief that a stranger is living in the patient's home) and delusions of infidelity. The imposter phenomenon is rare but can occur. Prevalence rates for delusions are reported to be 17% in PD patients overall [6, 9] and 25–30% in PD-D patients [4, 8, 10].

Agitation

PD-D patients may display agitation and other behavioural disturbances, often in the context of psychosis. While not as common as depression, anxiety, or apathy [1], a large treatment study found baseline agitation/aggression of some severity in 33% of PD-D patients, with a third of those experiencing clinically significant symptoms. Of patients who had some degree of agitation/aggression, half of caregivers reported clinically significant distress [4]. In addition, approximately 30% of PD-D patients were reported to have some irritability or emotional lability, over 20% had aberrant motor behaviour, and over 10% demonstrated disinhibited behaviours.

Disorders of sleep and wakefulness

Disorders of sleep and wakefulness may be the most common non-motor symptoms in PD. Up to 90% of patients report insomnia, hypersomnia, sleep fragmentation, sleep terrors, nightmares, nocturnal movements, or rapid eye movement (REM) sleep behaviour disorder (RBD) [6, 38–40]. The latter is characterized by loss of normal skeletal muscle atonia during REM sleep resulting in dream-enacting behaviour, with speaking, shouting, and prominent motor activity associated with vivid, frequently scary, dreams. Other sleep–wake cycle-related disorders in PD include restless legs syndrome (RLS) and periodic leg movements in sleep (PLMS). Patients with more advanced PD may have an increased frequency of obstructive or central sleep apnoea [41].

Excessive daytime sleepiness (EDS) or fatigue occurs in 15–50% of PD patients [42–44], and is more common in PD-D. Sudden-onset REM sleep (also known as daytime 'sleep attacks') may also occur. This has usually been reported in conjunction with dopamine agonist treatment [41, 45] and is expected to occur less in PD-D patients as they are generally not prescribed dopamine agonists.

A recent study suggests that not only is RBD associated with an increased risk of dementia, it may also predict the onset of PD-D. A group of 42 PD patients were given a polysomnogram at baseline and reassessed a mean of 4 years later. At baseline 27 patients had RBD, and at follow-up 48% of them had developed dementia while none of the remaining 13 patients without RBD at baseline had developed dementia. Loss of REM sleep atonia at baseline significantly predicted hallucinations and cognitive fluctuations, symptoms that commonly co-occur with PD-D, as well as the onset of dementia [46].

Compta et al. [47] compared sleep architecture in patients with PD and PD-D with controls and looked at levels of hypocretin-1 in the cerebrospinal fluid (CSF). Hypocretin cell loss in the hypothalamus was found in PD patients with advanced disease. Patients with PD and PD-D had higher scores on the Epworth Sleepiness Scale (ESS) [48] than controls, with PD-D patients more likely to score more than the cut-off score of 10. However, there were no differences in hypocretin-1 levels between the PD, PD-D, and control groups, and levels were unrelated to ESS scores or cognition. PD-D patients did exhibit slow dominant occipital frequency and/or loss of normal non-REM sleep architecture [47].

Pseudobulbar affect

Pseudobulbar affect (PBA), also known as involuntary emotional expression disorder (IEED) [49], is a specific form of affective lability that can occur in a variety of neurodegenerative diseases and neurological conditions, including PD. It is found in up to 10% of PD patients [50]; however, its prevalence in PD-D is not known. Clinically, PBA consists of repeated, brief episodes of involuntary expression of either crying or laughing, with the expressed emotion typically incongruent with the patient's underlying mood. If a stimulus is present, the emotional response is in excess of what would ordinarily be expected. For some patients, the episodes are embarrassing and distressing, and family members may mistakenly attribute crying episodes for an underlying depression.

Impulse control disorders

Impulse control disorders (ICDs), including pathological gambling, compulsive buying, compulsive sexual behaviour, and binge or compulsive eating, are increasingly recognized as common and clinically significant in PD [51, 52]. Case reports and cross-sectional studies have suggested an association between dopamine agonist treatment and ICDs in PD [53–55], and younger age is an additional risk factor [52]. Given that PD-D patients are typically older and not commonly prescribed dopamine agonists, it is expected that ICDs would be relatively uncommon in patients with PD-D, although formal research is needed.

Impact of deep brain stimulation

The impact of deep brain stimulation (DBS)—primarily bilateral subthalamic nucleus (STN) DBS—on NPS appears to be variable and complex [56]. Patients can experience transient post-operative neuropsychiatric abnormalities such as confusional states [57]. Recommendations to determine who is at increased risk of a poor post-operative prognosis include a neuropsychological evaluation prior to surgery and exclusion of those with significant baseline cognitive impairment [56].

The longer-term impact of DBS surgery includes executive dysfunction [58] and both overall improvement [56] and occasionally a worsening of depression, anxiety, psychosis, mania, and emotional lability [57, 59]. In general, post-surgical neuropsychological decline has shown no correlation with post-surgical motor status [58, 60], but it does appear to occur more often in patients with pre-existing neuropsychiatric disorders [59], a finding that further emphasizes the need for pre-surgical neuropsychological and psychiatric evaluation.

A recent study found that cortical lead point entry during DBS surgery may contribute to cognitive decline [61]. A group of 68 PD patients were randomized to have STN DBS or best medical treatment. Patients were administered a battery of neuropsychological tests at baseline and 6 months after treatment. If electrodes intersected with the caudate nuclei, primarily if the chronic stimulation lead passed through the head of the caudate, patients were at an increased risk for impairment of working memory and global cognition. For every 0.1-ml volume of the caudate nucleus that came in contact with the entering electrode, the odds ratio for global cognitive decline was 37.4 (confidence interval 2.1–371.8). Additionally, deficits in executive and working memory were found in patients in whom the active stimulating contact was not placed precisely within the STN.

Despite the potentially negative side effects of DBS, a recent study found that STN stimulation in PD may regulate neuropsychiatric complications [62]. A group of PD patients were administered a battery of neuropsychological assessments before and a year after STN DBS, having undergone on average a 73% reduction in dopaminergic medication post-surgery. Statistically significant improvements were found in verbal fluency, depression, anxiety, and apathy scores as well as hypomania and a host of hyperdopaminergic behaviours (i.e. dopamine dysregulation syndrome, behavioural addictions, and compulsive dopaminergic medication use), but patients experienced an increase in hypodopaminergic behaviours (i.e. apathy and decreased motivation and level of activity). This study highlights the important role that the level of dopamine replacement therapy plays in psychiatric functioning after DBS surgery.

Clinical impact

Co-morbid psychiatric symptoms in PD are predictive of caregiver stress, nursing home placement, more rapid cognitive decline, and mortality. In one study, caregivers of PD patients with depression, cognitive impairment, agitation, aberrant motor behaviour, or delusions experienced increased emotional or social distress [6]. In a subsequent study, these same researchers confirmed that agitation and depression are indicative of caregiver distress, and suggested that anxiety and apathy may contribute as well, with nearly 60% of caregivers reporting at least one NPI symptom causing at least moderate distress [4].

Regarding individual disorders, there is ample research demonstrating that depression in PD is associated with worse long-term outcomes, including cognitive decline, worse motor function, greater functional impairment, and increased mortality [63–65]. Hallucinations tend to be particularly predictive of greater cognitive decline and development of PD-D over time

[2, 11, 66, 67], caregiver stress and burden [4, 68, 69], nursing home placement [6, 68, 70, 71], and mortality [29, 71, 72]. One study in a population-based sample of PD patients found that the presence of dementia and hallucinations were independent predictors of nursing home placement [68, 69]. What remains unclear is whether psychosis is an independent risk factor for cognitive decline or simply a clinical correlate of cognitive impairment and more rapidly progressive disease.

Correlates and risk factors

In a study that used the NPI to assess NPS in PD-D patients [4], those with a Mini-Mental State Examination (MMSE) score of <20 and Hoehn and Yahr stage ≥3 had significantly higher overall NPI scores. Women were more likely to be in the mood cluster and men in the apathy cluster. The highest MMSE scores were found in the mood cluster and the lowest in the agitation and psychosis clusters. In addition, patients with more advanced disease were more likely to be in a cluster with significant NPS compared with those with mild disease. Other studies using the NPI have also reported that NPS in general are associated with increasing severity of both PD and cognitive impairment [5, 6, 8, 12]. While depression is common in all stages of PD, its prevalence has been reported to be higher in PD-D patients than in PD patients without dementia [1, 13]. In addition depression may be a risk factor for or a prodromal symptom of PD-D [12, 64, 65]. The relationship between severity of apathy and severity of PD is unclear [24, 25], but apathy has been associated with a range of cognitive deficits and dementia in PD [23, 25]. Although there is symptom overlap between depression and apathy, and patients meeting the criteria for one disorder often meet those for the other, these appear to be distinct clinical syndromes [23, 24].

Risk factors for or correlates of psychosis are a range of cognitive deficits [28, 69, 73, 74], older age, advanced disease [31, 32, 69, 75–79], and exposure to PD medication [69, 70, 74, 80, 81]. Until recently, exposure to dopaminergic therapy was implicated as the major cause of psychosis in PD [82]. Claims have been made that certain agents are less likely than others to induce psychosis, but evidence for this is anecdotal [83]. Despite the strong empirical association between exposure to medication and psychosis in PD, some recent studies have reported that the dosage and duration of anti-parkinsonian treatment are not directly correlated with psychosis [32, 75, 84, 85]. The aetiology of psychosis is complex and multifactorial, often including visual impairment and sleep disturbances [86, 87]. Hallucinations are often co-morbid with other NPS, including depression, anxiety, sleep disturbances, and apathy [33, 69].

Agitated patients on average have lower MMSE and higher Unified Parkinson's Disease Rating Scale (UPDRS) motor (primarily akinesia and rigidity) scores [75]. Agitation is often associated with other psychiatric symptoms, including delusions, hallucinations, and irritability [75]. In a factor analysis, irritability, hallucinations, and delusions clustered into one neuropsychiatric factor [6], and in a cluster analysis a small group of PD-D patients displayed high agitation and overall NPI scores [4].

Clinical factors that are associated with sleep disruption are immobility due to nocturnal bradykinesia and rigidity, tremor, dyskinesia, cramps, micturia, pain, and excessive sweating [40, 41, 88]. Sleep disturbances are also correlated with psychosis [89], depression [40], and cognitive impairment [88]. EDS, and perhaps fatigue as well, have been attributed variably to impairment in the striatal–thalamic–frontal cortical system, exposure to dopaminergic medication (especially dopamine agonists), and nocturnal sleep disturbances [41, 44, 88, 90]. Clinical correlates of EDS include advanced disease, depression, cognitive impairment, and psychosis [42, 43, 91].

Pathophysiology of neuropsychiatric symptoms

Although there is extensive literature on the pathophysiology of both NPS and cognitive impairment in PD, there has been almost no research on the pathophysiology of these symptoms in PD-D specifically.

In general, the high frequency of depression in PD has been explained by dysfunction in: (1) subcortical nuclei and the frontal lobes; (2) striatal–thalamic–frontal cortex circuits and limbic circuits; and (3) brainstem monoamine and indolamine systems (i.e. dopamine, serotonin, norepinephrine, and acetylcholine). Impairments in the pathways connecting subcortical structures and the frontal cortex also are thought to be important [92]. Functional brain imaging studies have reported simultaneous hypometabolism in the pan-frontal cortex and caudate in depressed PD patients, changes which are presumed to reflect neurodegeneration of the cortical–striatal–thalamic–cortical circuits [93, 94]. Regarding neurotransmitters, disproportionate degeneration of dopamine neurons in the ventral tegmental area (VTA) has been reported in PD patients with a history of depression [95]. Functional imaging studies in depressed PD patients have found both a decrease in signal intensity of neural pathways originating from monoaminergic brainstem nuclei [96] and a negative correlation between depression scores and dorsal midbrain serotonin transporter (5-HTT) densities [97].

Goal-directed behaviour is associated with dopaminergic and noradrenergic function as well as with activation of the prefrontal cortex and basal ganglia [98]. Supporting the role of the frontal cortical–striatal impairments in the development of diminished goal-directed behaviour (i.e. apathy), studies of apathy in PD have reported associations with executive deficits, impairment of verbal memory, and bradyphrenia [23, 99].

A recent study looking at cerebral metabolism and apathy found that areas involved in reward, emotion, and cognition are implicated in PD patients with apathy. Positive correlations were found between the following Brodmann areas (BA) and higher scores on the Apathy Evaluation Scale (AES): right inferior frontal gyrus (BA47), right middle frontal gyrus (BA10), right cuneus (BA18), and left anterior insula (BA13). The left and right cerebellum, posterior lobe, and inferior semilunar lobule were found to be negatively correlated with high AES scores [100].

As previously mentioned, the aetiology of psychosis in PD is complex and probably includes a complex interaction between medication exposure, PD pathology, aberrant REM-related phenomena, and co-morbid conditions, particularly cognitive impairment and visual disturbances. Dopaminergic medication may lead to excessive stimulation or hypersensitivity of mesocorticolimbic D2/D3 receptors and induce psychosis [101]. However, the association between psychosis, cognitive impairment, and mood disorders suggests more widespread involvement of other neurotransmitter systems or neural pathways. In this context, cholinergic deficits and serotonergic/dopaminergic imbalance have also been implicated in the development of psychosis in PD [82, 83, 101–104].

RBD and other sleep disturbances in PD have been attributed to both progressive degeneration of the cholinergic pedunculopontine nucleus [105] and reduced striatal dopaminergic activity [106]. With regard to the pathophysiology of PBA, a final common pathway seems to be disinhibition of the brainstem bulbar nuclei that control the expression of crying and laughing. PBA in PD probably results from impairment in neural pathways connecting the cortex and brainstem [107].

Assessment and diagnosis

As insight and memory can be impaired in patients with PD-D, it is important to include an informed other in the assessment of NPS; patient self-completed assessments are not appropriate for assessing such symptoms in PD-D. The new version of the UPDRS [108, 109] has individual questions that can be used to screen for symptoms that are common in PD-D, including depression, anxiety, psychosis, apathy, and disorders of sleep and wakefulness.

The most commonly used global instrument for assessing the presence and severity of NPS in PD-D is the NPI. The NPI was developed to overcome difficulties associated with assessing behavioural symptoms in patients with dementia, such as inaccurate reporting of symptom severity or frequency. The original NPI comprised a series of questions concerning 10 behavioural symptom domains: delusions, hallucinations, agitation/aggression, depression, anxiety, euphoria, apathy, disinhibition, irritability/lability, and aberrant motor behaviour. A 12-item version was subsequently developed, which includes additional questions on nighttime behavioural disturbances and appetite/eating changes. Domain-specific interview questions are administered to an informant, who is asked to assess the patient's behaviour in the past month. If a particular behaviour is endorsed, the severity (e.g. mild, moderate, or severe) and frequency (e.g. occasionally, often, frequently, or very frequently) are rated, and domain-specific scores are determined by multiplying severity and frequency. Subsequently, a brief caregiver-completed version of the NPI, the Neuropsychiatric Personality Inventory-Questionnaire (NPI-Q) [110] was also developed.

Management of neuropsychiatric symptoms

Depression and anxiety

There have been no controlled studies on the use of psychiatric medications for symptoms of depression and anxiety specifically in PD-D. Approximately 20–25% of PD patients in specialty care are taking an antidepressant at any given time, most commonly a selective serotonin reuptake inhibitor (SSRI) [111, 112], which is the recommended first-line antidepressant treatment type for depression in the elderly [113]. Results of numerous open-label trials using SSRIs and other newer antidepressants in PD suggest a positive effect and good tolerability [114]. Until recently, placebo-controlled studies with SSRIs reported negative findings [115–117]. However, a recent placebo-controlled study of SSRIs and serotonin–norepinephrine reuptake inhibitors (SNRIs) showed promising results for treating depression in PD with paroxetine and venlafaxine XR, respectively. Both medications were found to improve depression without worsening motor function. However, patients with PD-D were not included in this study, so results should be interpreted cautiously for the PD-D population [118]. In addition, although apparently rare, the combination of a SSRI and a monoamine oxidase inhibitor—used in the treatment of PD—can result in serotonin syndrome (i.e. development of symptoms such as mental confusion, hallucinations, agitation, headache, coma, shivering, sweating, hyperthermia, hypertension, tachycardia, nausea, diarrhoea, myoclonus, hyperreflexia, and tremor).

Two placebo-controlled studies with tricyclic antidepressants (TCA) were positive [117, 119]; however, TCAs can be difficult for PD patients to tolerate due to aggravation of PD-associated orthostatic hypotension, constipation, and cognitive problems [120], and they must be avoided in PD-D patients as they can cause cognitive worsening and increased confusion.

A commonly used dopamine agonist (pramipexole) for motor symptoms in PD was found to improve depressive symptoms as well. A 12-week placebo-controlled trial showed that participants (without dementia) taking 0.125–1.0 mg of pramipexole three times a day showed a 5.9 (+ 0.5) point decrease on the Beck Depression Inventory (BDI) as well as improvement on the Geriatric Depression Scale-15 (GDS-15). As was expected, patients also experienced an improvement in motor symptoms. Statistical analysis determined that 80% of the improvement was due to the effect of pramipexole on mood and 20% to improvements in motor functioning [121].

There have been no controlled studies on the treatment of anxiety in PD [122]. For patients who experience anxiety as part of an 'off' state, adjustments can be made to the PD medication in an attempt to decrease the duration and severity of these episodes. Anecdotally, newer antidepressants are commonly used for anxiety disorders, whether or not co-morbid depression is present. However, anxiety in PD responds variably to antidepressants, and many patients require treatment with benzodiazepines (most commonly low-dose lorazepam, alprazolam, and clonazepam). Given that PD-D patients are cognitively and frequently physically impaired, benzodiazepines must be used cautiously due to their propensity to worsen cognition, sedation, and gait/balance.

Apathy

Until recently there were no treatment studies for apathy in PD. Co-morbid psychiatric conditions (e.g. depression) were treated initially. Anecdotally, psychostimulants (e.g. methylphenidate) and stimulant-related compounds (e.g. modafinil) are used in clinical practice, but their effectiveness in PD-D patients is not known. In a small, randomized, placebo-controlled trial in PD patients with apathy but not dementia or depression, a rivastigmine patch significantly improved apathy compared with placebo [123]. Based on the proposed pathophysiology of apathy, antidepressants and other medications that increase dopamine or norepinephrine activity (e.g. dual reuptake inhibitor antidepressants, bupropion, and atomoxetine) may be beneficial [124]. In addition to pharmacological treatment, it is important to educate patients and families about the distinction between apathy and depression and to encourage steps that overcome patient inertia that may lead to improved functioning and quality of life [125].

Thobois et al. [126] found that symptoms of apathy occurring in PD patients after STN DBS surgery and withdrawal of dopaminergic therapy improved with piribedil (a D2/D3 receptor agonist) treatment in the context of a placebo-controlled study. Additionally, treatment with piribedil indicated a trend for improvement in depression, quality of life, and anhedonia. This clinical trial excluded PD-D patients, thus the results must be interpreted cautiously in this population.

Psychosis and agitation

Several studies have found a relationship between exposure to PD medication and the presence of some NPS, particularly psychosis and cognitive impairment [75, 80, 127–130]. If tolerated, a decrease in overall exposure to PD medication may lead to an improvement in mental status in PD-D patients. Based on expert opinion, medications are usually discontinued (if tolerated from a motor standpoint) in the following order: anticholinergics, selegiline, amantadine, dopamine agonists, catechol-O-methyltransferase (COMT) inhibitors, and, finally, a reduction in levodopa dosage [83, 131]. In a recent description of clinical outcomes in a small number of PD patients with psychosis, it was reported that a decrease in PD medications commonly led to improvement in psychosis, and the authors estimated that 30% of PD patients with psychosis may not require antipsychotic medication [132].

The effects of memantine, an N-methyl-D-aspartate (NMDA) receptor antagonist used in AD, has also been assessed in PD-D with mixed results; 20 mg of memantine daily was found to be safe and well-tolerated [133–135]. One double-blind, placebo-controlled, multicentre trial in a mixed population of DLB and PD-D patients found significant improvements in clinical global impressions of change (CGIC) scores; however, there were no improvements in NPI scores [134]. In contrast, a larger randomized, double-blind, placebo-controlled trial, also in a population of PD-D and DLB patients, found that memantine did not improve cognition or NPI scores in PD-D patients, although NPI scores for psychosis, sleep, and appetite in DLB patients did improve [133].

Cholinesterase inhibitors (donepezil, rivastigmine, and galantamine) have also been studied for their effect on cognitive impairment in PD-D, and indirectly for their effects on NPS [136]. In an open-label study examining the psychiatric benefits of donepezil in DLB and PD-D patients [137], 35 PD-D patients who completed at least 12 weeks of treatment had an average 12.0 point decrease in total NPI score (approximately a 50% decrease from the baseline NPI score) and reduced caregiver distress. In contrast, a small placebo-controlled crossover study of donepezil in PD-D did not report psychiatric benefits [138].

There is evidence that rivastigmine, approved for the treatment of PD-D based on the results of a large international study [139], may also have benefits for behavioural symptoms in this population. In that study, mean NPI scores decreased by 2.0 points in the rivastigmine-treated group over the course of treatment, compared with no change in the placebo-treated group. In addition, significantly more patients in the rivastigmine group had an improvement of at least 30% in NPI score (45.4 versus 34.6%). In a post hoc analysis of the data, it was found that those patients with visual hallucinations at baseline derived greater benefit from rivastigmine treatment relative to placebo treatment [140].

There is preliminary evidence that cholinesterase inhibitors may improve hallucinations in PD-D. A small open-label study of rivastigmine was conducted in PD patients with a range of NPS and significant cognitive impairment. Total NPI score, the hallucinations and sleep disturbance subscales specifically, improved significantly in those who completed the study (80% of the sample) over the course of 6 weeks of maximal treatment, and caregivers reported significantly less distress over time [141]. Similarly, a small open-label study of galantamine in PD-D found benefit for NPS overall and psychosis specifically [142].

When psychosis does not improve with the aforementioned clinical interventions, it is sometimes necessary to introduce antipsychotic treatment. Recent research shows that approximately a third of older PD patients newly treated with dopaminergic agents will be prescribed an antipsychotic within a 7-year period [143]. Four new-generation antipsychotics have been studied in the PD population: clozapine, risperidone, olanzapine, and quetiapine [80, 127, 128, 130]. Only clozapine has been shown to be efficacious for psychosis in PD, with few adverse motor effects [80, 127, 130]. Unfortunately, clozapine has a rare but serious side effect, agranulocytosis [80, 127, 130], which necessitates routine blood monitoring.

Risperidone and olanzapine are not recommended for use in PD, due to limited research and evidence that their use is associated with worsening parkinsonism [80, 127]. In one meta-analysis, worsening of motor symptoms was reported in 33% of PD patients treated with risperidone [144]; a similar meta-analysis found worsening of motor symptoms in 40% of patients treated with olanzapine [80, 145].

Quetiapine has become the first-line antipsychotic treatment for PD psychosis based on the results of open-label reporting of symptomatic improvement and good tolerability from a motor standpoint [80, 127, 130]. However, two randomized, placebo-controlled studies of quetiapine for psychosis in PD have been negative [146, 147]. In addition, a retrospective chart review of quetiapine for the treatment of hallucinations in PD found that PD-D patients were as likely as PD patients without dementia to experience a decrease in psychotic symptoms, but were more likely to report worsening of motor symptoms [148]. Another retrospective analysis found that while approximately 80% of the PD patients experienced at least partial remission of psychotic symptoms with quetiapine treatment, the presence of dementia was independently associated with non-response [149]. Finally, in an open-label study of quetiapine for psychosis in PD patients with and without dementia, those without dementia demonstrated a trend toward improvement on the Brief Psychiatric Rating Scale (BPRS) while PD-D patients showed no improvement. In addition, PD-D patients were more likely to experience motor worsening, required a longer titration period, and were eventually treated with a higher mean (SD) quetiapine dosage: 151 (90) versus 76 (59) mg/day [150].

In a recent study, a novel antipsychotic, pimavanserin [a serotonergic receptor (5-HT2A) inverse agonist] was found to be efficacious for the treatment of psychosis in PD in a randomized, placebo-controlled study [151]. Pimavanserin was superior to placebo on the primary psychosis outcome measure [change in the Scale for Assessment of Positive Symptoms (SAPS)-PD score], on several secondary outcome measures (caregiver impression ratings, symptoms of sleep and wakefulness, and caregiver burden), and was well tolerated from a motor standpoint. This drug may be approved for the treatment of psychosis in PD in the near future.

The use of antipsychotics in PD-D is potentially of particular concern. In 2005 the US Food and Drug Administration (FDA) issued an advisory letter warning regarding increased morbidity and mortality in patients with dementia associated with the use of atypical antipsychotics [152]. Specific causes of death reported were cardiovascular or infectious in nature, though prior studies did find significant linkages with cerebrovascular events [153, 154]. In 2008, the warning was extended to include conventional (i.e. typical) antipsychotics [155, 156]. One recent study suggests that the use of antipsychotics in PD may also be associated with increased mortality risk [157]. Thus, given the frequent occurrence of dementia in PD, the associated morbidity and mortality with use of antipsychotics in PD-D is likely to be higher than previously thought [158].

The effects of risperidone and citalopram on a group of hospitalized individuals with DLB and NPS were recently examined in a randomized study. Discontinuation rates in the DLB group were 65–75%, with no difference between patients randomized to risperidone versus citalopram; NPI and CGIC scores worsened in DLB patients compared with a comparison group of AD patients [159].

For the reasons mentioned there has been interest in exploring other treatment options for psychosis and agitation in patients with dementia. Cholinesterase inhibitors, antidepressants, benzodiazepines, and mood stabilizers have all been studied to varying degrees for these indications, but there are currently no clear pharmacological alternatives to antipsychotics [160, 161].

Disorders of sleep and wakefulness

Treatment depends on the specific disorder and its aetiology. Sleep disturbances that are due to nocturnal worsening of parkinsonism may respond to adjustments in the PD medication regimen. RLS and PLMS are commonly treated with dopaminergic medications, and RBD is typically treated with clonazepam; melatonin may also help. Preliminary studies suggest that EDS can be treated successfully with modafinil [162, 163], and psychostimulants are also used in clinical practice. The role of other hypnotic or psychiatric medications in the treatment of sleep disturbances in PD has not been evaluated.

Pseudobulbar affect

The combination of dextromethorphan hydrobromide and quinidine sulphate is FDA-approved for the treatment of PBA based on pivotal trials in patients with multiple sclerosis [164] and amyotrophic lateral sclerosis [165], but there have been no controlled studies in PD patients. Numerous small-scale studies have also found both TCAs and SSRIs to be efficacious in the treatment of PBA, although none included PD patients [166]. Anecdotally, SSRIs and mood stabilizers (e.g. valproic acid) appear to be effective for this syndrome in PD, but no reports specifically in PD-D patients are available. In addition, it is important to educate patients and family members on the distinction between PBA and depression.

Conclusion

Common psychiatric symptoms in PD-D range from disorders of affect to psychosis and agitation. The symptoms are problematic for both patients and caregivers alike, and are associated with

Table 5.1 Summary of neuropsychiatric symptoms in Parkinson's disease dementia (PD-D)

Symptoms or disorder	Clinical description	Prevalence estimates	Symptom management
Aggression/ agitation	Generally occurs in the context of psychosis	30–40%	Rule out acute medical or neurological disorder
	May be characterized by one of more the following: irritability, emotional lability, aberrant motor behaviours, and disinhibited behaviours		Consider decrease in PD medications
			Off-label use of antipsychotics, and benzodiazepines (should be used with caution in PD-D patients)
	Patients tend to have lower MMSE scores, and higher UPDRS and overall NPI scores		Off-label use of cholinesterase inhibitors and antidepressants
	Predictive of caregiver distress		
Anxiety	More likely to occur in women and in patients with non-motor fluctuations (e.g. slowness of thinking, fatigue, and dysphoria)	Common, but specific prevalence rates for anxiety not provided	Adjustments made to PD medications to minimize 'off' periods
			Antidepressants such as SSRIs
		Typically highly co-morbid with other affective disorders, especially depression	Low-dose benzodiazepines (should be used with caution in PD-D patients)
			STN DBS may improve symptoms
Apathy	More likely to occur in men	15–50%	Off-label use of medications that increase dopamine or norepinephrine activity (e.g. bupropion, SNRIs)
	Marked by diminished activity, motivation, and affect		The efficacy of psychostimulants and stimulant-related compounds in PD-D is unknown
	Associated with severity of cognitive impairment (executive and verbal memory deficits, bradyphrenia)		STN DBS may worsen symptoms if PD medication decreases
Depression	More likely to occur in women	30–60%	Use of second generation antidepressants (SSRIs and SNRIs)
	Occurs with increasing age and more severe disease		Tricyclic antidepressants should be avoided due to a potentially significant adverse event profile
	Risk factor for cognitive decline and development of PD-D		Beware of potential serotonin syndrome from combination of second generation antidepressants and monoamine oxidase B inhibitors
	Co-morbid with anxiety		May benefit from pharmacological dopaminergic stimulation of D2/D3 receptors. These medications should be used with caution as studies excluded patients with dementia STN DBS may improve symptoms

Table 5.1 (continued) Summary of neuropsychiatric symptoms in Parkinson's disease dementia (PD-D)

Symptoms or disorder	Clinical description	Prevalence estimates	Symptom management
PBA (involuntary emotional expression disorder)	Repeated brief episodes of involuntary expression of either crying or laughing, with expressed emotion typically incongruent with patient's mood May occur with or without a stimulus May be mistakenly attributed to underlying depression	5–10% of PD patients (prevalence in PD-D unknown)	No antidepressant studies with PD patients Anecdotally SSRIs and mood stabilizers effective in treating PBA Educate regarding the difference between PBA and depression
Psychosis	Correlates include older age, more advanced disease and exposure to PD medications Associated with cognitive decline and development of dementia, and worsening of motor symptoms Often co-morbid with depression, anxiety, sleep disturbances, and apathy Defined by either hallucinations or delusions Predictive of care-giver stress and nursing home placement	Hallucinations: 45–65% Delusions: 25–30%	Consider adjustment to PD medications Antipsychotic medications: quetiapine (first-line treatment in spite of lack of demonstrated efficacy), clozapine (efficacious but more adverse effects and more impractical to use) Indirect evidence supports introduction of cholinesterase inhibitor Pimavanserin is a novel, unapproved antipsychotic that has shown benefit in a recent clinical trial
Disorders of sleep and wakefulness	May be marked by one or more of the following: insomnia, hypersomnia, sleep fragmentation, sleep terrors, nightmares, nocturnal movements, RBD, RLS, PLMS, sleep apnoea and/or EDS, and sudden onset REM sleep Sudden onset REM sleep not common in PD-D patients as it is reported in conjunction with dopamin agonist treatment	90% of PD patients overall report some type of sleep disturbance 15–50% of PD-D patients experience EDS/fatigue	Insomnia—consider adjustment to PD medications, depending on specific disorder; consider sedative-hypnotic agent (must be used cautiously in PD-D patients) PLS and PLMS—dopaminergic medications RBD—clonazepam (must be used cautiously in PD-D patients) EDS—consider modafinil or psychostimulants

MMSE, Mini-Mental State Examination; UPDRS, Unified Parkinson's Disease Rating Scale; NPI, Neuropsychiatric Inventory; SSRI, selective serotonin reuptake inhibitor; STN DBS, subthalamic nucleus deep brain stimulation; SNRI, serotonin–norepinephrine reuptake inhibitor; PBA, pseudobulbar affect; RBD, rapid eye movement (REM) sleep behaviour disorder; RLS, restless legs syndrome; PLMS, periodic leg movements in sleep; EDS, excessive daytime sleepiness.

numerous adverse outcomes. Given recent evidence that dementia is a very common long-term outcome in PD, there needs to be greater attention devoted to the assessment, diagnosis, and clinical management of the range of NPS that occur in PD-D, including assessment of the role that PD treatments play either in the aetiology or treatment of these disorders. Table 5.1 summarizes the discussion in this chapter.

References

1. Emre M, Aarsland D, Brown R, et al. Clinical diagnostic criteria for dementia associated with Parkinson's disease. Mov Disord 2007; **22**: 1689–707.
2. Aarsland D, Andersen K, Larsen JP, et al. Prevalence and characteristics of dementia in Parkinson disease: an 8-year prospective study. Arch Neurol 2003; **60**: 387–92.
3. Cummings JL, Mega M, Gray K, et al. The Neuropsychiatric Inventory: comprehensive assessment of psychopathology in dementia. Neurology 1994; **44**: 2308–14.
4. Aarsland D, Brønnick K, Ehrt U, et al. Neuropsychiatric symptoms in patients with Parkinson's disease and dementia: frequency, profile and associated caregiver stress. J Neurol Neurosurg Psychiatry 2007; **78**: 36–42.
5. Bronnick K, Aarsland D, Larsen JP. Neuropsychiatric disturbances in Parkinson's disease clusters in five groups with different prevalence of dementia. Acta Psychiatr Scand 2005; **112**: 201–7.
6. Aarsland D, Larsen JP, Lim NG, et al. Range of neuropsychiatric disturbances in patients with Parkinson's disease. J Neurol Neurosurg Psychiatry 1999; **67**: 492–6.
7. Leroi I, Pantula H, McDonald K, et al. Neuropsychiatric symptoms in Parkinson's disease with mild cognitive impairment and dementia. Parkinson's Dis 2012; art ID 308097. doi: 10.1155/2012/308097
8. Aarsland D, Cummings JL, Larsen JP. Neuropsychiatric differences between Parkinson's disease with dementia and Alzheimer's disease. Int J Geriatr Psychiatry 2001; **16**: 184–91.
9. Aarsland D, Litvan I, Larsen JP. Neuropsychiatric symptoms of patients with progressive supranuclear palsy and Parkinson's disease. J Neuropsychiatry Clin Neurosci 2001; **13**: 42–9.
10. Aarsland D, Ballard C, Larsen JP, et al. A comparative study of psychiatric symptoms in dementia with Lewy bodies and Parkinson's disease with and without dementia. Int J Geriatr Psychiatry 2001; **16**: 528–36.
11. Galvin JE, Pollack J, Morris J. Clinical phenotype of Parkinson disease dementia. Neurology 2006; **67**: 1605–11.
12. Lieberman A. Are dementia and depression in Parkinson's disease related? Neurol Sci 2006; **248**: 138–42.
13. Giladi N, Treves TA, Paleacu D, et al. Risk factors for dementia, depression and psychosis in long-standing Parkinson's disease. J Neural Transm 2000; **107**: 59–71.
14. Emre M. What causes mental dysfunction in Parkinson's disease? Mov Disord 2003; **18**(Suppl. 6): S63–S71.
15. Hoehn MH, Yahr MD. Parkinsonism: onset, progression, and mortality. Neurology 1967; **17**: 427–42.
16. Menza MA, Robertson-Hoffman DE, Bonapace AS. Parkinson's disease and anxiety: comorbidity with depression. Biol Psychiatry 1993; **34**: 465–70.
17. Richard IH, Justus AW, Kurlan R. Relationship between mood and motor fluctuations in Parkinson's disease. J Neuropsychiatry Clin Neurosci 2001; **13**: 35–41.
18. Witjas T, Kaphan E, Azulay JP, et al. Nonmotor fluctuations in Parkinson's disease: frequent and disabling. Neurology 2002; **59**: 408–13.
19. Racette BA, Hartlein JM, Hershey T, et al. Clinical features and comorbidity of mood fluctuations in Parkinson's disease. J Neuropsychiatry Clin Neurosci 2002; **14**: 438–42.
20. Riedel O, Klotsche J, Spottke A, et al. Frequency of dementia, depression, and other neuropsychiatric symptoms in 1,449 outpatients with Parkinson's disease. J Neurol 2010; **257**: 1073–82.

21. **Hirono N, Mori E, Tanimukai S, et al.** Distinctive neurobehavioral features among neurodegenerative dementias. J Neuropsychiatry Clin Neurosci 1999; **11**: 498–503.

22. **Benoit M, Robert P, Staccini P, et al.** One-year longitudinal evaluation of neuropsychiatric symptoms in Alzheimer's disease. The REAL.FR Study. J Nutr Health Aging 2005; **9**: 134–9.

23. **Starkstein SE, Mayberg HS, Preziosi TJ, et al.** Reliability, validity, and clinical correlates of apathy in Parkinson's disease. J Neuropsychiatry Clin Neurosci 1992; **4**: 134–9.

24. **Pluck GC, Brown RG.** Apathy in Parkinson's disease. J Neurol Neurosurg Psychiatry 2002; **73**: 636–42.

25. **Dujardin K, Sockeel P, Devos D, et al.** Characteristics of apathy in Parkinson's disease. Mov Disord 2007; **22**: 778–84.

26. **Sockeel P, Dujardin K, Devos D, et al.** The Lille apathy rating scale (LARS), a new instrument for detecting and quantifying apathy: validation in Parkinson's disease. J Neurol Neurosurg Psychiatry 2006; **77**: 579–84.

27. **Dujardin K, Sockeel P, Delliaux M, et al.** Apathy may herald cognitive decline and dementia in Parkinson's disease. Mov Disord 2009; **24**: 2391–7.

28. **Santangelo G, Trojano L, Vitale C, et al.** A neuropsychological longitudinal study in Parkinson's patients with and without hallucinations. Mov Disord 2007; **22**: 2418–25.

29. **Goetz CG, Stebbins GT.** Risk factors for nursing home placement in advanced Parkinson's disease. Neurology 1993; **43**: 2227–9.

30. **Kulisevsky J, Pagonabarraga J, Pascual-Sedano B, et al.**, for the Trapecio Group Study. Prevalence and correlates of neuropsychiatric symptoms in Parkinson's disease without dementia. Mov Disord 2008; **23**: 1889–96.

31. **Fenelon G, Mahieux F, Huon R, et al.** Hallucinations in Parkinson's disease: prevalence, phenomenology and risk factors. Brain 2000; **123**: 733–45.

32. **Holroyd S, Currie L, Wooten GF.** Prospective study of hallucinations and delusions in Parkinson's disease. J Neurol Neurosurg Psychiatry 2001; **70**: 734–8.

33. **Mosimann UP, Rowan EN, Partington C, et al.** Characteristics of visual hallucinations in Parkinson's disease dementia and dementia with Lewy bodies. Am J Geriatr Psychiatry 2006; **14**: 153–60.

34. **Inzelberg R, Kipervasser S, Korczyn AD.** Auditory hallucinations in Parkinson's disease. J Neurol Neurosurg Psychiatry 1998; **64**: 533–5.

35. **Fenelon G, Thobois S, Bonnet AM, et al.** Tactile hallucinations in Parkinson's disease. J Neurol 2002; **249**: 1699–703.

36. **Tousi B, Frankel M.** Olfactory and visual hallucinations in Parkinson's disease. Parkinsonism Relat Disord 2004; **10**: 253–4.

37. **Goetz CG, Wuu J, Curgian L, et al.** Age-related influences on the clinical characteristics of new-onset hallucinations in Parkinson's disease patients. Mov Disord 2006; **21**: 267–70.

38. **Arnulf I, Bonnet A-M, Damier P, et al.** Hallucinations, REM sleep, and Parkinson's disease: a medical hypothesis. Neurology 2000; **55**: 281–8.

39. **Pappert E, Goetz C, Niederman F.** Hallucinations, sleep fragmentation and altered dream phenomena in Parkinson's disease. Mov Disord 1999; **14**: 117–21.

40. **Smith MC, Ellgring H, Oertel WH.** Sleep disturbances in Parkinson's disease patients and spouses. J Am Geriatr Soc 1997; **45**: 194–9.

41. **Stacy M.** Sleep disorders in Parkinson's disease. Drugs Aging 2002; **19**: 733–9.

42. **Tandberg E, Larsen JP, Karlsen K.** Excessive daytime sleepiness and sleep benefit in Parkinson's disease: a community-based study. Mov Disord 1999; **14**: 922–7.

43. **Friedman J, Friedman H.** Fatigue in Parkinson's disease. Neurology 1993; **43**: 2016–18.

44. **Hitten JJ, van Hoogland G, van der Velde EA, et al.** Diurnal effects of motor activity and fatigue in Parkinson's disease. J Neurol Neurosurg Psychiatry 1993; **56**: 874–7.

45. **Olanow CW, Schapira AH, Roth T.** Waking up to sleep episodes in Parkinson's disease. Mov Disord 2000; **15**: 212–15.

46. Postuma R, Bertrand J, Montplaisir J, et al. Rapid eye movement sleep behavior disorder and risk of dementia in Parkinson's disease: a prospective study. Mov Disord 2012; **27**: 720–6.

47. Compta Y, Santamaria J, Ratti L, et al. Cerebrospinal hypocretin, daytime sleepiness and sleep architecture in Parkinson's disease dementia. Brain 2009; **132**: 3308–17.

48. Johns M. A new method for measuring daytime sleepiness: the Epworth Sleepiness Scale. Sleep 1991; **14**: 540–5.

49. Cummings JL, Arciniegas DB, Brooks BR, et al. Defining and diagnosing involuntary emotional expression disorder. CNS Spectrums 2006; **11**: 1–7.

50. Phuong L, Garg S, Duda JE, et al. Involuntary emotional disorder in Parkinson's disease. Parkinsonism Relat Disord 2009; **15**: 511–15.

51. Galpern W, Stacy M. Management of impulse control disorders in Parkinson's disease. Curr Opin Neurol 2007; **9**: 189–97.

52. Voon V, Fox SH. Medication-related impulse control and repetitive behaviors in Parkinson disease. Arch Neurol 2007; **64**: 1089–96.

53. Weintraub D, Siderowf AD, Potenza MN, et al. Association of dopamine agonist use with impulse control disorders in Parkinson disease. Arch Neurol 2006; **63**: 969–73.

54. Voon V, Hassan K, Zurowski M, et al. Prospective prevalence of pathological gambling and medication association in Parkinson disease. Neurology 2006; **66**: 1750–2.

55. Voon V, Hassan K, Zurowski M, et al. Prevalence of repetitive and reward-seeking behaviors in Parkinson disease. Neurology 2006; **67**: 1254–7.

56. Voon V, Kubu C, Krack P, et al. Deep brain stimulation: neuropsychological and neuropsychiatric issues. Mov Disord 2006; **21**(Suppl. 14): S305–S326.

57. Herzog J, Volkmann J, Krack P, et al. Two-year follow-up of subthalamic deep brain stimulation in Parkinson's disease. Mov Disord 2003; **18**: 1332–7.

58. Smeding HM, Speelman JD, Koning-Haanstra M, et al. Neuropsychological effects of bilateral STN stimulation in Parkinson disease: a controlled study. Neurology 2006; **66**: 1830–6.

59. Houeto JL, Mesnage V, Mallet L, et al. Behavioral disorders, Parkinson's disease and subthalamic stimulation. J Neurol Neurosurg Psychiatry 2002; **72**: 701–7.

60. Berney A, Vingerhoets F, Perrin A, et al. Effect on mood of subthalamic DBS for Parkinson's disease: a consecutive series of 24 patients. Neurology 2002; **59**: 1427–9.

61. Witt K, Granert O, Daniels C, et al. Relation of lead trajectory and electrode position to neuropsychological outcomes of subthalamic neurostimulation in Parkinson's disease: results from a randomized trial. Brain 2013; **136**: 2109–19.

62. Lhommée E, Klinger H, Thobois S, et al. Subthalamic stimulation in Parkinson's disease: restoring the balance of motivated behaviors. Brain 2012; **135**: 1463–77.

63. Hughes TA, Ross HF, Mindham RH, et al. Mortality in Parkinson's disease and its association with dementia and depression. Acta Neurol Scand 2004; **110**: 118–23.

64. Starkstein SE, Bolduc PL, Mayberg HS, et al. Cognitive impairments and depression in Parkinson's disease: a follow up study. J Neurol Neurosurg Psychiatry 1990; **53**: 597–602.

65. Starkstein SE, Mayberg HS, Leiguarda R, et al. A prospective longitudinal study of depression, cognitive decline, and physical impairments in patients with Parkinson's disease. J Neurol Neurosurg Psychiatry 1992; **55**: 377–82.

66. Aarsland D, Andersen K, Larsen JP, et al. The rate of cognitive decline in Parkinson disease. Arch Neurol 2004; **61**: 1906–11.

67. Ramirez-Ruiz B, Junque C, Marti M, et al. Cognitive changes in Parkinson's disease patients with visual hallucinations. Dement Geriatr Cogn Disord 2007; **23**: 281–8.

68. Aarsland D, Larsen JP, Karlsen K, et al. Mental symptoms in Parkinson's disease are important contributors to caregiver distress. Int J Geriatr Psychiatry 1999; **14**: 866–74.

69. Marsh L, Williams JR, Rocco M, et al. Psychiatric comorbidities in patients with Parkinson disease and psychosis. Neurology 2004; **63**: 293–300.

70. Salter B, Andersen KE, Weiner WJ. Psychosis in Parkinson's disease: case studies. Neurol Clin 2006; **24**: 363–9.

71. Aarsland D, Larsen JP, Tandberg E, et al. Predictors of nursing home placement in Parkinson's disease: a population-based, prospective study. J Am Geriatr Soc 2000; **48**: 938–42.

72. Goetz CG, Tanner CM, Stebbins GT, et al. Risk factors for progression in Parkinson's disease. Neurology 1988; **38**: 1841–4.

73. Aarsland D, Andersen K, Larsen JP, et al. Risk of dementia in Parkinson's disease: a community-based, prospective study. Neurology 2001; **56**: 730–6.

74. Graham J, Grunewald R, Sager H. Hallucinosis in idiopathic Parkinson's disease. J Neurol Neurosurg Psychiatry 1997; **63**: 434–40.

75. Aarsland D, Larsen JP, Cummings JL, et al. Prevalence and clinical correlates of psychotic symptoms in Parkinson disease: a community-based study. Arch Neurol 1999; **56**: 595–601.

76. Weintraub D, Moberg PJ, Duda JE, et al. Effect of psychiatric and other non-motor symptoms on disability in Parkinson's disease. J Am Geriatr Soc 2004; **52**: 784–8.

77. Biglan KM, Holloway RG J, McDermott MP, et al. Risk factors for somnolence, edema, and hallucinations in early Parkinson disease. Neurology 2007; **69**: 187–95.

78. Biggins C, Boyd J, Harrop F, et al. A controlled, longitudinal study of dementia in Parkinson's disease. J Neurol Neurosurg Psychiatry 1992; **55**: 566–71.

79. Alves G, Larsen JP, Emre M, et al. Changes in motor subtype and risk for incident dementia in Parkinson's disease. Mov Disord 2006; **21**: 1123–30.

80. Wint DP, Okun MS, Fernandez HH. Psychosis in Parkinson's disease. J Geriatr Psychiatry Neurol 2004; **17**: 127–36.

81. Weintraub D, Morales KH, Duda JE, et al. Frequency and correlates of co-morbid psychosis and depression in Parkinson's disease. Parkinsonism Relat Disord 2006; **12**: 427–31.

82. Wolters ECh. Intrinsic and extrinsic psychosis in Parkinson's disease. J Neurol 2001; **248**(Suppl. 3): 22–7.

83. Henderson MJ, Mellers JDC. Psychosis in Parkinson's disease: 'between a rock and a hard place'. Int Rev Psychiatry 2000; **12**: 319–34.

84. Sanchez-Ramos JR, Ortoll R, Paulson GW. Visual hallucinations associated with Parkinson disease. Arch Neurol 1996; **53**: 1265–8.

85. Merims D, Shabtai H, Korczyn AD, et al. Antiparkinsonian medication is not a risk factor for the development of hallucinations in Parkinson's disease. J Neural Transm 2004; **111**: 1447–53.

86. Onofrj M, Thomas A, Bonanni L. New approaches to understanding hallucinations in Parkinson's disease: phenomenology and possible origins. Expert Rev Neurotherapeutics 2007; **7**: 1731–50.

87. Pacchetti C, Manni R, Zangaglia R, et al. Relationship between hallucinations, delusions, and rapid eye movement sleep behavior disorder in Parkinson's disease. Mov Disord 2005; **20**: 1439–48.

88. Phillips B. Movement disorders: a sleep specialist's perspective. Neurology 2004; **62**(Suppl. 2): S9–S16.

89. Comella CL, Tanner CM, Ristanovic RK. Polysomnographic sleep measures in Parkinson's disease patients with treatment-induced hallucinations. Ann Neurol 1993; **34**: 710–14.

90. Chaudhuri A, Behan PO. Fatigue and basal ganglia. J Neurol Sci 2000; **179**: 34–42.

91. Karlsen K, Larsen JP, Tandberg E, et al. Fatigue in patients with Parkinson's disease. Mov Disord 1999; **14**: 237–41.

92. Mayberg HS. Modulating dysfunctional limbic-cortical circuits in depression: towards development of brain-based algorithms for diagnosis and optimised treatment. Br Med Bull 2003; **65**: 193–207.

93. Mentis MJ, McIntosh AR, Perrine K, et al. Relationships among the metabolic patterns that correlate with mnemonic, visuospatial, and mood symptoms in Parkinson's disease. Am J Psychiatry 2002; **159**: 746–54.

94. Mayberg HS, Starkstein SE, Sadzot B, et al. Selective hypometabolism in the inferior frontal lobe in depressed patients with Parkinson's disease. Ann Neurol 1990; **28**: 57–64.

95. Brown AS, Gershon S. Dopamine and depression. J Neural Transm Gen Sect 1993; **91**: 75–109.

96. Berg D, Supprian T, Hofmann E, et al. Depression in Parkinson's disease: brainstem midline alteration on transcranial sonography and magnetic imaging. J Neurol 1999; **246**: 1186–93.

97. Murai T, Muller U, Werheid K, et al. In vivo evidence for differential association of striatal dopamine and midbrain serotonin systems with neuropsychiatric symptoms in Parkinson's disease. J Neuropsychiatry Clin Neurosci 2001; **13**: 222–8.

98. Duffy JD. The neural substrates of motivation. Psychiatr Ann 1997; **27**: 39–43.

99. Isella V, Melzi P, Grimaldi M, et al. Clinical, neuropsychological, and morphometric correlates of apathy in Parkinson's disease. Mov Disord 2002; **17**: 366–71.

100. Robert G, Le Jeune F, Lozachmeur C, et al. Apathy in patients with Parkinson disease without dementia or depression: a PET study. Neurology 2012; **79**: 1155–60.

101. Wolters ECh. Dopaminomimetic psychosis in Parkinson's disease patients: diagnosis and treatment. Neurology 1999; **52**(Suppl. 3): S10–S13.

102. Cheng A, Ferrier I, Morris C, et al. Cortical serotonin S-2 receptor-binding in Lewy body dementia, Alzheimer's and Parkinson's diseases. J Neurol Sci 1991; **106**: 50–5.

103. Perry E, Marshall E, Kerwin J. Evidence of monoaminergic-cholinergic imbalance related to visual hallucinations in Lewy body dementia. J Neurochem 1990; **55**: 1454–6.

104. Birkmayer W, Danielczyk W, Neumayer E, et al. Nucleus ruber and L-dopa psychosis: biochemical and post-mortem findings. J Neural Transm 1974; **35**: 93–116.

105. Jellinger K. The pedunculopontine nucleus in Parkinson's disease. J Neurol Neurosurg Psychiatry 1988; **51**: 540–3.

106. Eisensehr I, Linke R, Noachtar S, et al. Reduced striatal dopamine transporters in idiopathic rapid eye movement sleep behavior disorder. comparison with Parkinson's disease and controls. Brain 2000; **123**: 1155–60.

107. Green RL. Regulation of affect. Semin Clin Neuropsychiatry 1998; **3**: 195–200.

108. Gallagher DA, Goetz CG, Stebbins G, et al. Validation of the MDS-UPDRS Part I for nonmotor symptoms in Parkinson's disease. Mov Disord 2012; **27**: 79–83.

109. Goetz CG, Tilley BC, Shaftman SR, et al. Movement Disorder Society-sponsored revision of the Unified Parkinson's Disease Rating Scale (MDS-UPDRS): scale presentation and climimetric testing results. Mov Disord 2008; **23**: 2129–70.

110. Kaufer DI, Cummings JL, Ketchel P, et al. Validation of the NPI-Q, a brief clinical form of the Neuropsychiatric Inventory. J Neuropsychiatry Clin Neurosci 2000; **12**: 233–9.

111. Weintraub D, Moberg PJ, Duda JE, et al. Recognition and treatment of depression in Parkinson's disease. J Geriatr Psychiatry Neurol 2003; **16**: 178–83.

112. Richard IH, Kurlan R, Parkinson Study Group. A survey of antidepressant use in Parkinson's disease. Neurology 1997; **49**: 1168–70.

113. Alexopoulos GS, Katz IR, Reynolds CF III, et al. The expert consensus guideline series: pharmacotherapy of depressive disorders in older patients. Postgrad Med (Spec Rep) 2001; October: 1–86.

114. Weintraub D, Morales KH, Moberg PJ, et al. Antidepressant studies in Parkinson's disease: a review and meta-analysis. Mov Disord 2005; **20**: 1161–9.

115. Wermuth L, Sørensen PS, Timm S, et al. Depression in idiopathic Parkinson's disease treated with citalopram: a placebo-controlled trial. Nordic Journal of Psychiatry 1998; **52**:163–9.

116. Leentjens AF, Vreeling FW, Luijckx GJ, et al. SSRIs in the treatment of depression in Parkinson's disease. Int J Geriatr Psychiatry 2003; **18**: 552–4.

117. Menza M, Dobkin RD, Marin H, et al. A controlled trial of antidepressants in patients with Parkinson's disease and depression. Neurology 2009; **72**: 886–92.

118. **Richard I, McDermott M, Kurlan R, et al**. A randomized, double-blind, placebo-controlled trial of antidepressants in Parkinson's disease. Neurology 2012; **78**: 1229–36.

119. **Andersen J, Aabro E, Gulmann N, et al**. Anti-depressive treatment in Parkinson's disease: a controlled trial of the effect of nortriptyline in patients with Parkinson's disease treated with l-dopa. Acta Neurol Scand 1980; **62**: 210–19.

120. **Emre M**. Treatment of dementia associated with Parkinson's disease. Parkinsonism Relat Disord 2007; **13**(Suppl. 3): S457–S461.

121. **Barone P, Poewe W, Albrecht S, et al**. Pramipexole for the treatment of depressive symptoms in patients with Parkinson's disease: a randomised, double-blind, placebo-controlled trial. Lancet Neurol 2010; **9**: 573–80.

122. **Walsh K, Bennett G**. Parkinson's disease and anxiety. Postgrad Med J 2001; **77**: 89–93.

123. **Devos D, Moreau C, Maltete D, et al**. Rivastigmine in apathetic but dementia and depression-free patients with Parkinson's disease: a double-blind, placebo-controlled, randomized clinical trial. J Neurol Neurosurg Psychiatry 2014; **85**: 668–74.

124. **Marin RS, Fogel BS, Hawkins J, et al**. Apathy: a treatable syndrome. J Neuropsychiatry Clin Neurosci 1995; **7**: 23–30.

125. **Shulman LM**. Apathy in patients with Parkinson's disease. Int Rev Psychiatry 2000; **12**: 298–306.

126. **Thobois S, Lhommee E, Klinger H, et al**. Parkinsonian apathy responds to dopaminergic stimulation of D₂/D₃ receptors with piribedil. Brain 2013; **136**: 1568–77.

127. **Friedman JH, Factor SA**. Atypical antipsychotics in the treatment of drug-induced psychosis in Parkinson's disease. Mov Disord 2000; **15**: 201–11.

128. **Dewey RB, O'Suilleabhain PE**. Treatment of drug-induced psychosis with quetiapine and clozapine in Parkinson's disease. Neurology 2000; **55**: 1753–4.

129. **Weiner WJ, Minagar A, Shulman LM**. Quetiapine for l-dopa-induced psychosis in PD. Neurology 2000; **54**: 1538.

130. **Poewe W, Seppi K**. Treatment options for depression and psychosis in Parkinson's disease. J Neurol 2001; **248**(Suppl. 3): III12–III21.

131. **Olanow CW, Watts RL, Koller WC**. An algorithm (decision tree) for the management of Parkinson's disease (2001): treatment guidelines. Neurology 2001; **56** (Suppl. 5): S1–S88.

132. **Thomsen TR, Panisset M, Suchowersky O, et al**. Impact of standard of care for psychosis in Parkinson disease. J Neurol Neurosurg Psychiatry 2008; **79**: 1413–15.

133. **Emre M, Tsolaki M, Bonuccelli U, et al**. Memantine for patients with Parkinson's disease dementia or dementia with Lewy bodies: a randomized, double-blind, placebo-controlled trial. Lancet Neurol 2010; **9**: 969–77.

134. **Aarsland D, Ballard C, Walker Z, et al**. Memantine in patients with Parkinson's disease dementia or dementia with Lewy bodies: a double-blind, placebo-controlled, multicentre trial. Lancet Neurol 2009; **8**: 613–18.

135. **Leroi I, Overshott R, Byrne E, et al**. Randomized controlled trial of memantine in dementia associated with Parkinson's disease. Mov Disord 2009; **24**: 1217–40.

136. **Maidment I, Fox C, Boustani M**. Cholinesterase inhibitors for Parkinson's disease dementia. Cochrane Database Syst Rev 2006; CD004747.

137. **Thomas AJ, Burn DJ, Rowan EN, et al**. A comparison of the efficacy of donepezil in Parkinson's disease with dementia and dementia with Lewy bodies. Int J Geriatr Psychiatry 2005; **20**: 938–44.

138. **Ravina B, Putt M, Siderowf A, et al**. Donepezil for dementia in Parkinson's disease: a randomised, double blind, placebo controlled, crossover study. J Neurol Neurosurg Psychiatry 2005; **76**: 934–9.

139. **Emre M, Aarsland D, Albanese A, et al**. Rivastigmine for dementia associated with Parkinson's disease. N Engl J Med 2004; **351**: 2509–18.

140. Burn D, Emre M, McKeith I, et al. Effects of rivastigmine in patients with and without visual hallucinations in dementia associated with Parkinson's disease. Mov Disord 2006; **21**: 1899–907.

141. Reading PJ, Luce AK, McKeith IJ. Rivastigmine in the treatment of parkinsonian psychosis and cognitive impairment: preliminary findings from an open trial. Mov Disord 2001; **16**: 1171–95.

142. Aarsland D, Hutchinson M, Larsen JP. Cognitive, psychiatric and motor responses to galantamine in Parkinson's disease with dementia. Int J Geriatr Psychiatry 2003; **18**: 937–41.

143. Marras C, Kopp A, Qiu F, et al. Antipsychotic use in older adults with Parkinson's disease. Mov Disord 2007; **22**: 319–23.

144. Factor SA, Molho E, Friedman JH. Risperidone and Parkinson's disease. Mov Disord 2002; **17**: 221–2.

145. Fernandez HH, Trieschmann ME, Friedman.JH. Treatment of psychosis in Parkinson's disease: safety considerations. Drug Saf 2003; **26**: 643–59.

146. Ondo WG, Tintner R, Voung KD, et al. Double-blind, placebo-controlled, unforced titration parallel trial of quetiapine for dopaminergic-induced hallucinations in Parkinson's disease. Mov Disord 2005; **20**: 958–63.

147. Rabey JM, Prokhorov T, Miniovitz A, et al. Effect of quetiapine in psychotic Parkinson's disease patients: a double-blind labeled study of 3 months' duration. Mov Disord 2007; **22**: 313–18.

148. Reddy S, Factor SA, Molho E, et al. The effect of quetiapine on psychosis and motor function in parkinsonian patients with and without dementia. Mov Disord 2002; **17**: 676–81.

149. Fernandez HH, Trieschmann ME, Burke MA, et al. Long-term outcome of quetiapine use for psychosis among Parkinsonian patients. Mov Disord 2003; **18**: 510–14.

150. Prohorov T, Klein C, Miniovitz A, et al. The effect of quetiapine in psychotic Parkinsonian patients with and without dementia. An open-labeled study utilizing a structured interview. J Neurol 2006; **253**: 171–5.

151. Cummings J, Isaacson S, Mills R, et al. Pimavanserin for patients with Parkinson's disease psychosis: a randomised, placebo-controlled phase 3 trial. Lancet 2014; **383**: 533–40.

152. FDA Center for Drug Evaluation and Research. Information for healthcare professionals: conventional antipsychotics [16 June 2008]. <http://www.fda.gov/drugs/drugsafety/postmarketdrugsafetyinformationforpatientsandproviders/ucm124830.htm> (accessed 9 February 2009).

153. Schneider LS, Dagerman KS, Insel P. Risk of death with atypical antipsychotic drug treatment for dementia: meta-analysis of randomized placebo-controlled trials. J Am Med Assoc 2009; **294**: 1934–43.

154. Setoguchi S, Wang PS, Brookhart MA, et al. Potential causes of higher mortality in elderly users of conventional and atypical antipsychotic medications. J Am Geriatr Soc 2008; **56**: 1644–50.

155. Schneeweiss S, Setoguchi S, Brookhart A, et al. Risk of death associated with the use of conventional versus atypical antipsychotic drugs among elderly patients. Can Med Assoc J 2007; **176**: 627–32.

156. Gill SS, Bronskill SE, Normand S-LT, et al. Antipsychotic drug use and mortality in older adults with dementia. Ann Intern Med 2007; **146**: 775–86.

157. Marras C, Gruneir A, Wang X, et al. Antipsychotics and mortality in Parkinsonism. Am J Geriatr Psychiatry 2012; **20**: 149–58.

158. Friedman JH. Atypical antipsychotics in the elderly with Parkinson's disease and the 'black box' warning. Neurology 2006; **67**: 564–6.

159. Culo S, Mulsant B, Rosen J, et al. Treating neuropsychiatric symptoms in dementia with Lewy bodies: a randomized controlled-trial. Alzheimer Dis Assoc Disord 2010; **24**: 360–4.

160. APA Work Group on Alzheimer's Disease and Other Dementias. American Psychiatric Association Practice Guideline for the treatment of patients with Alzheimer's disease and other dementias. Second edition. Am J Psychiatry 2007; **164**(Suppl.): 5–56.

161. Howard RJ, Juszczak E, Ballard CG, et al. Donepezil for the treatment of agitation in Alzheimer's disease. N Engl J Med 2007; **357**: 1382–92.

162. **Nieves AV, Lang AE**. Treatment of excessive daytime sleepiness in patients with Parkinson's disease with modafinil. Clin Neuropharmacol 2002; **25**: 111–14.

163. **Adler CH, Caviness JN, Hentz JG, et al**. Randomized trial of modafinil for treating subjective daytime sleepiness in patients with Parkinson's disease. Mov Disord 2003; **18**: 287–93.

164. **Panitch HS, Thisted RA, Smith RA, et al**. Randomized, controlled trial of dextromethorphan/quinidine for pseudobulbar affect in multiple sclerosis. Ann Neurol 2006; **59**: 780–7.

165. **Brooks BR, Thisted RA, Appel SH, et al**. Treatment of pseudobulbar affect in ALS with dextromethorphan/quinidine: a randomized trial. Neurology 2004; **63**: 1364–70.

166. **Arciniegas DB, Topkoff J**. The neuropsychiatry of pathologic affect: an approach to evaluation and treatment. Semin Clin Neuropsychiatry 2000; **5**: 290–306.

Chapter 6

Interaction between affect and executive functions in Parkinson's disease

Paolo Barone and Gabriella Santangelo

Introduction

The relationship between affect and cognition is a topic of continuing interest [1]. Affect and cognition are processes that are interconnected, related, and mediated by a circuitry that is widely distributed throughout the brain and includes subcortical areas typically considered to be 'affective' (e.g. the amygdala and nucleus accumbens) as well as portions of the cortex that are typically considered 'cognitive' (e.g. the ventromedial prefrontal cortex/anterior cingulate and orbitofrontal cortex) [2] (Fig. 6.1).

Cognitive impairment in Parkinson's disease (PD) can be found in all stages of the disease and may precede the development of dementia. It includes impairments in attention, encoding memory, and visuospatial and executive functions, the latter being mainly attributed to the disruption of the fronto-striatal circuitry (see Chapter 4) [3]. Affective disorders in PD include depression, apathy, and anhedonia. Prevalence rates for depression in PD vary from 2.7% to more than 90% [4], whereas the prevalence rates for apathy range from 13.9 to 70%, the mean prevalence being 35% [5]. This variability may be in part due to differences in study methods, the presence of substantial overlap between symptoms of PD and symptoms of depression, and the criteria used to diagnose depression and apathy [4]. There is a particular problem when using the Diagnostic and Statistical Manual of Mental Disorders, fourth edition (DSM-IV), because of the ambiguity between depression, apathy, and dementia [6]. Furthermore, apathy and anhedonia, which are both included in DSM Criterion A.2, may be independent of depression and may reflect the decreased involvement of PD patients in their usual activities rather than being the consequence of a depressive disorder.

Classically, dopamine denervation is associated with motor symptoms in PD. However, dopamine neurotransmission seems to have a relevant role in controlling both the cognitive and the emotional aspects of the disease. Depression in PD is associated with the loss of dopamine and noradrenaline innervation in the limbic system [7], and may fluctuate along with motor functions, improving during the 'on' state and worsening during the 'off' state [8]. Similar fluctuations are reported for apathy in PD, suggesting that apathy is at least partly a dopamine-dependent syndrome [9]. Finally, the neural substrate of anhedonia is suggested to be due to dysfunction of the dopaminergic–mesolimbic reward circuit involving the ventral striatum and prefrontal cortex [10]. Along with the above observations that support a role in controlling affect in PD, the dopamine system also seems to be deeply involved in controlling cognition related to frontal lobe functions. In particular, mesocortical dopamine inputs to the prefrontal cortex regulate working memory function, planning, and attention, suggesting that dopamine alterations may at least be partly responsible for executive dysfunctions in PD [11].

Fig. 6.1 Circuitry interconnections between affective and cognitive functions. GPE, external global pallidus; STN, subthalamic nucleus; VP, ventral pallidum; AMY, amygdala; GPi-SNpr, internal globus pallidus and substantia nigra pars reticulata; DA, dopamine; CX, cortex.

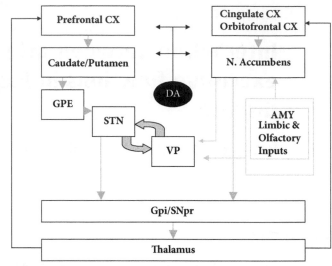

This review analyses the association between affective disorders and cognitive impairment in PD, with a special focus on the relationship between executive dysfunction, depression, anhedonia, and apathy.

Depression and executive functions in PD

There is controversy about the relationship between depression and cognitive dysfunction in PD patients (Table 6.1). Three possible patterns emerge: (1) depression influences cognition in PD—in this case depression would mainly influence the severity (quantity) of cognitive impairment [12–23]; (2) depression and cognitive impairment are independently induced, though many symptoms of the two conditions might overlap in PD [24–28]; (3) cognitive dysfunctions that are related to PD neuropathology are the substrate of a depressive disorder in PD—in this case a distinct pattern of cognitive impairment (quality) would be associated with depression.

Evidence that depression affects cognition derives from both epidemiological studies that indicate depression to be a risk factor for dementia [29] and from the observation that severely depressed PD (dPD) patients are more cognitively impaired than patients with mild depression. In particular, Starkstein et al. [14] found that PD patients with major depression (MD) reported a significantly worse performance in tasks assessing frontal lobe functions such as verbal fluency, set-shifting, and attention compared with PD patients without MD. No significant difference in cognitive profile between PD patients with minor depression and non-depressed PD patients was found. Consistently, Tröster et al. [23] found that depression exacerbates memory and language impairment in PD. However, differences in cognitive performance between dPD and non-dPD patients disappeared when patients were matched for total Mattis Dementia Rating Scale (MDRS) score, suggesting that depression influences the severity rather than the profile of cognitive impairment in PD. One limitation of the two studies mentioned above was the absence of a comparison group including patients with MD but without PD.

Kuzis et al. [15] compared the cognitive profile of dPD and non-dPD patients and depressed patients without PD and found that all depressed patients (with and without PD) reported poorer performance on tasks assessing verbal fluency and auditory attention than non-depressed PD

Table 6.1 Cognitive functions as assessed in Parkinson's disease (PD) patients with and without depression

Study and cognitive task	PD patients with depression	PD patients without depression	Depressed patients without PD
Starkstein et al. (1989) [13]			
Wisconsin Card Sorting Test	+	−	
Controlled word association	+	−	
Digit Span:			
Forwards	−	−	
Backwards	−	−	
Trail Making Test	+	−	
Design Fluency Test	+	−	
Symbol Digit Modalities	+	−	
MMSE	+	−	
Troster et al. (1995) [23]			
MDRS	+	−	
Wisconsin Card Sorting Test	−	−	
Boston Naming Test	+	−	
Controlled word association	+	−	
Animal naming test	+	−	
WAIS-R			
Digit Span	−		
Logical Memory I	+	−	
Logical Memory II	−	−	
When groups matched for mean MDRS:			
Wisconsin Card Sorting Test	−	−	
Boston Naming Test	−	−	
Controlled word association	−	−	
Animal naming test	−	−	
WAIS-R:			
Digit Span	−	−	
Logical Memory I	−	−	
Logical Memory II	−	−	
Kuzis et al. (1997) [15]			
Raven Progressive Matrices	+	−	−
Wisconsin Card Sorting Test		−	−

Table 6.1 (continued) Cognitive functions as assessed in Parkinson's disease (PD) patients with and without depression

Study and cognitive task	PD patients with depression	PD patients without depression	Depressed patients without PD
Categories	+	–	–
Perseverations	+	–	+
Verbal fluency:			
Buschke Total Recall Test	+	–	–
Buschke Delayed Recall Test	–	–	–
Benton Visual Retention Test	–	–	–
Digit Span:			
Forwards	–	–	–
Backwards	+	–	+
Costa et al. (2006) [21]			
Digit Span:			
Forwards	–	–	
Backwards	–	–	
Corsi Test:			
Forwards	–	–	
Backwards	–	–	
Immediate visual memory	+	–	
Word list recall:			
Immediate recall	–	–	
Delayed recall	+	–	
Word list recognition: correct items	+	–	
Prose recall			
Immediate recall	–	–	
Delayed recall	–	–	
Rey's figure:			
Immediate reproduction	–	–	
Delayed reproduction	–	–	
Freehand copying of drawings	–	–	
Copying drawings with landmarks	–	–	
Copying Rey's figure	–	–	
Sentence construction	+	–	

Table 6.1 (continued) Cognitive functions as assessed in Parkinson's disease (PD) patients with and without depression

Study and cognitive task	PD patients with depression	PD patients without depression	Depressed patients without PD
Raven's Progressive Matrices 47	+	−	
Modified Card Sorting Test			
Categories achieved	+	−	
Perseverative errors	+	−	
Non-perseverative errors	−	−	
Lexical verbal fluency	+	−	
Uekermann et al. (2003) [19]			
Digit Span:			
Forwards	−	−	−
Backwards	+	−	−
Benton Visual Retention Test	−	−	−
Word list recall:			−
Immediate	−	−	−
Delayed	−	−	−
Semantic verbal fluency	−	−	−
Lexical verbal fluency	+	−	−
Hayling Test	−	−	
Stefanova et al. (2006) [20]			
WAIS-R:			
Verbal IQ	−	−	
Performance of IQ	+	−	
Rey Auditory Verbal Learning Test:			
Recall	−	−	
Delayed recall	−	−	
Letter (lexical) fluency	+	−	
Category (semantic) fluency	+	−	
Boston Naming Task	+	−	
Hooper Test	−	−	
Trail Making Test:			
Form A	−	−	
Form B	−	−	

Table 6.1 (continued) Cognitive functions as assessed in Parkinson's disease (PD) patients with and without depression

Study and cognitive task	PD patients with depression	PD patients without depression	Depressed patients without PD
Silberman et al. (2006) [28]			
Stroop Test	–	–	
Emotional Stroop Test	–	–	

MMSE, Mini-Mental State Examination; MDRS, Mattis Dementia Rating Scale; WAIS-R, Wechsler Adult Intelligence Scale–Revised.

+, altered performance on cognitive tasks; –, normal performance on cognitive tasks.

patients. Moreover, dPD patients showed a significantly worse performance on frontal tasks evaluating concept formation and set-shifting compared with non-depressed PD patients, patients with depression alone, and normal subjects of a control group. This finding suggests that alteration of frontal lobe functions, such as concept formation and set-shifting, may result from an interaction between PD neuropathology and the mechanism of MD. Consistently, Costa et al. [21] found that PD patients with MD performed worse than non-depressed PD patients on long-term verbal episodic memory tasks, abstract reasoning tasks, and tasks assessing executive functioning. They concluded that MD in PD is specifically associated with a qualitatively distinct neuropsychological profile that may be related to the alteration of prefrontal and limbic cortical areas.

Since the duration of PD might be an important factor for both neuropathological and cognitive changes, Uekermann et al. [19] explored cognitive functions in early PD, finding poorer performance on short-term memory and lexical fluency tasks in dPD patients compared with non-dPD patients, depressed patients without PD, and control subjects. Similarly in early PD patients, Stefanova et al. [20] found that MD in PD patients was associated with cognitive impairment of specific domains (visuospatial memory, spatial working memory, language) and more profound executive and visuospatial deficits, whereas dysthymic disorder was associated only with a quantitative increase in executive dysfunctions observed in non-dPD. They concluded that cognitive impairment in early PD may be predicted by the severity of depression. Since depression is reported to be associated with right-side disease onset and disease duration, Foster et al. [30] explored whether mood disturbances are associated with side of onset and disease duration in patients with PD and affect cognitive functioning. They found that parkinsonian patients with right hemibody onset of motor symptoms experienced more depression as the PD progressed and that they showed more severe alterations of cognitive functioning than PD patients with left hemibody onset.

Evidence that depression and cognitive dysfunctions are independent derives from a variety of studies mainly focusing on general screening tools for dementia, such as the Mini-Mental State Examination [24–27]. In one study, executive dysfunction, as explored by the Stroop and Emotional Stroop Tests, was related neither to depression nor to the severity of PD [28].

The relationship between depression and executive dysfunction is generally thought to be one of depression affecting the severity of cognitive impairment. Conversely, executive dysfunction, which is related to neuropathology of PD, might be responsible for depressive symptoms, especially considering that the DSM-IV criteria for diagnosis of MD do not separate anhedonia from apathy (DSM-IVA, Criterion 2). Santangelo et al. [31] subtyped PD patients with MD according to the occurrence of apathy/anhedonia (DSM-IVA, Criterion 2). They found that dPD patients with high levels of apathy and/or anhedonia scored significantly worse on frontal tasks than patients with depressed mood (DSM-IVA, Criterion 1) and non-depressed patients. These findings suggest that the combination of apathy, anhedonia, and frontal lobe dysfunction might contribute to the overdiagnosis of depression in PD. More recently, Varanese et al. [32] found that depression, unlike apathy, was not associated with executive impairment in PD patients. These findings indirectly support the idea that apathy and depression are two independent non-motor symptoms of PD.

Subthreshold depression (SD) is characterized by depressive symptoms not meeting the criteria for MD. SD is not associated with objective cognitive deficits (assessed by means of screening tools for dementia) [33–36] but is related to subjective cognitive complaints [36]. Therefore, it should be investigated accurately because it might reduce quality of life and might be a predictor of development of MD in PD, as demonstrated in the general population [37].

Apathy and executive functions in PD

Apathy is a primary loss of motivation, interest, and effortful behaviour. Studies in PD patients have shown that the presence of apathy is specifically associated with frontal lobe dysfunction. Starkstein et al. [38] found that PD patients with apathy performed worse than PD without apathy on part B of the Trail Making Test and lexical fluency task. Consistently, Pluck and Brown [39] found that PD patients with apathy showed decreased performance compared with PD patients without apathy on tasks evaluating specific frontal lobe functions including verbal fluency, changing mental categories, and inhibition. Isella et al. [40] confirmed the relationship between apathy and frontal lobe dysfunction in PD patients; they found that PD patients with apathy showed a poorer performance than PD patients without apathy on tasks assessing verbal fluency set-shifting, sensitivity to interference, and ability to inhibit automatic behaviour. More recently, Zgaljardic et al. [41] demonstrated that patients with significant levels of apathy performed worse than patients with low apathy scores on measures of verbal fluency and verbal and non-verbal conceptualization. Low performance on cognitive tasks assessing verbal fluency, working memory, verbal abstraction, and executive dysfunction significantly predicts both the presence and the worsening of apathy. More recently, Varanese et al. [32] found that apathy was associated with deficits in implementing efficient cognitive strategies: patients with apathy had poorer performance than patients without apathy in immediate recall and executive tasks. Grossi et al. [42] found that apathy is characterized by a similar neuropsychological profile in patients with dementia regardless of the pathology (PD or Alzheimer's) responsible for the dementia. In both diseases apathy was found to be associated with defects on frontal tasks, thus strongly supporting the existence of an 'apathetic syndrome'.

Although apathy is generally considered to occur in advanced disease stages, studies have found a prevalence rate of 22.9% in de novo PD patients [43]. In a longitudinal study, apathy was found to be a predictor of the development of dementia. Conversely, dementia at baseline, a more rapid decline in speech and axial impairment [44], and poor performance on the interference task of the Stroop Test [45] may predict development of incident apathy in PD patients.

Anhedonia and executive functions in PD

Anhedonia is an inability to experience pleasure from normally pleasurable life events such as eating, exercise, or social or sexual interaction. Findings about the relationship between anhedonia and frontal lobe dysfunctions are discordant. Isella et al. [46] carried out a study to formally assess the prevalence and correlates of physical anhedonia in PD patients compared with normal controls. They found higher levels of anhedonia in PD patients with respect to controls and no significant association of physical anhedonia with clinical or neuroradiological features or frontal lobe dysfunction. However, others found that in both PD and progressive supranuclear palsy, anhedonia assessed using the Snaith–Hamilton Pleasure Scale was associated with frontal lobe dysfunction as evaluated by means of the Frontal Assessment Battery [47, 48], a short neuropsychological tool that assesses executive functions at the bedside. In 2013 a study reported that in patients with MD anhedonia was associated with impaired divided attention and also with a degree of apraxia and impairment of verbal memory [49]. Since current findings about the relationship between anhedonia and frontal lobe dysfunction are conflicting, this question needs further investigation.

Conclusion

In PD, executive dysfunction is associated with depression, apathy, and anhedonia, though there is no clear-cut agreement on the causative relationship between cognitive and affective disorders. It is conceivable that they share a common neurochemical and neuroanatomical background consisting of degeneration of the mesocortical and mesolimbic dopaminergic projections. In the PD population a subgroup of patients may be identified as having specific characteristics: more severe executive dysfunction associated with apathy/anhedonia and depression, and increased risk for dementia. Thus, evaluations of both neuropsychological profile and the presence of depressed mood, apathy, and anhedonia should be regarded as a routine procedure for predicting prognosis and decision-making with regard to treatment.

References

1. Forgas JP. *Affect in social thinking and behavior*. New York: Psychology Press, 2006.
2. Duncan S, Barrett LF. Affect is a form of cognition: a neurobiological analysis. Cogn Emot 2007; **21**: 1184–211.
3. Zgaljardic DJ, Borod JC, Foldi NS, et al. A review of the cognitive and behavioral sequelae of Parkinson's disease: relationship to frontostriatal circuitry. Cogn Behav Neurol 2003; **16**: 193–210.
4. Reijnders JS, Ehrt U, Weber WE, et al. A systematic review of prevalence studies of depression in Parkinson's disease. Mov Disord 2008; **23**: 183–9.
5. Santangelo G, Trojano L, Barone P, et al. Apathy in Parkinson's disease: diagnosis, neuropsychological correlates, pathophysiology and treatment. Behav Neurol 2013; **27**: 501–13.
6. Marsh L, McDonald WM, Cummings J, et al. [NINDS/NIMH Work Group on Depression and Parkinson's Disease]. Provisional diagnostic criteria for depression in Parkinson's disease: report of NINDS7NIMH Work Group. Mov Disord 2006; **21**: 148–58.
7. Remy P, Doder M Lees A, et al. Depression in Parkinson's disease: dopamine and noradrenaline innervation in the limbic system. Brain 2005; **128**: 1314–22.
8. Kulisevsky J, Pascual-Sedano B, Barbanoj M, et al. Acute effects of immediate and controlled-release levodopa on mood in Parkinson's disease: a double-blind study. Mov Disord 2007; **22**: 62–7.
9. Czernecki V, Pillon B, Houeto JL, et al. Motivation, reward, and Parkinson's disease: influence of dopatherapy. Neuropsychologia 2002; **40**: 2257–67.
10. Robbins T, Evritt B. Neurobehavioural mechanisms of reward and motivation. Curr Opin Neurobiol 1996; **6**: 228–36.
11. Seamans JK, Yang CR. The principal features and mechanism of dopamine modulation in the prefrontal cortex. Prog Neurobiol 2004; **74**: 1–58.
12. Mayeux R, Stern Y, Rosen J, et al. Depression, intellectual impairment, and Parkinson disease. Neurology 1981; **31**: 645–50.

13. **Starkstein SE, Preziosi TJ, Berthier ML, et al.** Depression and cognitive impairment in Parkinson's disease. Brain 1989; **112**: 1141–53.

14. **Starkstein SE, Preziosi TJ, Bolduc PL, et al.** Depression in Parkinson's disease. J Nerv Ment Dis 1990; **178**: 27–31.

15. **Kuzis G, Sabe L, Tiberti C, et al.** Cognitive functions in major depression and Parkinson disease. Arch Neurol 1997; **54**: 982–6.

16. **Cubo E, Bernard B, Leurgans S, et al.** Cognitive and motor function in patients with Parkinson's disease with and without depression. Clin Neuropharmacol 2000; **23**: 331–4.

17. **Anguenot A, Loll PY, Neau JP, et al.** Depression and Parkinson's disease: study of a series of 135 Parkinson's patients. Can J Neurol Sci 2002; **29**: 139–46.

18. **Norman S, Troster AI, Fields JA, et al.** Effects of depression and Parkinson's disease on cognitive functioning. J Neuropsychiatry Clin Neurosci 2002; **14**: 31–6.

19. **Uekermann J, Daum I, Peters S, et al.** Depressed mood and executive dysfunction in early Parkinson's disease. Acta Neurol Scand 2003; **107**: 341–8.

20. **Stefanova E, Potrebic A, Ziropadja L, et al.** Depression predicts the pattern of cognitive impairment in early Parkinson's disease. J Neurol Sci 2006; **248**: 131–7.

21. **Costa A, Peppe A, Carlesimo GA, et al.** Major and minor depression in Parkinson's disease: a neuropsychological investigation. Eur J Neurol 2006; **13**: 972–80.

22. **Tröster AI, Paolo AM, Lyons KE, et al.** The influence of depression on cognition in Parkinson's disease: a pattern of impairment distinguishable from Alzheimer's disease. Neurology 1995; **45**: 672–6.

23. **Tröster AI, Stalp LD, Paolo AM, et al.** Neuropsychological impairment in Parkinson's disease with and without depression. Arch Neurol 1995; **52**: 1164–9.

24. **Beliauskas LA, Glantsz RH.** Depression type in Parkinson's disease. J Clin Exp Neuropsychol 1989; **11**: 597–604.

25. **Santamaria J, Tolosa E, Valles A.** Parkinson's disease with depression: a possible subgroup of idiopathic parkinsonism. Neurology 1986; **36**: 1130–3.

26. **Taylor AE, Saint-Cyr JA, Lang AE, et al.** Parkinson's disease and depression: a critical reevaluation. Brain 1986; **109**: 279–92.

27. **Huber SJ, Paulson GW, Shuttleworth EC.** Relationship of motor symptoms, intellectual impairment, and depression in Parkinson's disease. J Neurol Neurosurg Psychiatry 1988; **51**: 855–8.

28. **Silberman CD, Laks J, Capitão CF, et al.** Frontal functions in depressed and nondepressed Parkinson's disease patients: impact of severity stages. Psychiatry Res 2007; **149**: 285–9.

29. **Stern Y, Marder K, Tang MX, et al.** Antecedent clinical features associated with dementia in Parkinson's disease. Neurology 1993; **43**: 1690–2.

30. **Foster PS, Drago V, Mendez K, et al.** Mood disturbances and cognitive functioning in Parkinson's disease: the effects of disease duration and side of onset of motor symptoms. J Clin Exp Neuropsychol 2013; **35**: 71–82.

31. **Santangelo G, Vitale C, Trojano L, et al.** Relationship between depression and cognitive dysfunctions in Parkinson's disease without dementia. J Neurol 2009; **256**: 632–8.

32. **Varanese S, Perfetti B, Ghilardi MF, et al.** Apathy, but not depression, reflects inefficient cognitive strategies in Parkinson's disease. PLoS ONE 2011; **6**(3): e17846.

33. **Reiff J, Schmidt N, Riebe B, et al.** Subthreshold depression in Parkinson's disease. Mov Disord 2011; **26**: 1741–4.

34. **Nation DA, Katzen HL, Papapetropoulos S, et al.** Subthreshold depression in Parkinson's disease. Int J Geriatr Psychiatry 2009; **24**: 937–43.

35. **Ehrt U, Brønnick K, De Deyn PP, et al.** Subthreshold depression in patients with Parkinson's disease and dementia-clinical and demographic correlates. Int J Geriatr Psychiatry 2007; **22**: 980–5.

36. **Santangelo G, Vitale C, Trojano L, et al.** Subthreshold depression and subjective cognitive complaints in Parkinson's disease. Eur J Neurol. 2014; **21**: 541–4.

37. Meeks TW, Vahia IV, Lavretsky H, et al. A tune in 'A minor' can be 'B major': a review of epidemiology, illness course, and public health implications of subthreshold depression in older adults. J Affect Disord 2011; **129**: 126–42.

38. Starkstein SE, Mayberg HS, Preziosi TJ, et al. Reliability, validity, and clinical correlates of apathy in Parkinson's disease. J Neuropsychiatry Clin Neurosci 1992; **4**: 134–9.

39. Pluck GC, Brown RG. Apathy in Parkinson's disease. J Neurol Neurosurg Psychiatry 2002; **73**: 636–42.

40. Isella V, Melzi P, Grimaldi M, et al. Clinical, neuropsychological, and morphometric correlates of apathy in Parkinson's disease. Mov Disord 2002; **17**: 366–71.

41. Zgaljardic DJ, Borod JC, Foldi NS, et al. Relationship between self-reported apathy and executive dysfunction in nondemented patients with Parkinson disease. Cogn Behav Neurol 2007; **20**: 184–92.

42. Grossi D, Santangelo G, Barbarulo AM, et al. Apathy and related executive syndromes in dementia associated with Parkinson's disease and in Alzheimer's disease. Behav Neurol 2013; **27**: 515–22.

43. Pedersen KF, Alves G, Brønnick K, et al. Apathy in drug-naïve patients with incident Parkinson's disease: the Norwegian ParkWest study. J Neurol 2010; **257**: 217–23.

44. Pedersen KF, Alves G, Aarsland D, et al. Occurrence and risk factors for apathy in Parkinson disease: a 4-year prospective longitudinal study. J Neurol Neurosurg Psychiatry 2009; **80**: 1279–82.

45. Santangelo G, Vitale C, Picillo M, et al. Relationship between apathy and cognitive dysfunctions in de novo, untreated Parkinson's disease: a prospective longitudinal study. Eur J Neurol 2014; doi: 10.1111/ene.12467.

46. Isella V, Iurlaro S, Piolti R, et al. Physical anhedonia in Parkinson's disease. J Neurol Neurosurg Psychiatry 2003; **74**: 1308–11.

47. Dubois B, Slachevsky A, Litvan I, Pillon B. The FAB: a Frontal Assessment Battery at bedside. Neurology 2000; **12**: 1621–6.

48. Santangelo G, Morgante L, Savica R, et al., on behalf of the PRIAMO study group. Anhedonia and cognitive impairment in Parkinson's disease: Italian validation of the Snaith–Hamilton Pleasure Scale and its application in the clinical routine practice during the PRIAMO study. Parkinsonism Relat Disord 2009; **15**: 576–81.

49. Spalletta G, Fagioli S, Meco G, et al. Hedonic tone and its mood and cognitive correlates in Parkinson's disease. Depress Anxiety 2013; **30**: 85–91.

Chapter 7

Motor symptoms and phenotype in patients with Parkinson's disease dementia

David J. Burn and Alison J. Yarnall

Introduction

Although considered primarily a disorder of movement, non-motor complications are now rec‐ ognized to precede and accompany the bradykinesia, rigidity, and tremor of Parkinson's disease (PD). Given the frequency of these non-motor complications, they are assumed to be an intrinsic part of the pathophysiological process of PD, and presumably reflect multifocal cell dysfunction and loss in strategic subcortical and cortical structures. It therefore seems reasonable to expect that expression of the motor and non-motor phenotype in any individual with PD is unlikely to be an independent process, and that some interrelationship may exist between the two.

This chapter specifically considers the association between motor phenotype and dementia associated with PD (PD-D). It will also briefly address related features as part of this phenotype. The issue of motor phenotype as a predictive factor for incident dementia will be discussed, as well as the evidence for levodopa responsiveness and motor complications in PD-D. Finally, the rate of progression of the extrapyramidal symptoms in PD-D will be described.

Motor phenotype in patients with PD-D

The notion of certain motor features being overrepresented in people with PD and cognitive impairment is not new. The DATATOP study, which included 800 patients with early untreated PD, reported that bradykinesia and postural instability and gait disturbance (PIGD) were more common at onset in patients with a rapid rate of disease progression compared with those having a relatively slow rate of progression [1]. This was substantiated in a study from 2011 describing the natural evolution of PD, where PIGD phenotype at disease presentation was a predictor of pro‐ gression to Hoehn and Yahr Stage 3 in a multivariate model [2]. In the former study, the authors described a means of classifying patients into tremor-dominant (TD), PIGD-dominant, and inde‐ terminate phenotypes on the basis of an equation derived from items in the Unified Parkinson's Disease Rating Scale (UPDRS) Parts II and III (this classification has been extensively revised subsequent to its initial publication). Comparisons of TD PD ($n = 441$) with the PIGD-dominant type ($n = 233$) provided support for the existence of clinical subtypes, with the latter group report‐ ing significantly greater subjective intellectual, motor, and occupational impairment than the TD group. In the same year, Ebmeier et al. [3] assessed a whole population cohort of 157 patients with parkinsonism to determine prevalence figures for dementia and to examine the relationship between dementia, cognitive impairment, and extrapyramidal signs. Dementia, defined accord‐ ing to DSM-III-R criteria, was present in 23.3% of all patients. The authors reported that dementia and cognitive impairment were associated with overall measures of motor impairment and rigidity, but not tremor, also after controlling for age, gender, and education. Gnanalingham et al. [4] compared motor and cognitive function in patients with dementia with Lewy bodies (DLB), PD, or Alzheimer's disease. PD-D cases were not specifically identified in this study. Compared with patients with PD, DLB patients had greater scores for rigidity and deficits in a finger-tapping test, but rest tremor and left/right asymmetry in extrapyramidal signs were more evident in PD. DLB patients were also less likely to present with left/right asymmetry in motor symptoms at the onset of their parkinsonism. In a later cross-sectional study specifically aimed at comparing extrapyramidal features in PD, PD-D, and DLB patients, the PIGD phenotype was found to be more common in PD-D (88% of cases) and DLB (69% of cases) groups compared with the PD group (38% of cases), in which TD and PIGD phenotypes were more equally represented ($P < 0.001$) [5].

Poorer cognitive performance in PD is associated with greater impairment in motor and non-motor domains. Papapetropoulos et al. [6] evaluated the impact of cognitive impairment on disease severity and motor function in 82 PD patients, 41 and 41 of whom, respectively, did and did not have cognitive impairment, matched for age at onset and duration of the disease. Those patients with cognitive impairment had overall poorer motor function, worse rigidity (both axial and limb) and bradykinesia, as well as worse performance in activities of daily living compared with PD patients without cognitive impairment. In a cohort study of 400 PD patients, more severe cognitive impairment was associated with significantly more impairment in motor, autonomic, depressive, and psychotic domains [7]. Furthermore, patients with a PIGD-dominant phenotype showed more cognitive impairment than patients with a TD phenotype. This is in keeping with a more recent study, which also demonstrated that the PIGD motor phenotype led to a greater decline specifically in attentional function over 3 years of follow-up [8].

In contrast to most previous studies which reported a greater risk for dementia in PD patients with predominant rigidity and akinesia, Vingerhoets et al. [9] reported in their retrospective cohort analysis that older age and tremor at onset were significant predictors of poor cognitive performance. Although the reasons for this disparity are unclear, it should be appreciated that tremor has uncommonly been related to PD-D and is not recognized per se as a risk factor for incident dementia.

Studies attempting to relate cognitive impairment to asymmetry of motor symptoms in PD have found contradictory results. Thus, Tomer et al. [10] examined 88 patients with unilateral onset of PD and found that patients whose motor signs began on the left side of their body consistently performed more poorly on a battery of cognitive measures than did patients with right-sided onset. In a later study, PD patients with right-sided tremor onset performed significantly better than other PD subgroups in a neuropsychological battery and comparably to controls [11]. Williams et al. [12] applied multiple regression analysis to examine UPDRS subscore contributions to cognitive function in 108 PD patients. They found that right-sided symptoms (for laterality), axial symptoms (for region), and bradykinesia (for type of symptoms) were the best predictors of cognitive function in this patient group. In contrast, St Clair et al. [13] found no difference in neuropsychological functioning between two groups of PD patients with either predominant left- or right-sided motor signs, matched for disease duration, severity of motor signs, and degree of lateralized motor deficits. The results of these studies are therefore confusing and conclusions are limited in most cases by sample size, the battery of tests chosen (hemispheric predilection), and the natural hand dominance of patients tested versus the side of symptom dominance. The most parsimonious explanation would be that side of symptom dominance does not have a major influence upon cognitive function in PD or PD-D.

A data-driven approach to motor phenotype and cognition

The relationship between motor phenotype and dementia may also be examined by exploring heterogeneity within cohorts of PD patients using a data-driven approach. This approach is non-hypothesis driven and avoids arbitrary a priori subclassifications. Graham and Sagar [14] explored heterogeneity in 176 patients with PD by using comprehensive demographic, motor, mood, and cognitive information. Cluster analysis revealed three subgroups of patients—one subgroup with a disease duration of 5.6 years and two subgroups with one of 13.4 years. A 'motor only' subtype was characterized by motor symptom progression in the absence of intellectual impairment. Equivalent motor symptom progression was shown by a 'motor and cognitive' subtype which was accompanied by deficits in executive function progressing to global cognitive impairment. A 'rapid progression' subtype was characterized by an older age at disease onset and rapidly progressive motor and cognitive disability. Lewis et al. [15] subsequently investigated the heterogeneity of PD using a similar approach in a cohort of 120 patients in the early disease phase (Hoehn and Yahr Stages I–III). The analysis revealed four main subgroups: (1) patients with a younger disease onset; (2) a TD subgroup of patients; (3) a non-TD subgroup with significant levels of cognitive impairment and mild depression; and (4) a subgroup with rapid disease progression but no cognitive impairment. Both studies suggest that, at least in cross-sectional analyses, distinct motor–cognitive phenotypes exist in PD, although these studies do not permit the assessment of change over time. In other words, motor phenotype is not necessarily stable, and patients who are initially TD may not remain so throughout their disease.

These clinical findings were corroborated in part by a large retrospective clinico-pathological study of 242 pathologically confirmed cases of PD from the Queen Square Brain Bank [16]. Selikhova and colleagues [16] confirmed that those with early onset shared similar characteristics to those classified by Lewis et al. [15], with greater time to falls and cognitive decline, but pathologically similar Lewy body (LB) burden to TD phenotypes. Interestingly, those with TD disease did not have significantly longer disease duration than those with non-TD presentations. The latter group was strongly associated with the development of cognitive impairment, had more extensive LB disease, and had greater deposition of amyloid-beta plaque plus neurofibrillary tangles than other subtypes. Participants with rapid disease progression tended to be older at disease onset, were more likely to have early midline motor deficits plus early depression, and to present with TD disease. The burden of LB disease was lower than in those who were non-TD, but similar to those with early onset and TD disease.

Expanding the motor phenotype

PD-D is also an independent risk factor for falls. In a prospective study of 109 subjects with PD evaluated over 12 months, falls occurred in 68% of patients [18]. Previous falls, disease duration, loss of arm swing, and notably dementia were independent predictors of falling. A subsequent meta-analysis of falling in PD was unable to include cognitive impairment and dementia as a predictive variable because this had not been quantified in all of the six studies included [19]. A more recent prospective study determined whether measures of attention were associated with falls in 164 PD patients [20]. A total of 103 (63%) subjects fell once or more during the 12-month study period. Regression analysis revealed an association of fall frequency with poorer attentional scores, which was retained after correcting for UPDRS score. The close association between cognition and falls in PD may in part relate to cholinergic dysfunction [21, 22]; this has implications for the identification of those PD patients most at risk of falling, and for the management and prevention of falls in this patient group. Indeed a small study of PD patients without dementia who had a fall demonstrated a reduction in falls by almost half in those who were taking cholinesterase inhibitors compared with placebo, supporting further work in this area [23].

The PIGD phenotype has also been associated with more frequent excessive daytime sleepiness (EDS) in PD-D, although this association was lost over a 2-year follow-up period, suggesting that the pathophysiology of EDS and motor phenotype is anatomically and/or temporally distinct [24]. Intriguingly, in PD patients without dementia, rapid eye movement sleep behaviour disorder (RBD) is more common in patients with a PIGD phenotype and is associated with greater frequency of falls and reduced levodopa responsiveness [25, 26]. Moreover, the presence of RBD in PD has been strongly associated with more severe symptoms and signs of orthostatic hypotension [26–28]. A phenotypic pattern of PD associated with PD-D is thus emerging, characterized by a PIGD motor disturbance, RBD, EDS, greater autonomic disturbance, and increased frequency of falls.

Early cognitive impairment and motor function

In addition to motor phenotype in established PD-D, what evidence is there for differences in extrapyramidal signs in PD patients with mild cognitive impairment (PD-MCI)? Establishing differences at this point in the disease process could give greater insight into the underlying pathophysiological process. In a community study of 159 patients with incident PD, 36% subjects had some cognitive impairment at baseline assessment, defined as scores of less than one standard deviation (SD) below normative values [29]. Those with global or frontal impairments were significantly older and had more severe motoric disease and lower pre-morbid intelligence than those who were cognitively normal. Longitudinal assessment of the same cohort confirmed that a non-TD phenotype at baseline assessment was a predictor of cognitive decline independent of age, in addition to impairments in more posteriorly mediated cognitive tasks [30]. A cross-sectional study of patients in the Netherlands with early PD found that participants with MCI (defined at a score of 2 SD below the mean score of matched controls in three or more neuropsychological tests) were older, more likely to be male, and had greater disease severity, greater depression scores, and more severe axial and speech symptoms than those who were cognitively normal [31]. However, only age remained a significant predictor of cognitive dysfunction in logistic regression modelling. More recently, in a large study of 121 early, drug-naïve PD participants and 100 healthy controls, Poletti et al. [32] reported that bradykinesia, axial impairment, and absence of tremor were associated with an increased risk of MCI, and that patients with PIGD-dominant disease had a higher proportion of MCI diagnoses than those who with TD disease (23.2 versus 6.3%). In contrast, other studies in early PD have not demonstrated differences between axial impairment [33] or proportion of PIGD phenotype [34] in those with MCI or normal cognition, suggesting that motor phenotype becomes more important as the disease progresses. This has been demonstrated in studies of prevalent PD [35, 36], where subtypes of PD-MCI may be important in further classifying the disorder. In particular, non-amnestic multiple-domain MCI has been found to be linked with motor impairment, with axial functioning/gait making a significant contribution to multinominal logistic regression models of PD-MCI subtype [35].

Taken together, these observations suggest that the pathological processes determining motor phenotype may be dissociated from those determining cognition, either in temporal or spatial evolution or both. By their cross-sectional nature, however, most of these studies were unable to address whether motor phenotype may be an independent risk factor for incident dementia in PD (this is addressed in the next section 'Motor phenotype as a risk factor for dementia').

Motor phenotype as a risk factor for dementia

Although a number of risk factors have been reported for incident dementia in PD, three have been consistently found in almost all studies: advanced age, motor phenotype, and baseline cognitive performance [30, 41–47]. Advanced age is the single most significant risk factor, in both cross-sectional and prospective studies, although older age and more severe motor symptoms are synergistic in predicting dementia [48]. When a cohort of patients was divided into four groups by dichotomizing around their median age and UPDRS motor scores, the group with older age and severe disease had a 12-fold increased risk for incident dementia compared with the younger patients with mild disease [48]. As younger patients with greater disease severity and older patients with less severe motor symptoms did not show a significantly increased risk, a combined effect of age and disease severity was assumed. In addition to the overall severity of extrapyramidal features influencing the likelihood of developing PD-D, a non-TD motor phenotype also predicts a greater risk for incident dementia. In one prospective study of 40 PD patients, 25% of 16 patients with the PIGD phenotype developed dementia over 2 years, compared with none of 18 patients with the TD phenotype or six with indeterminate phenotype [49].

As mentioned, the predominant motor phenotype may not necessarily remain stable throughout the disease course. Thus a patient may evolve from a TD to a PIGD phenotype, presumably reflecting the underlying pathological progression. This, in turn, may influence the risk of developing dementia. In a Norwegian community-based sample of 171 PD patients without dementia followed prospectively over 8 years, logistic regression was used to analyse the relationship between subtype of parkinsonism and dementia [50]. The transition from the TD to PIGD subtype was associated with a more than three-fold increase in the rate of decline measured by the Mini-Mental State Examination (MMSE). Compared with patients with a persistent TD or indeterminate subtype, the odds ratio for dementia was 56.7 [95% confidence interval (CI): 4.0–808] for patients changing from a TD or indeterminate subtype to the PIGD subtype, and 80.0 (95% CI: 4.6–1400) for patients with a persistent PIGD subtype. Furthermore, patients with a TD subtype at baseline did not develop dementia until they developed a PIGD motor subtype, and dementia did not occur among patients with persistent tremor dominance. Although the CIs were wide for these estimates, reflecting relatively small numbers, this work emphasizes the importance of current motor phenotype and associated risk of dementia.

In a community-based study performed in Cambridgeshire, UK, incident cases of PD were recruited, thereby removing much of the bias associated with selective mortality in prevalence cohorts [30, 47]. Bivariate comparisons of baseline demographic, clinical, and neuropsychological variables versus rate of cognitive decline showed that, in addition to older age, a non-TD motor phenotype, a higher UPDRS motor score, and below average performance on tests of semantic fluency, pentagon copying, spatial recognition memory, and the Tower of London test were associated with a more rapid rate of cognitive decline. Multivariate analysis revealed that a non-TD motor phenotype together with poor semantic fluency and inaccurate pentagon copying were the most significant predictors of cognitive decline, independent of age. Patients with a non-TD phenotype were 4.1 times more likely to develop dementia than TD patients.

Axial symptoms and PD-D may have an overlapping pathogenesis, with distinct loci of dysfunction different from those underlying TD PD. Specifically, the postural instability of PD tends to be refractory to dopaminergic therapy, and may relate to the loss of subcortical neurons within the cholinergic system which also plays an important role in the cognitive and neuropsychiatric symptoms of PD-D [22]. In addition, recent work [51] that examined cerebrospinal fluid (CSF) in de novo PD has suggested that neurotransmitter dysfunction may not be the only overlapping pathophysiological process between cognition and motor phenotype. Alves et al. [51] looked at the CSF of 99 untreated patients with PD and 46 age-matched controls. Those with PD and a PIGD phenotype (*n* = 39) had significantly lower amyloid-beta markers than those who had TD disease (*n* = 60); there were no significant differences in CSF marker levels between the TD PD group and controls. Furthermore, multivariate linear regression models with adjustments for age, white matter hyperintensities, and cognition demonstrated significant associations of CSF amyloid-beta with PIGD score and lower limb bradykinesia, highlighting that abnormal deposition of amyloid-beta may contribute to motoric disease beyond its effect on cognition.

Response to levodopa and motor complications

The axial symptoms of PD are commonly viewed as being less responsive to levodopa. They may be caused by 'non-dopaminergic' lesions, for example in the pedunculopontine nucleus. Levodopa responsiveness could therefore be expected to be reduced in PD-D with a predominant PIGD phenotype. One possibility, of course, is that previously levodopa-responsive symptoms become refractory as dementia develops [52]. To date, a majority of cross-sectional and longitudinal studies have failed to directly assess levodopa response in PD-D versus PD patients without dementia. Using a 200 mg single-dose levodopa challenge, one study failed to detect significant differences in mean improvement on UPDRS motor score, although more patients without dementia experienced an improvement of >20% compared with those with PD-D (90 versus 65%) [53]. A later study included patients with DLB, PD, and PD-D and failed to detect differences in levodopa responsiveness between PD and PD-D [54]. Given the clinical (including motor phenotype) and pathological similarity between PD-D and DLB, it is also of potential relevance to consider the results of a study in 19 DLB subjects in whom levodopa was increased and motor response assessed a mean of 3 months later [55]. Motor improvement was found in only 6 of the 19 patients, despite a mean daily increase of 111 mg levodopa. A longitudinal study found greater cognitive decline over a 3-year period in those PD patients with less than 50% improvement in their UPDRS score after a levodopa test performed at baseline [56]. More recently, a prospective study of 34 PD patients assessed annually over a mean follow-up of 11.4 years from the point of commencement of levodopa found that the patients who developed dementia had a more rapid decline in motor function [57]. Moreover, further follow-up of the same participants at a mean of 14.8 years showed that although the magnitude of levodopa response was well preserved over disease progression in all participants (*n* = 17), those with dementia had worse motor scores and diminished levodopa response [58]. Similarly, at 18.2 years (*n* = 8), most of these patients were at an advanced stage of the disease, with those who had developed dementia demonstrating more rapid motor decline [59].

Overall, it is not possible to draw firm conclusions about differences in the degree of levodopa responsiveness between PD subjects with and without dementia. The limited evidence available to date would suggest, however, an attenuated or diminished response in those with PD-D.

Levodopa-induced motor complications

Whereas fewer dyskinesias were reported in PD-D patients in a cross-sectional study [60], a longitudinal study found greater mental deterioration in those patients exhibiting dystonic levodopa-induced dyskinesias at baseline [56]. Clissold et al [57] reported fluctuator versus non-fluctuator status in a longitudinal study of levodopa responsiveness in 22 surviving PD patients, in addition to their latest MMSE score. When considering fluctuator status in those subjects with a MMSE score of ≤24, compared with those above this level (a threshold previously suggested to support a diagnosis of PD-D), only 15% of the fluctuators were classified as PD-D versus 44% of the non-fluctuators. Although these data are insufficient to infer differences in the occurrence of levodopa-induced motor complications in PD-D, they lend some support to the notion that fluctuations may be less frequent.

Neuroleptic sensitivity

Although placebo-controlled studies have previously excluded patients with PD-D, open-label studies with clozapine in PD-related psychosis have included PD-D subjects and found that the drug was similarly well-tolerated in PD-D and PD patients without dementia. Sedation and hypotension are the main side effects described. One study evaluated severe neuroleptic sensitivity reactions (NSRs) according to an operationalized definition, blind to clinical and neuropathological diagnoses, in prospectively studied patients exposed to neuroleptics from two centres [61]. Severe NSR only occurred in patients with DLB—in 53% DLB, 39% PDD, and 27% PD patients—and did not occur in Alzheimer's disease. No other clinical or demographic features predicted severe NSR. This high frequency of NSR in PD-D clearly has important implications for clinical practice, particularly as even so-called 'atypical neuroleptics' such as risperidone, olanzapine, and aripiprazole are not exempt from causing this problem in the closely related DLB [62].

Rate of progression of motor symptoms in PD-D

The development of dementia may be associated with a more aggressive course of motor disease [14, 57, 60]. Jankovic and Kapadia [63] determined the overall rate of functional decline in 297 PD patients, followed up for an average of 6.4 (range 3–17) years. Patients were categorized as having TD or PIGD-dominant PD and the two categories were compared for progression of their total UPDRS scores. Patients with an older age at onset had more rapid progression of PD than those with a younger age at onset, while cognitive deterioration was greater in the older-onset group. Regression analysis of 108 patients whose symptoms were rated during their 'off' state showed a faster rate of cognitive decline as age at onset increased, and the annual rate of decline in the UPDRS scores, when adjusted for age at initial visit, was steeper for the PIGD-dominant group compared with the TD group. Dementia at baseline was associated with more rapid motor decline in two studies [64, 65], but this remained significant in only one study after adjusting for other baseline factors, where PD-D patients had a 7.9-point higher annual decline in UPDRS motor scores than those without dementia at baseline [65]. In a longitudinal study, a more rapid decline in UPDRS III scores was reported in PD-D compared with PD patients over 2 years (9.7 versus 5.1 points, respectively) [49]. Although not statistically significant, the absolute deterioration at 2 years was greater in the PIGD than the TD PD subgroup. Rate of motor decline in the PD-D patients was independent of baseline disease duration. In a study of 232 PD patients followed for 8 years, population-averaged logistic regression models were used to describe annual disease progression and to analyse the influence of potential risk factors on functional decline [66]. Age, age at onset, disease duration, and EDS at baseline were strong and independent predictors of greater impairment in motor function and disability, while cognitive impairment at baseline predicted higher disability and a higher Hoehn and Yahr score. Age at disease onset was, however, the main predictor of motor decline, indicating a slower and more restricted pathological process in patients with younger-onset PD.

Conclusion

A consistent motor phenotype associated with PD-D has emerged from observational studies. These patients are more likely to have symmetric disease and fewer tremors than their counterparts without dementia. The phenotype may be expanded to include a higher frequency of falls, sleep disorders (RBD and possibly EDS), and autonomic impairment. The PD-D patient may be less likely to experience levodopa-related dyskinesias and be more refractory to levodopa treatment overall, although more work is required to clarify these points and to control for potential confounders, including age, cumulative doses of levodopa received, and disease duration. Neuroleptics, including so-called 'atypical' agents, should be used with caution in PD-D, as the patients may be sensitized to potentially life-threatening extrapyramidal side effects associated with these drugs. The PIGD phenotype is a robust predictor of incident dementia in PD, and conversion to this phenotype during the disease course appears to have sinister portent with regard to deterioration in cognition. Finally, the presence of dementia seems to herald a more rapid deterioration in motor function, which may contribute to the increased mortality observed in PD-D patients.

References

1. Jankovic J, McDermott M, Carter J., et al. Variable expression of Parkinson's disease: a base-line analysis of the DATATOP cohort. The Parkinson Study Group. Neurology 1990; **40**: 1529–34.
2. Evans JR, Mason SL, Williams-Gray CH, et al. The natural history of treated Parkinson's disease in an incident, community based cohort. J Neurol Neurosurg Psychiatry 2011; **82**: 1112–18.
3. Ebmeier KP, Calder SA, Crawford JR, et al. Clinical features predicting dementia in idiopathic Parkinson's disease: a follow-up study. Neurology 1990; **40**: 1222–4.
4. Gnanalingham KK, Byrne EJ, Thornton A, et al. Motor and cognitive function in Lewy body dementia: comparison with Alzheimer's and Parkinson's diseases. J Neurol Neurosurg Psychiatry 1997; **62**: 243–52.
5. Burn DJ, Rowan EN, Minett T, et al. Extrapyramidal features in Parkinson's disease with and without dementia and dementia with Lewy bodies: a cross-sectional comparative study. Mov Disord 2003; **18**: 884–9.
6. Papapetropoulos S, Ellul J, Polychronopoulos P, et al. A registry-based, case-control investigation of Parkinson's disease with and without cognitive impairment. Eur J Neurol 2004; **11**: 347–51.
7. Verbaan D, Marinus J, Visser M, et al. Cognitive impairment in Parkinson's disease. J Neurol Neurosurg Psychiatry 2007; **78**: 1182–7.
8. Taylor JP, Rowan EN, Lett D, et al. Poor attentional function predicts cognitive decline in patients with non-demented Parkinson's disease independent of motor phenotype. J Neurol Neurosurg Psychiatry 2008; **79**: 1318–23.
9. Vingerhoets G, Verleden S, Santens P, et al. Predictors of cognitive impairment in advanced Parkinson's disease. J Neurol Neurosurg Psychiatry 2003; **74**: 793–6.
10. Tomer R, Levin BE, Weiner WJ. Side of onset of motor symptoms influences cognition in Parkinson's disease. Ann Neurol 1993; **34**: 579–84.
11. Katzen HL, Levin BE, Weiner W. Side and type of motor symptom influence cognition in Parkinson's disease. Mov Disord 2006; **21**: 1947–53.
12. Williams LN, Seignourel P, Crucian GP, et al. Laterality, region, and type of motor dysfunction correlate with cognitive impairment in Parkinson's disease. Mov Disord 2007; **22**: 141–5.
13. St Clair J, Borod JC, Sliwinski M, et al. Cognitive and affective functioning in Parkinson's disease patients with lateralized motor signs. J Clin Exp Neuropsychol 1998; **20**: 320–7.
14. Graham JM, Sagar HJ. A data-driven approach to the study of heterogeneity in idiopathic Parkinson's disease: Identification of three distinct subtypes. Mov Disord 1999; **14**: 10–20.

15. **Lewis SJG, Foltynie T, Blackwell AD, et al**. Heterogeneity of Parkinson's disease in the early clinical stages using a data driven approach. J Neurol Neurosurg Psychiatry 2005; **76**: 343–8.

16. **Selikhova M, Williams DR, Kempster PA, et al**. A clinico-pathological study of subtypes in Parkinson's disease. Brain 2009; **132**: 2947–57.

17. **Wood BH, Bilclough JA, Bowron A, et al**. Incidence and prediction of falls in Parkinson's disease: a prospective multidisciplinary study. J Neurol Neurosurg Psychiatry 2002; **72**: 721–5.

18. **Pickering, R.M., et al.**, A meta-analysis of six prospective studies of falling in Parkinson's disease. Movement Disorders, 2007. **22**(13): p. 1892–900.

19. **Allcock LM, Rowan EN, Steen IN, et al**. Impaired attention predicts falling in Parkinson's disease. Parkinsonism Relat Disord 2009; **15**: 110–15.

20. **Bohnen NI, Müller ML, Koeppe RA, et al**. History of falls in Parkinson disease is associated with reduced cholinergic activity. Neurology 2009; **73**: 1670–6.

21. **Yarnall AJ, Rochester L, Burn DJ**. The interplay of cholinergic function, attention, and falls in Parkinson's disease. Mov Disord 2011; **26**: 2496–503.

22. **Chung KA, Lobb BM, Nutt JG, et al**. Effects of a central cholinesterase inhibitor on reducing falls in Parkinson disease. Neurology 2010; **75**: 1263–9.

23. **Boddy F, Rowan EN, Lett D, et al**. Subjectively reported sleep quality and excessive daytime somnolence in Parkinson's disease with and without dementia, dementia with Lewy bodies and Alzheimer's disease. Int J Geriatr Psychiatry 2007; **22**: 529–35.

24. **Postuma RB, Gagnon JF, Vendette M, et al**. REM sleep behaviour disorder in Parkinson's disease is associated with specific motor features. J Neurol Neurosurg Psychiatry 2008; **79**: 1117–21.

25. **Romenets SR, Gagnon JF, Latreille V, et al**. Rapid eye movement sleep behavior disorder and subtypes of Parkinson's disease. Mov Disord 2012; **27**: 996–1003.

26. **Allcock LM, Kenny RA, Burn DJ**. Clinical phenotype of subjects with Parkinson's disease and orthostatic hypotension: autonomic symptom and demographic comparison. Mov Disord 2006; **21**: 1851–5.

27. **Postuma RB, Gagnon JF, Vendette M, et al**. Manifestations of Parkinson disease differ in association with REM sleep behavior disorder. Mov Disord 2008; **23**: 1665–72.

28. **Foltynie T, Brayne CE, Robbins TW, et al**. The cognitive ability of an incident cohort of Parkinson's patients in the UK. The CamPaIGN study. Brain 2004; **127**: 550–60.

29. **Williams-Gray CH, Foltynie T, Brayne CEG, et al**. Evolution of cognitive dysfunction in an incident Parkinson's disease cohort. Brain 2007; **130**: 1787–98.

30. **Muslimovic D, Post B, Speelman JD, et al**. Cognitive profile of patients with newly diagnosed Parkinson disease. Neurology 2005; **65**: 1239–45.

31. **Poletti M, Frosini D, Pagni C, et al**. Mild cognitive impairment and cognitive-motor relationships in newly diagnosed drug-naive patients with Parkinson's disease. J Neurol Neurosurg Psychiatry 2012; **83**: 601–6.

32. **Elgh E, Domellöf M, Linder J, et al**. Cognitive function in early Parkinson's disease: a population-based study. Eur J Neurol 2009; **16**: 1278–84.

33. **Yarnall AJ, Breen DP, Duncan GW, et al**. Characterizing mild cognitive impairment in incident Parkinson's disease: the ICICLE-PD study Neurology 2014; **82**: 1–9.

34. **Goldman JG, Weis H, Stebbins G, et al**. Clinical differences among mild cognitive impairment subtypes in Parkinson's disease. Mov Disord 2012; **27**: 1129–36.

35. **Sollinger AB, Goldstein FC, Lah JJ, et al**. Mild cognitive impairment in Parkinson's disease: Subtypes and motor characteristics. Parkinsonism Relat Disord 2010; **16**: 177–80.

36. **Hughes TA, Ross HF, Musa S, et al**. A 10-year study of the incidence of and factors predicting dementia in Parkinson's disease. Neurology 2000; **54**: 1596–602.

37. Levy G, Tang MX, Cote LJ, et al. Motor impairment in PD: relationship to incident dementia and age. Neurology 2000; **55**: 539–44.

38. Aarsland D, Andersen K, Larsen JP, et al. Risk of dementia in Parkinson's disease—a community-based, prospective study. Neurology 2001; **56**: 730–6.

39. Aarsland D, Kvaløy JT, Andersen K, et al. The effect of age of onset of PD on risk of dementia. J Neurol 2007; **254**: 38–45.

40. Hobson P, Meara J. Risk and incidence of dementia in a cohort of older subjects with Parkinson's disease in the United Kingdom. Mov Disord 2004; **19**: 1043–9.

41. Uc EY, McDermott MP, Marder KS, et al. Incidence of and risk factors for cognitive impairment in an early Parkinson disease clinical trial cohort. Neurology 2009; **73**: 1469–77.

42. Williams-Gray CH, Evans JR, Goris A, et al. The distinct cognitive syndromes of Parkinson's disease: 5 year follow-up of the CamPaIGN cohort. Brain 2009; **132**: 2958–69.

43. Levy G, Schupf N, Tang MX, et al. Combined effect of age and severity on the risk of dementia in Parkinson's disease. Ann Neurol 2002; **51**: 722–9.

44. Burn DJ, Rowan EN, Allan LM, et al. Motor subtype and cognitive decline in Parkinson's disease, Parkinson's disease with dementia, and dementia with Lewy bodies. J Neurol Neurosurg Psychiatry 2006; **77**: 585–9.

45. Alves G, Larsen JP, Emre M, et al. Changes in motor subtype and risk for incident dementia in Parkinson's disease. Mov Disord 2006; **21**: 1123–30.

46. Alves G, Pedersen KF, Bloem BR, et al. Cerebrospinal fluid amyloid-beta and phenotypic heterogeneity in de novo Parkinson's disease. J Neurol Neurosurg Psychiatry 2013; **84**: 537–43.

47. Joyce JN, Ryoo HL, Beach TB, et al. Loss of response to levodopa in Parkinson's disease and co-occurrence with dementia: role of D3 and not D2 receptors. Brain Res 2002; **955**: 138–52.

48. Bonelli SB, Ransmayr G, Steffelbauer M, et al. L-dopa responsiveness in dementia with Lewy bodies, Parkinson disease with and without dementia. Neurology 2004; **63**: 376–8.

49. Molloy S, McKeith IG, O'Brien JT, et al. The role of levodopa in the management of dementia with Lewy bodies. J Neurol Neurosurg Psychiatry 2005; **76**: 1200–3.

50. Goldman JG, Goetz CG, Brandabur M, et al. Effects of dopaminergic medications on psychosis and motor function in dementia with Lewy bodies. Mov Disord 2008; **23**: 2248–50.

51. Caparros-Lefebvre D, Pécheux N, Petit V, et al. Which factors predict cognitive decline in Parkinson's disease? J Neurol Neurosurg Psychiatry 1995; **58**: 51–5.

52. Clissold BG, McColl CD, Reardon KR, et al. Longitudinal study of the motor response to levodopa in Parkinson's disease. Mov Disord 2006; **21**: 2116–21.

53. Alty JE, Clissold BG, McColl CD, et al. Longitudinal study of the levodopa motor response in Parkinson's disease: relationship between cognitive decline and motor function. Mov Disord 2009; **24**: 2337–43.

54. Ganga G, Alty JE, Clissold BG, et al. Longitudinal study of levodopa in Parkinson's disease: effects of the advanced disease phase. Mov Disord 2013; **28**: 476–81.

55. Elizan TS, Sroka H, Maker H, et al. Dementia in idiopathic Parkinson's disease. Variables associated with its occurrence in 203 patients. J Neural Transm 1986; **65**: 285–302.

56. Aarsland D, Perry R, Larsen JP, et al. Neuroleptic sensitivity in Parkinson's disease and parkinsonian dementias. J Clin Psychiatry 2005; **66**: 633–7.

57. Burn DJ, McKeith IG. Current treatment of dementia with Lewy bodies and dementia associated with Parkinson's disease. Mov Disord 2003; **18**(Suppl. 6): S72–S79.

58. Jankovic J, Kapadia AS. Functional decline in Parkinson disease. Arch Neurol 2001; **58**: 1611–15.

59. **Hely MA, Morris JG, Reid WG, et al.** Age at onset: the major determinant of outcome in Parkinson's disease. Acta Neurol Scand 1995; **92**: 455–63.

60. **Louis ED, Tang MX, Cote L, et al.** Progression of parkinsonian signs in Parkinson disease. Arch Neurol 1999; **56**: 334–7.

61. **Alves G, Wentzel-Larsen T, Aarsland D, et al.** Progression of motor impairment and disability in Parkinson disease: a population-based study. Neurology 2005; **65**: 1436–41.

Chapter 8

Interaction between cognition and gait in patients with Parkinson's disease

Jeffrey M. Hausdorff, Jenny Zitser, Anat Mirelman, and Nir Giladi

Introduction

Gait disturbances and falls are a frequent cause of morbidity and mortality in patients with Parkinson's disease (PD) [1–4]. Within 3 years of diagnosis, over 85% of people with clinically probable PD develop gait problems [5]. This stems, in part, from the pathology of the basal ganglia and dopamine dysregulation [6] that causes impaired execution of automatic and repetitive movements such as those that are critical to walking. In addition to its effects on these so-called motor systems, PD also affects cognition, most notably executive function and attention [7–11] (see also Chapter 4). Criteria have recently been proposed for mild cognitive impairment in PD (PD-MCI) [12], and it is becoming increasingly recognized that MCI can already occur in the early stages of the disease. In this chapter, we describe the evidence demonstrating that these cognitive deficits have a profound impact on many of the gait changes that are commonly seen in PD.

Gait disturbances and fall risk

Gait disturbances in PD may be divided into two types: continuous and episodic or paroxysmal [13–15]. Continuous changes refer to alterations in the walking pattern that are more or less consistent from one step to the next, i.e., they persist and are apparent all the time. In contrast, episodic gait disturbances occur occasionally, emerging in an apparently random, inexplicable manner. Both types of gait disturbances may be influenced by the cognitive changes associated with PD and both are associated with an increased risk of falls. The estimated prevalence of falls in PD ranges from 40 to 90% and generally increases with disease duration [4, 16–22]. In parallel, cognitive impairment also usually worsens as the disease progresses; often, it may progress to dementia in advanced PD. The question that we address in further detail is: how do these cognitive changes impact and exacerbate the gait impairments?

The continuous gait disturbances include slowed ambulation with decreased or absent arm swing, longer double limb support [3, 23–25], and impaired postural control [26–29]. One of the keys to these gait problems is the inability of patients with PD to generate a sufficient stride length [3, 24, 30]. Gait disturbances in PD also include features that are not always visible in routine clinical observation but become apparent when gait is evaluated quantitatively with a gait analysis system, e.g., gait asymmetry, diminished left–right coordination [31], and a loss of consistency in someone's ability to produce a steady gait rhythm, resulting in higher stride-to-stride variability [26, 32–34]. These changes can be detected even in patients with very mild disease [32]. In particular, gait stability, as evaluated by either quantitative gait assessment [7, 35–55] or Unified

Parkinson's Disease Rating Scale (UPDRS) sub-items [53, 55], is consistently associated with visuospatial abilities. Visual sampling (saccadic frequency) may contribute to this relationship in PD [56, 57]. These symptoms, in turn, often lead to a self-imposed restriction of daily activities [16, 58] which exacerbates reduced mobility, causes a further loss of independence, and deprives patients of social contacts, leading to isolation, depression [59], and an overall reduced quality of life [60].

Recent research further supports the association between cognitive changes in PD and continuous gait changes. Several studies suggest that older adults who perform poorly under dual-task gait conditions are at increased risk for falls [61–63]. Similarly, a number of investigations have demonstrated a relationship between attentional abilities, gait, and fall risk in PD [64, 65]. Indeed, Allock et al. [66] demonstrated that attentional deficits are prospectively associated with future falls in patients with PD. Deficits in attention and executive function apparently play an important role in the high fall risk observed in patients with PD.

The episodic gait disturbances include festination, start hesitation, and freezing of gait (FOG) [2, 16, 17]. The latter is a debilitating phenomenon that is commonly experienced by patients with advanced PD [2, 67–69]. FOG is typically a paroxysmal gait disturbance [67, 70] of a 'sudden and transient' nature [71]. Patients who experience FOG frequently report that during the freezing episode their feet are inexplicably 'glued' to the ground. FOG has been referred to as a motor block and has been associated with executive dysfunction [51, 72] and with a worse progression of cognitive decline [7]. Furthermore, different aspects of FOG in PD correlate with visuospatial deficits in combination with executive dysfunction [52]. Shine and colleagues [73] compared 'freezers' with 'non-freezers' under different cognitive loading conditions while participants were in a MRI scanner. During increased cognitive loading, the dorsolateral prefrontal cortex, posterior parietal cortices, pre-supplementary motor area (SMA), and extra-striate visual areas were recruited. These regions are known to comprise a neural network, termed the 'cognitive control network', which has been shown to co-activate in the presence of a variety of executive tasks, as well as during goal-directed behaviour [73–75]. After controlling for motor and affective symptoms, differences still remained between freezers and non-freezers. One explanation is that these differences were due to impairment in the mechanisms underlying dual-task performance caused by the same pathophysiological mechanism that is responsible for the presence of FOG [76].

Changes in cognition, attention, and executive function

Cognitive decline in PD patients occurs even in the early stages of the disease [77] and includes deficits in several cognitive domains [78, 79]. It is estimated that 19–30% of newly diagnosed PD patients present with cognitive impairments [80–82], and these impairments worsen with disease progression [83]. In 2011, a study [55] investigated the relationship between cognitive performance and motor dysfunction in newly diagnosed drug-naïve PD patients, reporting correlations between bradykinesia and set-shifting and between axial signs and memory and visuospatial functions.

Other studies suggest that PD patients whose motor dysfunction is not principally characterized by tremor, i.e., patients classified as having the postural instability and gait disturbance (PIGD) phenotype, present increased rates of cognitive impairment and dementia [84–87]. These studies have been performed on PD patients under dopaminergic treatment and presented two main confounding factors: the unknown effect of therapy on cognition and the different effect of dopaminergic treatment on different motor symptoms [88].

Executive function and attention are two of the most notable functions impaired by PD [8, 77, 89]. Executive function refers to a group of higher cognitive processes by which performance is optimized in situations requiring the operation of multiple cognitive functions [90–92]. Consequently, PD patients show diminished performance in tasks demanding planning, set-shifting, and inhibition of responses, suggesting mental inflexibility or rigidity, slow generation of ideas, and reduced performance on tasks that involve attentional processes or divided attention [77, 89, 93, 94]. People with PD are often taught conscious strategies to improve their gait pattern, such as focusing on walking with longer steps. The type and severity of the cognitive impairment may, however, limit the ability to use such strategies to compensate for the gait abnormalities.

Impaired executive function might also result in inappropriate or unsafe prioritization of tasks when walking under dual-task conditions. In general, dual-tasking relies on frontal lobe function, in particular executive function and the ability to divide attention [95, 96]. The rationale behind using dual-tasking paradigms is, therefore, that if a gait feature is automated and does not require cognitive function, performance of a second task should not alter that aspect of gait. Alternatively, if that feature depends on cognitive function then performance of one or both of the tasks will be affected [97].

To better understand the role of attention on gait in PD, Hausdorff et al. [98] evaluated the effects of a cognitively challenging task on gait variability. This gait feature is a marker of fall risk that also reflects the consistency and automaticity of walking. Subjects with PD walked under normal conditions and while performing another task simultaneously (serial seven subtractions). When walking while cognitively challenged, gait variability increased significantly, more than two-fold ($p < 0.002$) (see Fig. 8.1). Dual tasking also has a negative impact on left–right coordination (see

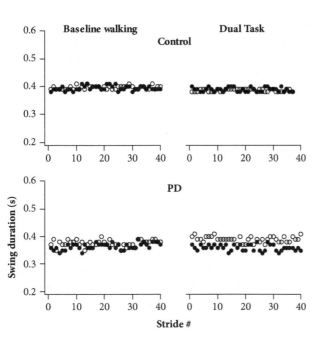

Fig. 8.1 Swing times for each foot in a control subject and a Parkinson's disease (PD) patient. The left and right columns show swing time and asymmetry during usual walking and during dual-tasking, respectively. The effect of dual-tasking is clearly apparent for the PD patient where right-foot values (full black dots) become further separated from the left-foot values (open dots). Such an effect was not present for the control subject, whose gait asymmetry values were 0.3 and 1.0 in the usual walking and the dual-tasking conditions, respectively. The corresponding values were 3.0 and 7.0 for the PD patient.

Springer and Exp Brain Res, Gait asymmetry in patients with Parkinson's disease and elderly fallers: when does the bilateral coordination of gait require attention? 177, 2007, 336–346, Yogev G, Plotnik M, Peretz C, Giladi N, Hausdorff JM, Fig. 1 ©2007 with kind permission from Springer Science and Business Media.

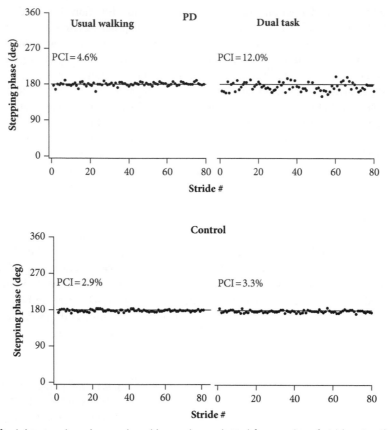

Fig. 8.2 Left–right stepping phase values (degrees) are plotted for a series of strides. For the Parkinson's disease (PD) patient (top panels), the phase values became more scattered and more distanced from the 180° line during dual-tasking (right panel) as compared with the usual walking (left panel). The data from the control subject showed only minor changes in the left–right stepping phase pattern in the presence of dual-tasking (lower panels). PCI, phase coordination index.

Reproduced from Bilateral coordination of gait and Parkinson's disease: the effects of dual tasking, Plotnik M, Giladi N, Hausdorff JM, 80, 347–350, ©2009 with permission from BMJ Publishing Group Ltd.

Fig. 8.2). These results highlight the profound effects of attention and dual-tasking on walking, exacerbating gait variability and impairing the ability of patients with PD to maintain a stable walk.

In parallel, a number of studies have demonstrated that the dual-tasking effect is larger in subjects with cognitive impairment than in controls [37–40, 101]. Furthermore, dual-tasking affects certain aspects of gait differentially in specific populations. An increase in the complexity of the dual task further worsens several gait properties [39, 40]. Moreover, when comparing different grades of cognitive impairment [e.g. subjects with MCI and patients with Alzheimer's disease (AD)], more severe cognitive impairment (i.e. AD) is associated with more detrimental dual-tasking effects on gait [40]. These associations in other populations should be kept in mind when considering the relationship between cognitive function and gait in PD.

It is also important to add that the majority of studies in PD have examined the impact of concurrent task performance during the on-medication state, though a small number examined dual-task walking in the off-medication state only [10, 102]. Studies that examined the effects of medication demonstrated improvements in dual-task walking performance on-medication compared with off-medication [102, 103]. A recent meta-analysis reported that changes in gait performance during dual-tasking were also associated with increased risk for falling among healthy older adults and, to a considerable extent, among frail older adults [104].

In a follow-up study, Yogev et al. [29] examined 30 patients with idiopathic PD (mean age 70.9 years) with moderate disease severity (Hoehn and Yahr Stages 2–3) and 28 age- and gender-matched healthy controls. Gait variability was measured under single- and dual-tasking conditions (with different levels of cognitive loading). Compared with the controls, gait variability was significantly increased in the PD group under all conditions ($p < 0.01$; see Fig. 8.3). Further, as the degree of cognitive loading increased, so did gait variability, compared with usual walking, but only in the PD patients. Thus, the gap between the gait variability of the healthy controls and the patients grew as the level of cognitive loading increased (see Fig. 8.4).

Consistent with previous reports, executive function was significantly worse in the PD group ($p < 0.0002$) than in aged-matched controls. However, memory, information processing, and

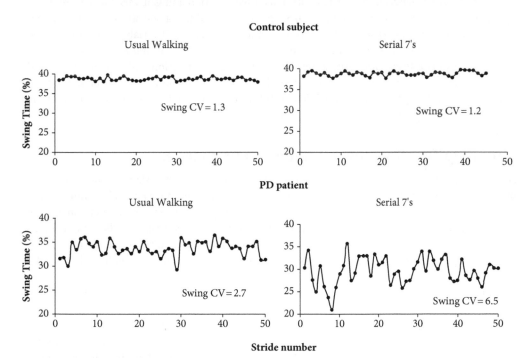

Fig. 8.3 Example of a swing time series from a patient with Parkinson's disease (PD) and a control, under usual walking conditions and when performing serial seven subtractions. Under usual walking conditions, variability is greater in the patient with PD [coefficient of variation (CV) = 2.7%] compared with the control (CV = 1.3%). Variability increases during dual-tasking in the subject with PD (CV = 6.5%), but not in the control (CV = 1.2%).

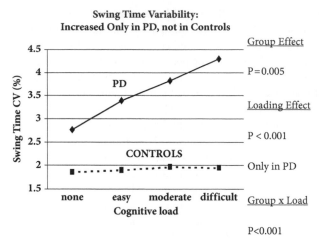

Swing Time Variability:
Increased Only in PD, not in Controls

Fig. 8.4 For all levels of dual-tasking difficulty, values for gait variability among the Parkinson's disease (PD) subjects were significantly increased compared with the controls. In PD but not in controls, variability increased with the level of difficulty of the dual task. In contrast, gait speed (not shown) responded similarly in both groups.

Group Effect
$P = 0.005$
Loading Effect
$P < 0.001$
Only in PD
Group x Load
$P < 0.001$

Dual tasking, gait rhythmicity, and Parkinson's disease: which aspects of gait are attention demanding?/Yogev G, Giladi N, Peretz C, Springer S, Simon ES, Hausdorff JM/Eur J Neurosci 22/ Copyright © 2005.

scores on the Mini-Mental State Examination (MMSE), a general measure of cognitive function, were not different between the participants. Executive function and gait variability were moderately related during usual walking ($r = -0.39$; $p = 0.007$), and this association became stronger during cognitive loading ($r = 0.49$; $p = 0.002$). On the other hand, gait variability was not related to memory or to information processing abilities during any of the walking conditions. These findings demonstrate specific associations between executive function and gait variability and also suggest a cause-and-effect relationship. In the presence of the impaired executive function in patients with PD, greater attentional demands lead to greater reliance on executive function, and subsequently greater effects on gait variability.

Cognitive function and continuous gait changes

A growing body of research links gait to cognitive function [105–109]. Many studies have demonstrated an association between poor executive/attention performance and gait dysfunction in older adults [35, 106, 107, 110–114]. For example, a recent systematic review and meta-analysis of 27 prospective studies conducted in healthy older adults with at least 1 year of follow-up reported a significant relationship between executive dysfunction and increased risk of falling [36]. Thus, it is not altogether surprising that dual-tasking also affects the gait of patients with PD [42, 44–46, 98–100]. The simultaneous performance of two attention-demanding tasks not only causes competition for attention resources but also challenges the brain to decide how to prioritize the two tasks [115].

The 'posture first' strategy claims that healthy subjects spontaneously prioritize postural and walking stability over success on a 'secondary' cognitive task when no specific instructions are given about task prioritization [44, 116, 117]. Several reports have also described this concept of 'wrong prioritization' (first task and then posture) as an explanation for the increased risk of falling in PD patients [44, 117]. However, PD patients with intact cognition have shown an ability to prioritize tasks similar to that of healthy older adults [45]. Nonetheless, executive function and attention, two closely related cognitive domains, may play an important role in prioritization, gait, and fall risk in PD.

Gait impairments in PD that become worse under dual-task conditions include reduced gait speed and stride length [10, 43, 64, 65, 118–120], decreased symmetry and coordination between left and right steps [99, 100], and increased stride-to-stride variability [29, 43, 98]. PD patients also walk with greater gait asymmetry [99], reduced bilateral coordination, and increased gait variability compared with age-matched controls during dual-tasking conditions [42, 43, 45, 98, 100]. They may, therefore, use compensatory strategies to achieve a more normal gait by recruiting attentional resources to correct for the reduced automaticity and to compensate for the continuous gait changes [24, 121].

Automaticity refers to the ability to perform a skilled movement with no or minimal conscious or executive control or attention directed toward the movement [122, 123]. The basal ganglia are believed to play a role in the automatic control of movement [124]. The ability to circumvent the impaired basal ganglia using cortical inputs is, however, limited because it may depend on higher-level cognitive functions, like executive function and attention; however, these are also impaired in PD [125–127]. As a result, the overall effects of dual-tasking in PD patients generally exceed those seen in healthy subjects.

Another mechanism that could contribute to impaired walking during dual tasks in PD is dopaminergic dysfunction in the basal ganglia [128]. The degeneration of dopaminergic neurons in PD appears to affect both motor and cognitive circuits within the basal ganglia. Pathology of the basal ganglia circuits that project to the dorsolateral prefrontal cortex may contribute to the deficits in executive function that are prominent in PD [128–130]. Dual-task walking deficits are improved by antiparkinsonian medication [131], supporting the idea that motor and cognitive impairments are due in part to dopaminergic deficits. However, the impact of antiparkinsonian medication may be limited to those impairments mediated by dopamine dysfunction, and many studies also demonstrate dual-task walking deficits in people with PD in the on-medication state.

In addition to dopaminergic deficits, there is now increasing evidence supporting the importance of cholinergic loss in the pathophysiology of non-motor symptoms in PD. The nucleus basalis of Meynert supplies the majority of cholinergic input to the cerebral cortex, with the pedunculopontine nucleus providing many subcortical structures with acetylcholine. Both these structures undergo degeneration in PD, with more severe loss associated with cognitive impairment [132]. The nucleus basalis of Meynert is important for cognition and attentional processes [133, 134]. Imaging studies have demonstrated degeneration of the cholinergic system in PD, PD dementia, and dementia with Lewy bodies, with improvements in attention seen following the introduction of cholinesterase inhibitors [135, 136]. Neuropathological studies confirm marked degeneration of the cholinergic pedunculopontine nucleus in PD [132]; this nucleus has been associated with motor control, gait, and possibly balance [137]. Conversely, anticholinergic drugs are associated with cognitive decline and increase the risk of falling in the elderly. In addition, these drugs are also known to precipitate visual hallucinations, lending support to a cholinergic basis for visual hallucinations in PD [136].

Bohnen et al. [138, 139] examined the relationship between gait speed, falls, and cholinergic function in PD. In a positron emission tomography (PET) imaging study of 44 patients with PD, they found that cholinergic hypofunction was associated with falls while nigrostriatal dopaminergic denervation was not. In a follow-up study, they compared gait speed among PD patients with relatively isolated nigrostriatal degeneration, healthy control subjects, and PD patients with co-morbid basal forebrain cholinergic degeneration, also accounting for the degree of nigrostriatal denervation. The results revealed that gait speed is not significantly slower than normal in PD patients with relatively isolated nigrostriatal dopaminergic denervation. They suggested that co-morbid cortical cholinergic denervation is a more robust marker of slowing of gait in PD than nigrostriatal denervation alone; this may reflect declining capacity for cognitive compensation of motor performance during ambulation. Cumulatively, these findings provide evidence for the involvement of non-dopaminergic pathways and dopamine-resistant features of impaired motor function in PD [138–140].

Findings from acetylcholinesterase PET studies also show that cholinergic denervation is associated with poorer performance on cognitive tasks [141]; cognitive performance was more impaired among PD patients whose cortical cholinergic innervation levels were below normal compared with those within normal ranges. In addition, an independent effect of nigrostriatal dopaminergic denervation on cognition was described. These in vivo and neuropathological findings support the 'dual-syndrome' hypothesis of cognitive impairment in PD proposed by Kehagia et al. [142]. This hypothesis suggests independent contributions of dopaminergic denervation on fronto-striatal cognitive (including executive) impairments and of cholinergic denervation on visuospatial and attentional impairments in PD [140]. One could speculate that this dual-syndrome hypothesis applies not only to cognition but also to gait and their interdependence in PD.

These studies lead to the question: might augmentation of cholinergic neurotransmission reduce fall risk in PD, and if yes by which mechanisms? First, the role of optimal cognitive input in maintaining balance and avoiding falls is becoming increasingly apparent [143]. While it is recognized that cognitive deficits and falling are associated, the specific links remain to be delineated. It could be postulated that attention to the surrounding environment is important for maintaining balance and avoiding falls. Impaired attentional processes have been described in PD [144, 145], and these may be improved by cholinergic stimulation [146].

Alternative explanations for the association of anticholinergics with increased fall risk might also be possible. The use of anticholinergic drugs might represent a surrogate marker for conditions associated with imbalance [147, 148]. Much clinical experience with anticholinergics in PD over the years has not suggested worsened balance as a side effect. Anticholinergics were the primary class of medication used to treat PD for decades before levodopa. If falls were a side effect of anticholinergics this might have had an impact on clinical practice [149].

A number of studies have evaluated the effectiveness of cognitive training for improving gait and balance and reducing the risk of falls in older adults, patients with dementia, or parkinsonian patients [150]. Although the results of these preliminary studies on gait measures are encouraging [57], traditional gait training generally fails to fully address complex gait activities [151]. Still, the results suggest that training improves dual-task gait in older adults with balance impairment, in patients with dementia, and in patients with PD [151, 152].

Freezing of gait and cognitive deficits

Only a limited number of studies have directly examined the relationship between the transient, episodic gait changes and the cognitive deficits in PD. Still, several lines of work suggest that there is indeed a connection and perhaps even a cause and effect relationship, with the cognitive alterations exacerbating or leading to these deficits. This work largely focuses on one of the episodic gait disturbances in PD, i.e. FOG.

FOG affects 50–80% of patients with PD and leads to a high risk of falls and reduced quality of life [2, 100, 153–155]. As noted, the mechanisms underlying FOG are largely unknown. Some have suggested that internal or external triggers (e.g. emotional reaction, change in the walking environment) may operate on the background of an altered gait pattern to cause a further transient deterioration in locomotion control, which leads to FOG [69, 156, 157]. One possibility is that mental capacity and affect may play a role as triggers of FOG [69]. Indeed, 'panic attacks' have been associated with FOG [158], and Amboni et al. [72] observed that

FOG was correlated with lower scores in cognitive tests related to frontal lobe and executive functions in patients with PD. In the study by Amboni et al., PD patients who suffered from FOG (PD + FOG) scored lower on tests of executive functions including verbal fluency, the clock test, and the frontal assessment battery, whereas scores on the MMSE and the Unified Parkinson's Disease Rating Scale (UPDRS) motor scores were no different in the subjects with and without FOG. Other studies also suggest that executive function is especially impaired among PD + FOG patients [74, 75]. These findings support a possible role of frontal-cognitive impairment in PD + FOG patients.

How might frontal-cognitive impairment induce FOG? It is helpful to examine the inter-ictal gait pattern of PD + FOG patients and compare it with that of PD patients who do not experience FOG (PD – FOG). Although the walking pattern of both groups appeared to be similar between freezing episodes (e.g. inter-ictal stride time and gait speed are no different in PD – FOG and PD + FOG [159–161]), subtle changes in the gait pattern of PD + FOG patients have been observed. These include an increased stride-to-stride variability [159], increased gait asymmetry [156], and altered bilateral coordination in walking periods isolated from freezing episodes [31] in PD + FOG compared with PD – FOG patients (see Fig. 8.5). The findings regarding asymmetry and bilateral coordination might contribute to the relatively high incidence of FOG during turns [28], as turning is a task that demands a high level of bilateral coordination.

Support for the idea that turns are especially sensitive to cognitive loading comes from our analysis of data from 213 community-living, relatively healthy older adults (mean age 76.6 ± 5.8 years) [162]. Subjects walked for 2 minutes at a self-selected pace, back and forth along a 25-m-long corridor, including 180° turns at each end with and without dual-tasking (serial seven subtractions). During turns, but not during straight-line walking, stride-to-stride time variability was significantly higher ($p < 0.008$) in the dual-tasking condition compared with the baseline walking [162]. We have also reported that turning ability was associated with specific cognitive functions [163]. Turns require more attention and cognitive resources than straight-line walking. This may help to explain, in part, why turns are associated with FOG.

Three gait attributes (i.e. gait variability, gait asymmetry, and bilateral coordination of walking) are more impaired in PD + FOG than in PD – FOG patients [100, 156, 159]. Changes in gait variability, gait asymmetry, and the bilateral coordination of walking therefore appear to be associated with FOG. Taken together, these studies suggest that irregular central timing mechanisms of gait motor programmes are associated with freezing. Since dual-tasking is known to have a large impact on these three aspects of gait in PD, one can speculate further that the dual-task effect will be even greater in PD + FOG patients with executive function impairments that are apparently even greater than those seen in PD – FOG patients [72]. In one of the few studies on the effect of dual-tasking on gait with reference to susceptibility to FOG in PD, Camicioli et al. [101] found that PD + FOG patients exhibited a greater increase in the number of steps needed to complete walking during dual-tasking. The findings suggest that PD + FOG may be more dependent on attention, and supports idea that the dual-task effects on gait are larger in PD + FOG than in PD – FOG.

Dagan et al. [164] investigated this issue in a study of 30 PD patients with motor response fluctuations during the 'on' state. Twenty patients had a history of FOG and 10 were non-freezers. Patients walked 80 m at a comfortable pace and then repeated the walking task while performing serial seven subtractions. Gait variability, gait asymmetry, and the phase coordination index tended to increase (i.e. become worse) in the PD + FOG patients during usual walking and became much worse during dual-tasking. The changes were accompanied by a marked reduction in gait speed during dual-tasking. Multivariable regression showed that executive function and anxiety made a significant contribution to this 'dual-task cost' in gait variability and gait speed.

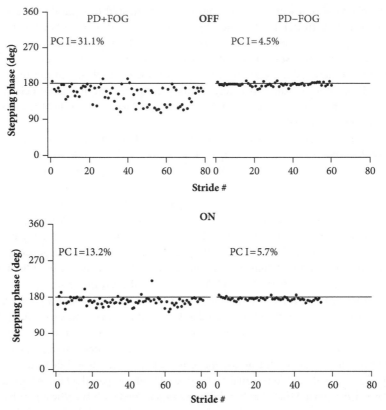

Fig. 8.5 Stepping phase values are plotted for one patient with Parkinson's disease (PD) + freezing of gait (FOG) and one patient from the PD – FOG group, both in the 'off' and 'on' states. A marked inability to consistently generate a 180° phase is observed in PD + FOG, but not in PD – FOG, during the 'off' state. The deviation in the phase (ϕ), from 180° (ϕ_{ABS}), was 29° for the PD + FOG patient and 3.8° for the PD – FOG patient. During the 'off' state, the PD + FOG patient was more inconsistent in phase generation (ϕ_{CV} = 15%) in comparison with the PD – FOG patient (ϕ_{CV} = 2.4%). In these examples, improvement is seen during the 'on' state for the PD + FOG patient, but not for the PD – FOG patient. PCI, phase coordination index.

Springer and Exp Brain Res, A new measure for quantifying the bilateral coordination of human gait: effects of aging and Parkinson's disease 181, 2007, 561–570, Plotnik M, Giladi N, Hausdorff JM, Fig. 2 ©2007 with kind permission from Springer Science and Business Media.

These findings further suggest that in advanced PD, a poor emotional state and reduced executive function aggravate the effects of dual-tasking, especially in patients susceptible to FOG [164].

Some of the most intriguing evidence linking attention to FOG comes from the study by Devos et al. [165]. They examined the effects of methylphenidate (MPH; Ritalin®), a drug extensively used in the therapy of attention deficits, mainly in children but also in older adults [166–168]. Although the mechanism underlying the efficacy of MPH is not fully understood [169], its effect on attention has been well established. In addition to other changes in motor function and gait in response to the 3-month pilot study of the effects of MPH in patients with advanced PD, Devos et al. [165] observed a reduction in the number of FOG episodes in response to MPH. This reported reduction in the frequency of FOG episodes could be explained in a number of different ways; one possibility is that MPH improved attentional abilities and that this in turn led to a reduction in FOG, perhaps by enabling patients to better allocate resources among competing tasks. Other mechanisms, however, could also account for this improvement. Nevertheless, this finding and the results of a subsequent randomized controlled trial [170] with similar results further support the association between executive function and FOG.

The idea that disease-related alterations in executive function and attention influence the continuous gait changes and fall risk in PD is also supported by preliminary work using pharmacological interventions [171]. Assuming that executive function and attention deficits alter gait, enhancement of these cognitive domains could improve gait. An open-label pilot study examined this idea, testing the hypothesis that MPH may improve gait and reduce fall risk in patients with PD [172]. Auriel et al. [172] evaluated the effect of a single dose (20 mg) of MPH on cognitive function, gait performance, and markers of fall risk in 21 patients with PD (mean age 70.2 ± 9.2 years). Patients took their antiparkinsonian medications in the morning, performed baseline testing, received a single dose of MPH, and were then re-tested about 2 hours later. Significant increases in a computerized battery index of attention ($p < 0.013$) and executive function ($p < 0.05$) were observed in response to MPH. In contrast, scores of memory, visuospatial orientation, and hand–eye coordination were unchanged. Significant improvements were also observed in the Timed Up and Go test, a classic measure of fall risk ($p < 0.001$), gait speed ($p < 0.005$), and stride time variability ($p < 0.013$) (see Table 8.1). The dual-tasking effect on stride-to-stride variability was also significantly reduced ($p < 0.05$), demonstrating that a single dose (20 mg) of MPH not only significantly improved attention and executive function in patients with PD, but also resulted in improvements in gait speed, gait variability, and markers of fall risk. A similar study in healthy older adults where a placebo was also administered supported this finding [173]. In addition, a 3-month open-label pilot study of MPH in patients with advanced PD found marked improvement in stride length and other measures of mobility [165]. These findings support the idea that gait disturbances in PD are related to executive function and attention. Moreau et al. [170] have also confirmed the effectiveness of MPH in improving slow gait and freezing in advanced PD patients receiving subthalamic nucleus stimulation in a multicentre random control trial.

In patients with mild PD, recruitment of attentional resources may serve as a compensatory mechanism to improve gait [121, 174]. This may be sufficient to help restore, to some degree, a functional gait pattern. In patients with advanced PD, however, both motor and cognitive functions deteriorate further, potentially limiting the ability to utilize cognitive resources and attention to compensate for the impaired motor function. Gait may become even more 'fragile' and sensitive to external perturbations, increasing the demand for attentional resources. The potential

Table 8.1 Effects of methylphenidate (MPH) on gait and mobility in patients with Parkinson's disease

	Before MPH	**After MPH**	*p*-**value**
Timed up and go (s)	11.9 ± 3.8	10.6 ± 2.3	0.0001
Gait speed (m/s)	1.07 ± 0.19	1.13 ± 0.21	0.005
Average stride time (ms)	1114 ± 85	1100 ± 79	0.068
Stride time variability (%)	2.28 ± 0.63	2.00 ± 0.47	0.013

Auriel E, Hausdorff JM, Herman T, Simon ES, Giladi N, Effects of methylphenidate on cognitive function and gait in patients with Parkinson's disease: a pilot study, Clin Neuropharmacol, 29, 15–17, ©2006.

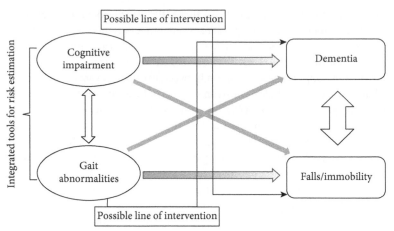

Fig. 8.6 Cognitive impairment commonly leads to and predicts dementia, whereas gait abnormalities increase the risk for falling (horizontal arrows). Cognitive impairment and gait abnormalities, as well as dementia and falls, have been found to be associated with each other (diagonal arrows). Moreover, according to recent evidence, gait abnormalities predict dementia and cognitive impairment increases fall risk (grey arrows). Based on the close relationship between cognition and gait, on the one hand, integrated tools for risk estimation are needed (bracket), but on the other hand possible lines of intervention (black arrows) could include enhancing cognition to improve gait and reduce fall risk and gait training to reduce dementia risk.

protective effect of cognitive compensation strategies against decline in gait speed is greater in subjects with a higher cognitive reserve [170]. This might suggest that cognitive reserve plays a pivotal role in regulating changes in both age-related and disease-related gait impairment [57, 175]. Perhaps this explains why cognitive challenges (i.e. dual-tasking) impact on gait, especially during gait conditions known to be associated with FOG (e.g. turns) and how they combine to determine the likelihood that FOG will occur [100, 157, 176, 177].

Conclusion

Patients with PD suffer from cognitive deficits, especially in executive functions and attention. Gait disturbances, both continuous and episodic, are also common in PD. While many questions remain about the relationship between these symptoms, it appears that these are not independent. Rather, cognitive deficits seem to exacerbate motor dysfunction in both the continuous and episodic gait disturbances, increasing the risk of falls R. As summarized in Fig. 8.6, recognition of this interrelationship may help to improve the management of gait disturbances in PD.

References

1. **Balash Y, Peretz C, Leibovich G, et al.** Falls in outpatients with Parkinson's disease: frequency, impact and identifying factors. J Neurol 2005; **252**: 1310–15.
2. **Bloem BR, Hausdorff JM, Visser JE, et al.** Falls and freezing of gait in Parkinson's disease: a review of two interconnected, episodic phenomena. Mov Disord 2004; **19**: 871–84.

3. **Morris ME, Iansek R, Matyas TA, et al**. The pathogenesis of gait hypokinesia in Parkinson's disease. Brain 1994; **117**: 1169–81.

4. **Pickering RM, Grimbergen YA, Rigney U, et al**. A meta-analysis of six prospective studies of falling in Parkinson's disease. Mov Disord 2007; **22**: 1892–900.

5. **Kang GA, Bronstein JM, Masterman DL, et al**. Clinical characteristics in early Parkinson's disease in a central California population-based study. Mov Disord 2005; **20**: 1133–42.

6. **Ouchi Y, Kanno T, Okada H, et al**. Changes in dopamine availability in the nigrostriatal and mesocortical dopaminergic systems by gait in Parkinson's disease. Brain 2001; **124**: 784–92.

7. **Amboni M, Barone P, Picillo M, et al**. A two-year follow-up study of executive dysfunctions in parkinsonian patients with freezing of gait at on-state. Mov Disord 2010; **25**: 800–2.

8. **Hausdorff JM, Doniger GM, Springer S, et al**. A common cognitive profile in elderly fallers and in patients with Parkinson's disease: the prominence of impaired executive function and attention. Exp Aging Res 2006; **32**: 411–29.

9. **Herman T, Weiss A, Brozgol M, et al**. Identifying axial and cognitive correlates in patients with Parkinson's disease motor subtype using the instrumented Timed Up and Go. Exp Brain Res 2014; **232**: 713–21.

10. **Lord S, Rochester L, Hetherington V, et al**. Executive dysfunction and attention contribute to gait interference in 'off' state Parkinson's disease. Gait Posture 2010; **31**: 169–74.

11. **Yogev-Seligmann G, Hausdorff JM, Giladi N**. The role of executive function and attention in gait. Mov Disord 2008; **23**: 329–42.

12. **Litvan I, Goldman JG, Tröster AI, et al**. Diagnostic criteria for mild cognitive impairment in Parkinson's disease: Movement Disorder Society Task Force guidelines. Mov Disord 2012; **27**: 349–56.

13. **Giladi N, Balash J**. Paroxysmal locomotion gait disturbances in Parkinson's disease. Neurol Neurochir Pol 2001; **35**(Suppl. 3): 57–63.

14. **Giladi N, Hausdorff JM, Balash Y**. Episodic and continuous gait disturbances in Parkinson's disease. In: Galvez-Jimenez N (ed.) *Scientific basis for the treatment of Parkinson's disease*, 2nd edn. London: Taylor and Francis, 2005; pp. 321–2.

15. **Giladi N, Horak FB, Hausdorff JM**. Classification of gait disturbances: distinguishing between continuous and episodic changes. Mov Disord 2013; **28**: 1469–73.

16. **Bloem BR, Grimbergen YA, Cramer M, et al**. Prospective assessment of falls in Parkinson's disease. J Neurol 2001; **248**: 950–8.

17. **Gray P, Hildebrand K**. Fall risk factors in Parkinson's disease. J Neurosci Nurs 2000; **32**: 222–8.

18. **Ashburn A, Stack E, Pickering RM, et al**. A community-dwelling sample of people with Parkinson's disease: characteristics of fallers and non-fallers. Age Ageing 2001; **30**: 47–52.

19. **Koller WC, Glatt S, Vetere-Overfield B, et al**. Falls and Parkinson's disease. Clin Neuropharmacol 1989; **12**: 98–105.

20. **Wood BH, Bilclough JA, Bowron A, et al**. Incidence and prediction of falls in Parkinson's disease: a prospective multidisciplinary study. J Neurol Neurosurg Psychiatry 2002; **72**: 721–5.

21. **Hely MA, Reid WG, Adena MA, et al**. The Sydney multicenter study of Parkinson's disease: the inevitability of dementia at 20 years. Mov Disord 2008; **23**: 837–44.

22. **Kerr GK, Worringham CJ, Cole MH, et al**. Predictors of future falls in Parkinson disease. Neurology 2010; **75**: 116–24.

23. **Ebersbach G, Sojer M, Valldeoriola F, et al**. Comparative analysis of gait in Parkinson's disease, cerebellar ataxia and subcortical arteriosclerotic encephalopathy. Brain 1999; **122**: 1349–55.

24. **Morris ME, Iansek R, Matyas TA, et al**. Stride length regulation in Parkinson's disease. Normalization strategies and underlying mechanisms. Brain 1996; **119**: 551–68.

25. **Morris ME, Huxham FE, McGinley J, et al**. Gait disorders and gait rehabilitation in Parkinson's disease. Adv Neurol 2001; **87**: 347–61.

26. **Blin O, Ferrandez AM, Serratrice G.** Quantitative analysis of gait in Parkinson patients: increased variability of stride length. J Neurol Sci 1990; **98**: 91–7.

27. **Hausdorff JM, Rios DA, Edelberg HK.** Gait variability and fall risk in community-living older adults: a 1-year prospective study. Arch Phys Med Rehabil 2001; **82**: 1050–6.

28. **Schaafsma JD, Giladi N, Balash Y, et al.** Gait dynamics in Parkinson's disease: relationship to Parkinsonian features, falls and response to levodopa. J Neurol Sci 2003; **212**: 47–53.

29. **Yogev G, Giladi N, Peretz C, et al.** Dual tasking, gait rhythmicity, and Parkinson's disease: which aspects of gait are attention demanding? Eur J Neurosci 2005; **22**: 1248–56.

30. **Morris ME, Iansek R, Matyas TA, et al.** Ability to modulate walking cadence remains intact in Parkinson's disease. J Neurol Neurosurg Psychiatry 1994; **57**: 1532–4.

31. **Plotnik M, Giladi N, Hausdorff JM.** A new measure for quantifying the bilateral coordination of human gait: effects of aging and Parkinson's disease. Exp Brain Res 2007; **181**: 561–70.

32. **Baltadjieva R, Giladi N, Gruendlinger L, et al.** Marked alterations in the gait timing and rhythmicity of patients with de novo Parkinson's disease. Eur J Neurosci 2006; **24**: 1815–20.

33. **Frenkel-Toledo S, Giladi N, Peretz C, et al.** Treadmill walking as an external pacemaker to improve gait rhythm and stability in Parkinson's disease. Mov Disord 2005; **20**: 1109–14.

34. **Hausdorff JM, Cudkowicz ME, Firtion R, et al.** Gait variability and basal ganglia disorders: stride-to-stride variations of gait cycle timing in Parkinson's disease and Huntington's disease. Mov Disord 1998; **13**: 428–37.

35. **Martin KL, Blizzard L, Wood AG, et al.** Cognitive function, gait, and gait variability in older people: a population-based study. J Gerontol A Biol Sci Med Sci 2013; **68**: 726–32.

36. **Muir SW, Gopaul K, Montero Odasso MM.** The role of cognitive impairment in fall risk among older adults: a systematic review and meta-analysis. Age Ageing 2012; **41**: 299–308.

37. **Theill N, Martin M, Schumacher V, et al.** Simultaneously measuring gait and cognitive performance in cognitively healthy and cognitively impaired older adults: the Basel motor-cognition dual-task paradigm. J Am Geriatr Soc 2011; **59**: 1012–18.

38. **Sheridan PL, Solomont J, Kowall N, et al.** Influence of executive function on locomotor function: divided attention increases gait variability in Alzheimer's disease. J Am Geriatr Soc 2003; **51**: 1633–7.

39. **Montero-Odasso M, Muir SW, Speechley M.** Dual-task complexity affects gait in people with mild cognitive impairment: the interplay between gait variability, dual tasking, and risk of falls. Arch Phys Med Rehabil 2012; **93**: 293–9.

40. **Muir SW, Speechley M, Wells J, et al.** Gait assessment in mild cognitive impairment and Alzheimer's disease: the effect of dual-task challenges across the cognitive spectrum. Gait Posture 2012; **35**: 96–100.

41. **Hausdorff JM.** Gait dynamics in Parkinson's disease: common and distinct behavior among stride length, gait variability, and fractal-like scaling. Chaos 2009; **19**: 026113.

42. **Plotnik M, Giladi N, Dagan Y, et al.** Postural instability and fall risk in Parkinson's disease: impaired dual tasking, pacing, and bilateral coordination of gait during the 'ON' medication state. Exp Brain Res 2011; **210**: 529–38.

43. **Plotnik M, Dagan Y, Gurevich T, et al.** Effects of cognitive function on gait and dual tasking abilities in patients with Parkinson's disease suffering from motor response fluctuations. Exp Brain Res 2011; **208**: 169–79.

44. **Bloem BR, Valkenburg VV, Slabbekoorn M, et al.** The multiple tasks test. Strategies in Parkinson's disease. Exp Brain Res 2001; **137**: 478–86.

45. **Yogev-Seligmann G, Rotem-Galili Y, Dickstein R, et al.** Effects of explicit prioritization on dual task walking in patients with Parkinson's disease. Gait Posture 2012; **35**: 641–6.

46. **Yogev-Seligmann G, Giladi N, Gruendlinger L, et al.** The contribution of postural control and bilateral coordination to the impact of dual tasking on gait. Exp Brain Res 2013; **226**: 81–93.

47. **Rochester L, Nieuwboer A, Baker K, et al.** Walking speed during single and dual tasks in Parkinson's disease: which characteristics are important? Mov Disord 2008; **23**: 2312–18.

48. **Al-Yahya E, Dawes H, Smith L, et al.** Cognitive motor interference while walking: a systematic review and meta-analysis. Neurosci Biobehav Rev 2011; **35**: 715–28.

49. **Beauchet O, Annweiler C, Dubost V, et al.** Stops walking when talking: a predictor of falls in older adults? Eur J Neurol 2009; **16**: 786–95.

50. **Smulders K, Esselink RA, Weiss A, et al.** Assessment of dual tasking has no clinical value for fall prediction in Parkinson's disease. J Neurol 2012; **259**: 1840–7.

51. **Naismith SL, Shine JM, Lewis SJ.** The specific contributions of set-shifting to freezing of gait in Parkinson's disease. Mov Disord 2010; **25**: 1000–4.

52. **Nantel J, McDonald JC, Tan S, et al.** Deficits in visuospatial processing contribute to quantitative measures of freezing of gait in Parkinson's disease. Neuroscience 2012; **221**: 151–6.

53. **Uc EY, Rizzo M, Anderson SW, et al.** Visual dysfunction in Parkinson disease without dementia. Neurology 2005; **65**: 1907–13.

54. **Amboni M, Barone P, Iuppariello L, et al.** Gait patterns in Parkinsonian patients with or without mild cognitive impairment. Mov Disord 2012; **27**: 1536–43.

55. **Domellof ME, Elgh E, Forsgren L.** The relation between cognition and motor dysfunction in drug-naive newly diagnosed patients with Parkinson's disease. Mov Disord 2011; **26**: 2183–9.

56. **Galna B, Lord S, Daud D, et al.** Visual sampling during walking in people with Parkinson's disease and the influence of environment and dual-task. Brain Res 2012; **1473**: 35–43.

57. **Amboni M, Barone P, Hausdorff JM.** Cognitive contributions to gait and falls: evidence and implications. Mov Disord 2013; **28**: 1520–33.

58. **Adkin AL, Frank JS, Jog MS.** Fear of falling and postural control in Parkinson's disease. Mov Disord 2003; **18**: 496–502.

59. **Schrag A, Jahanshahi M, Quinn NP.** What contributes to depression in Parkinson's disease? Psychol Med 2001; **31**: 65–73.

60. **Chapuis S, Ouchchane L, Metz O, et al.** Impact of the motor complications of Parkinson's disease on the quality of life. Mov Disord 2005; **20**: 224–30.

61. **Faulkner KA, Redfern MS, Cauley JA, et al.** Multitasking: association between poorer performance and a history of recurrent falls. J Am Geriatr Soc 2007; **55**: 570–6.

62. **Verghese J, Buschke H, Viola L, et al.** Validity of divided attention tasks in predicting falls in older individuals: a preliminary study. J Am Geriatr Soc 2002; **50**: 1572–6.

63. **Zijlstra A, Ufkes T, Skelton DA, et al.** Do dual tasks have an added value over single tasks for balance assessment in fall prevention programs? A mini-review. Gerontology 2008; **54**: 40–9.

64. **O'Shea S, Morris ME, Iansek R.** Dual task interference during gait in people with Parkinson disease: effects of motor versus cognitive secondary tasks. Phys Ther 2002; **82**: 888–97.

65. **Bond JM, Morris M.** Goal-directed secondary motor tasks: their effects on gait in subjects with Parkinson disease. Arch Phys Med Rehabil 2000; **81**: 110–16.

66. **Allcock LM, Rowan EN, Steen IN, et al.** Impaired attention predicts falling in Parkinson's disease. Parkinsonism Relat Disord 2009; **15**: 110–15.

67. **Fahn S.** The freezing phenomenon in parkinsonism. Adv Neurol 1995; **67**: 53–63.

68. **Giladi N.** Freezing of gait. Clinical overview. Adv Neurol 2001; **87**: 191–7.

69. **Giladi N, Hausdorff JM.** The role of mental function in the pathogenesis of freezing of gait in Parkinson's disease. J Neurol Sci 2006; **248**: 173–6.

70. **Giladi N, McDermott MP, Fahn S, et al.** Freezing of gait in PD: prospective assessment in the DATA-TOP cohort. Neurology 2001; **56**: 1712–21.

71. **Lamberti P, Armenise S, Castaldo V, et al.** Freezing gait in Parkinson's disease. Eur Neurol 1997; **38**: 297–301.

72. **Amboni M, Cozzolino A, Longo K, et al.** Freezing of gait and executive functions in patients with Parkinson's disease. Mov Disord 2008; **23**: 395–400.

73. Shine JM, Matar E, Ward PB, et al. Differential neural activation patterns in patients with Parkinson's disease and freezing of gait in response to concurrent cognitive and motor load. *PLoS ONE* 2013; **8**: e52602.

74. Kostic VS, Agosta F, Pievani M, et al. Pattern of brain tissue loss associated with freezing of gait in Parkinson disease. Neurology 2012; **78**: 409–16.

75. Tessitore A, Amboni M, Esposito F, et al. Resting-state brain connectivity in patients with Parkinson's disease and freezing of gait. Parkinsonism Relat Disord 2012; **18**: 781–7.

76. Herman T, Giladi N, Hausdorff JM. Neuroimaging as a window into gait disturbances and freezing of gait in patients with Parkinson's disease. Curr Neurol Neurosci Rep 2013; **13**: 411.

77. Dubois B, Pillon B. Cognitive deficits in Parkinson's disease. J Neurol 1997; **244**: 2–8.

78. Goldman JG, Litvan I. Mild cognitive impairment in Parkinson's disease. Minerva Med 2011; **102**: 441–59.

79. Palavra NC, Naismith SL, Lewis SJ. Mild cognitive impairment in Parkinson's disease: a review of current concepts. Neurol Res Int 2013; **2013**: 576091.

80. Aarsland D, Bronnick K, Larsen JP, et al. Cognitive impairment in incident, untreated Parkinson disease: the Norwegian ParkWest study. Neurology 2009; **72**: 1121–6.

81. Elgh E, Domellof M, Linder J, et al. Cognitive function in early Parkinson's disease: a population-based study. Eur J Neurol 2009; **16**: 1278–84.

82. Muslimovic D, Post B, Speelman JD, et al. Cognitive profile of patients with newly diagnosed Parkinson disease. Neurology 2005; **65**: 1239–45.

83. Muslimovic D, Schmand B, Speelman JD, et al. Course of cognitive decline in Parkinson's disease: a meta-analysis. J Int Neuropsychol Soc 2007; **13**: 920–32.

84. Burn DJ, Rowan EN, Allan LM, et al. Motor subtype and cognitive decline in Parkinson's disease, Parkinson's disease with dementia, and dementia with Lewy bodies. J Neurol Neurosurg Psychiatry 2006; **77**: 585–9.

85. Sollinger AB, Goldstein FC, Lah JJ, et al. Mild cognitive impairment in Parkinson's disease: subtypes and motor characteristics. Parkinsonism Relat Disord 2010; **16**: 177–80.

86. Taylor JP, Rowan EN, Lett D, et al. Poor attentional function predicts cognitive decline in patients with non-demented Parkinson's disease independent of motor phenotype. J Neurol Neurosurg Psychiatry 2008; **79**: 1318–23.

87. Uc EY, McDermott MP, Marder KS, et al. Incidence of and risk factors for cognitive impairment in an early Parkinson disease clinical trial cohort. Neurology 2009; **73**: 1469–77.

88. Poletti M, Frosini D, Pagni C, et al. Mild cognitive impairment and cognitive-motor relationships in newly diagnosed drug-naive patients with Parkinson's disease. J Neurol Neurosurg Psychiatry 2012; **83**: 601–6.

89. Caballol N, Marti MJ, Tolosa E. Cognitive dysfunction and dementia in Parkinson disease. Mov Disord 2007; **22**(Suppl. 17): S358–S366.

90. Goethals I, Audenaert K, Van de WC, et al. The prefrontal cortex: insights from functional neuroimaging using cognitive activation tasks. Eur J Nucl Med Mol Imaging 2004; **31**: 408–16.

91. Lezak M. *Executive function.* New York: Oxford University Press, 1983.

92. Stuss DT, Bisschop SM, Alexander MP, et al. The Trail Making Test: a study in focal lesion patients. Psychol Assess 2001; **13**: 230–9.

93. Nieoullon A. Dopamine and the regulation of cognition and attention. Prog Neurobiol 2002; **67**: 53–83.

94. Stam CJ, Visser SL, Op de Coul AA, et al. Disturbed frontal regulation of attention in Parkinson's disease. Brain 1993; **116**: 1139–58.

95. Della Sala S, Baddeley A, Papagno C, et al. Dual-task paradigm: a means to examine the central executive. Ann NY Acad Sci 1995; **769**: 161–71.

96. Szameitat AJ, Schubert T, Muller K, et al. Localization of executive functions in dual-task performance with fMRI. J Cogn Neurosci 2002; **14**: 1184–99.

97. Pashler H. Dual-task interference in simple tasks: data and theory. Psychol Bull 1994; **116**: 220–44.

98. Hausdorff JM, Balash J, Giladi N. Effects of cognitive challenge on gait variability in patients with Parkinson's disease. J Geriatr Psychiatry Neurol 2003; **16**: 53–8.

99. Yogev G, Plotnik M, Peretz C, et al. Gait asymmetry in patients with Parkinson's disease and elderly fallers: when does the bilateral coordination of gait require attention? Exp Brain Res 2007; **177**: 336–46.

100. Plotnik M, Giladi N, Hausdorff JM. Bilateral coordination of gait and Parkinson's disease: the effects of dual tasking. J Neurol Neurosurg Psychiatry 2009; **80**: 347–50.

101. Camicioli R, Howieson D, Lehman S, et al. Talking while walking: the effect of a dual task in aging and Alzheimer's disease. Neurology 1997; **48**: 955–8.

102. Camicioli R, Oken BS, Sexton G, et al. Verbal fluency task affects gait in Parkinson's disease with motor freezing. J Geriatr Psychiatry Neurol 1998; **11**: 181–5.

103. Spildooren J, Vercruysse S, Desloovere K, et al. Freezing of gait in Parkinson's disease: the impact of dual-tasking and turning. Mov Disord 2010; **25**: 2563–70.

104. Beauchet O, Annweiler C, Lecordroch Y, et al. Walking speed-related changes in stride time variability: effects of decreased speed. J Neuroeng Rehabil 2009; **6**: 32.

105. Alexander NB, Hausdorff JM. Guest editorial: linking thinking, walking, and falling. J Gerontol A Biol Sci Med Sci 2008; **63**: 1325–8.

106. Hausdorff JM, Yogev G, Springer S, et al. Walking is more like catching than tapping: gait in the elderly as a complex cognitive task. Exp Brain Res 2005; **164**: 541–8.

107. Hausdorff JM, Schweiger A, Herman T, et al. Dual-task decrements in gait: contributing factors among healthy older adults. J Gerontol A Biol Sci Med Sci 2008; **63**: 1335–43.

108. Marquis S, Moore MM, Howieson DB, et al. Independent predictors of cognitive decline in healthy elderly persons. Arch Neurol 2002; **59**: 601–6.

109. Verghese J, Lipton RB, Hall CB, et al. Abnormality of gait as a predictor of non-Alzheimer's dementia. N Engl J Med 2002; **347**: 1761–8.

110. Coppin AK, Shumway-Cook A, Saczynski JS, et al. Association of executive function and performance of dual-task physical tests among older adults: analyses from the InChianti study. Age Ageing 2006; **35**: 619–24.

111. Herman T, Mirelman A, Giladi N, et al. Executive control deficits as a prodrome to falls in healthy older adults: a prospective study linking thinking, walking, and falling. J Gerontol A Biol Sci Med Sci 2010; **65**: 1086–92.

112. Mirelman A, Herman T, Brozgol, M et al. Executive function and falls in older adults: new findings from a five-year prospective study link fall risk to cognition. PLoS ONE 2012; **7**: e40297.

113. Springer S, Giladi N, Peretz C, et al. Dual-tasking effects on gait variability: the role of aging, falls, and executive function. Mov Disord 2006; **21**: 950–7.

114. van Iersel MB, Kessels RP, Bloem BR, et al. Executive functions are associated with gait and balance in community-living elderly people. J Gerontol A Biol Sci Med Sci 2008; **63**: 1344–9.

115. Yogev-Seligmann G, Hausdorff JM, Giladi N. Do we always prioritize balance when walking? Towards an integrated model of task prioritization. Mov Disord 2012; **27**: 765–70.

116. Schwenk M, Zieschang T, Oster P, et al. Dual-task performances can be improved in patients with dementia: a randomized controlled trial. Neurology 2010; **74**: 1961–8.

117. Bloem BR, Grimbergen YA, van Dijk JG, et al. The 'posture second' strategy: a review of wrong priorities in Parkinson's disease. J Neurol Sci 2006; **248**: 196–204.

118. Brown LA, de Bruin N, Doan JB, et al. Novel challenges to gait in Parkinson's disease: the effect of concurrent music in single- and dual-task contexts. Arch Phys Med Rehabil 2009; **90**: 1578–83.

119. **Galletly R, Brauer SG.** Does the type of concurrent task affect preferred and cued gait in people with Parkinson's disease? Aust J Physiother 2005; **51**: 175–80.

120. **Rochester L, Hetherington V, Jones D, et al.** Attending to the task: interference effects of functional tasks on walking in Parkinson's disease and the roles of cognition, depression, fatigue, and balance. Arch Phys Med Rehabil 2004; **85**: 1578–85.

121. **Rubinstein TC, Giladi N, Hausdorff JM.** The power of cueing to circumvent dopamine deficits: a review of physical therapy treatment of gait disturbances in Parkinson's disease. Mov Disord 2002; **17**: 1148–60.

122. **Poldrack RA, Sabb FW, Foerde K, et al.** The neural correlates of motor skill automaticity. J Neurosci 2005; **25**: 5356–64.

123. **Wu T, Kansaku K, Hallett M.** How self-initiated memorized movements become automatic: a functional MRI study. J Neurophysiol 2004; **91**: 1690–8.

124. **Takakusaki K, Oohinata-Sugimoto J, Saitoh K, et al.** Role of basal ganglia-brainstem systems in the control of postural muscle tone and locomotion. Prog Brain Res 2004; **143**: 231–7.

125. **Brown RG, Marsden CD.** Dual task performance and processing resources in normal subjects and patients with Parkinson's disease. Brain 1991; **114**: 215–31.

126. **Rowe J, Stephan KE, Friston K, et al.** Attention to action in Parkinson's disease: impaired effective connectivity among frontal cortical regions. Brain 2002; **125**: 276–89.

127. **Uekermann J, Daum I, Bielawski M, et al.** Differential executive control impairments in early Parkinson's disease. J Neural Transm Suppl 2004; **68**: 39–51.

128. **Kelly VE, Eusterbrock AJ, Shumway-Cook A.** A review of dual-task walking deficits in people with Parkinson's disease: motor and cognitive contributions, mechanisms, and clinical implications. Parkinsons Dis 2012; **2012**: 918719.

129. **Zgaljardic DJ, Borod JC, Foldi NS, et al.** A review of the cognitive and behavioral sequelae of Parkinson's disease: relationship to frontostriatal circuitry. Cogn Behav Neurol 2003; **16**: 193–210.

130. **Zgaljardic DJ, Borod JC, Foldi NS, et al.** An examination of executive dysfunction associated with frontostriatal circuitry in Parkinson's disease. J Clin Exp Neuropsychol 2006; **28**: 1127–44.

131. **Doumas M, Smolders C, Krampe RT.** Task prioritization in aging: effects of sensory information on concurrent posture and memory performance. Exp Brain Res 2008; **187**: 275–81.

132. **Hirsch EC, Graybiel AM, Duyckaerts C, et al.** Neuronal loss in the pedunculopontine tegmental nucleus in Parkinson disease and in progressive supranuclear palsy. Proc Natl Acad Sci USA 1987; **84**: 5976–80.

133. **Harati H, Barbelivien A, Cosquer B, et al.** Selective cholinergic lesions in the rat nucleus basalis magnocellularis with limited damage in the medial septum specifically alter attention performance in the five-choice serial reaction time task. Neuroscience 2008; **153**: 72–83.

134. **Sarter M, Gehring WJ, Kozak R.** More attention must be paid: the neurobiology of attentional effort. Brain Res Rev 2006; **51**: 145–60.

135. **Bohnen NI, Albin RL.** The cholinergic system and Parkinson disease. Behav Brain Res 2011; **221**: 564–73.

136. **Yarnall A, Rochester L, Burn DJ.** The interplay of cholinergic function, attention, and falls in Parkinson's disease. Mov Disord 2011; **26**: 2496–503.

137. **Jenkinson N, Nandi D, Muthusamy K, et al.** Anatomy, physiology, and pathophysiology of the pedunculopontine nucleus. Mov Disord 2009; **24**: 319–28.

138. **Bohnen NI, Muller ML, Koeppe RA, et al.** History of falls in Parkinson disease is associated with reduced cholinergic activity. Neurology 2009; **73**: 1670–6.

139. **Bohnen NI, Frey KA, Studenski S, et al.** Gait speed in Parkinson disease correlates with cholinergic degeneration. Neurology 2013; **81**: 1611–16.

140. **Muller ML, Bohnen NI.** Cholinergic dysfunction in Parkinson's disease. Curr Neurol Neurosci Rep 2013; **13**: 377.

141. **Bohnen NI, Kaufer DI, Hendrickson R, et al.** Cognitive correlates of cortical cholinergic denervation in Parkinson's disease and parkinsonian dementia. J Neurol 2006; **253**: 242–7.

142. **Kehagia AA, Barker RA, Robbins TW.** Cognitive impairment in Parkinson's disease: the dual syndrome hypothesis. Neurodegener Dis 2013; **11**: 79–92.

143. **Woollacott M, Shumway-Cook A.** Attention and the control of posture and gait: a review of an emerging area of research. Gait Posture 2002; **16**: 1–14.

144. **Dujardin K, Degreef JF, Rogelet P, et al.** Impairment of the supervisory attentional system in early untreated patients with Parkinson's disease. J Neurol 1999; **246**: 783–8.

145. **Woodward TS, Bub DN, Hunter MA.** Task switching deficits associated with Parkinson's disease reflect depleted attentional resources. Neuropsychologia 2002; **40**: 1948–55.

146. **Chung KA, Lobb BM, Nutt JG, et al.** Effects of a central cholinesterase inhibitor on reducing falls in Parkinson disease. Neurology 2010; **75**: 1263–9.

147. **Ensrud KE, Blackwell TL, Mangione CM, et al.** Central nervous system-active medications and risk for falls in older women. J Am Geriatr Soc 2002; **50**: 1629–37.

148. **Thapa PB, Gideon P, Cost TW, et al.** Antidepressants and the risk of falls among nursing home residents. N Engl J Med 1998; **339**: 875–82.

149. **Ahlskog JE.** Think before you leap: donepezil reduces falls? Neurology 2010; **75**: 1226–7.

150. **Segev-Jacubovski O, Herman T, Yogev-Seligmann G, et al.** The interplay between gait, falls and cognition: can cognitive therapy reduce fall risk? Expert Rev Neurother 2011; **11**: 1057–75.

151. **Mirelman A, Maidan I, Herman T, et al.** Virtual reality for gait training: can it induce motor learning to enhance complex walking and reduce fall risk in patients with Parkinson's disease? J Gerontol A Biol Sci Med Sci 2011; **66**: 234–40.

152. **Silsupadol P, Shumway-Cook A, Lugade V, et al.** Effects of single-task versus dual-task training on balance performance in older adults: a double-blind, randomized controlled trial. Arch Phys Med Rehabil 2009; **90**: 381–7.

153. **Giladi N, Nieuwboer A.** Understanding and treating freezing of gait in parkinsonism, proposed working definition, and setting the stage. Mov Disord 2008; **23**(Suppl. 2): S423–S425.

154. **Moore O, Peretz C, Giladi N.** Freezing of gait affects quality of life of peoples with Parkinson's disease beyond its relationships with mobility and gait. Mov Disord 2007; **22**: 2192–5.

155. **Nutt JG, Bloem BR, Giladi N, et al.** Freezing of gait: moving forward on a mysterious clinical phenomenon. Lancet Neurol 2011; **10**: 734–44.

156. **Plotnik M, Giladi N, Balash Y, et al.** Is freezing of gait in Parkinson's disease related to asymmetric motor function? Ann Neurol 2005; **57**: 656–63.

157. **Plotnik M, Hausdorff JM.** The role of gait rhythmicity and bilateral coordination of stepping in the pathophysiology of freezing of gait in Parkinson's disease. Mov Disord 2008; **23**(Suppl. 2): S444–S450.

158. **Lieberman A.** Are freezing of gait (FOG) and panic related? J Neurol Sci 2006; **248**: 219–22.

159. **Hausdorff JM, Schaafsma JD, Balash Y, et al.** Impaired regulation of stride variability in Parkinson's disease subjects with freezing of gait. Exp Brain Res 2003; **149**: 187–94.

160. **Willems AM, Nieuwboer A, Chavret, F et al.** The use of rhythmic auditory cues to influence gait in patients with Parkinson's disease, the differential effect for freezers and non-freezers, an explorative study. Disabil Rehabil 2006; **28**: 721–8.

161. **Willems AM, Nieuwboer A, Chavret F, et al.** Turning in Parkinson's disease patients and controls: the effect of auditory cues. Mov Disord 2007; **22**: 1871–8.

162. **Weiss A, Gruendlinger L, Plotnik M, et al.** Is turning during walking an automated motor task, or is it a complex cognitive action? Parkinsonism Relat Disord 2008; **14**: 123.

163. **Mirelman A, Heman T, Yasinovsky K, et al.** Fall risk and gait in Parkinson's disease: the role of the LRRK2 G2019S mutation. Mov Disord 2013; **28**: 1683–90.

164. **Dagan Y, Plotnik M, Gruendlinger L, et al.** Emotion, cognition, freezing of gait and dual tasking in patients with advanced Parkinson's disease: a volatile mixture. Mov Disord 2008; **23**(Suppl. 1): S327.

165 Devos D, Krystkowiak P, Clement F, et al. Improvement of gait by chronic, high doses of methylphenidate in patients with advanced Parkinson's disease. J Neurol Neurosurg Psychiatry 2007; **78**: 470–5.

166. Galynker I, Ieronimo C, Miner C, et al. Methylphenidate treatment of negative symptoms in patients with dementia. J Neuropsychiatry Clin Neurosci 1997; **9**: 231–9.

167. Homsi J, Walsh D, Nelson KA, et al. Methylphenidate for depression in hospice practice: a case series. Am J Hosp Palliat Care 2000; **17**: 393–8.

168. Whyte J, Hart T, Vaccaro M, et al. Effects of methylphenidate on attention deficits after traumatic brain injury: a multidimensional, randomized, controlled trial. Am J Phys Med Rehabil 2004; **83**: 401–20.

169. Auriel E, Hausdorff JM, Giladi N. Methylphenidate for the treatment of Parkinson disease and other neurological disorders. Clin Neuropharmacol 2009; **32**: 75–81.

170. Moreau C, Delval A, Defebvre L, et al. Methylphenidate for gait hypokinesia and freezing in patients with Parkinson's disease undergoing subthalamic stimulation: a multicentre, parallel, randomised, placebo-controlled trial. Lancet Neurol 2012; **11**: 589–96.

171. Vale S. Current management of the cognitive dysfunction in Parkinson's disease: how far have we come? Exp Biol Med 2008; **233**: 941–51.

172. Auriel E, Hausdorff JM, Herman T, et al. Effects of methylphenidate on cognitive function and gait in patients with Parkinson's disease: a pilot study. Clin Neuropharmacol 2006; **29**: 15–17.

173. Ben-Itzhak R, Giladi N, Gruendlinger L, et al. Can methylphenidate reduce fall risk in community-living older adults? A double-blind, single-dose cross-over study. J Am Geriatr Soc 2008; **56**: 695–700.

174. Rochester L, Hetherington V, Jones D, et al. The effect of external rhythmic cues (auditory and visual) on walking during a functional task in homes of people with Parkinson's disease. Arch Phys Med Rehabil 2005; **86**: 999–1006.

175. Holtzer R, Wang C, Lipton R, et al. The protective effects of executive functions and episodic memory on gait speed decline in aging defined in the context of cognitive reserve. J Am Geriatr Soc 2012; **60**: 2093–8.

176. Moreau C, Defebvre L, Bleuse S, et al. Externally provoked freezing of gait in open runways in advanced Parkinson's disease results from motor and mental collapse. J Neural Transm 2008; **115**: 1431–6.

177. Plotnik M, Bartsch R, Yogev G, et al. Synchronization of right–left stepping while walking is compromised in patients with Parkinson's disease during mental loading. Mov Disord 2006; **21**: S592.

178. Montero-Odasso M, Verghese J, Beauchet O, et al. Gait and cognition: a complementary approach to understanding brain function and the risk of falling. J Am Geriatr Soc 2012; **60**: 2127–36.

Chapter 9

Disorders of sleep and autonomic function in Parkinson's disease dementia

Eduardo Tolosa, Judith Navarro-Otano, and Alex Iranzo

Introduction

Cognitive deterioration is common in Parkinson's disease (PD) and many patients develop dementia with disease progression. Dementia generally occurs late in PD, as is the case for other symptoms not responsive to levodopa. These symptoms include motor features such as motor blocks (also known as freezing of gait), dysarthria, disequilibrium, and falls as well as non-motor ones such as sleep disturbances and dysautonomia. Some of these symptoms are thought to be disease related, a consequence of the nervous system pathology that occurs in PD. They may also present as adverse effects of antiparkinsonian medication or a manifestation of co-morbidities, frequent in the elderly.

In this chapter we will review sleep disturbances and dysautonomia occurring in PD patients with dementia (PD-D). Although both types of disturbances are known to also occur in early stages of PD, even in the prodromal phases, they can be particularly prominent in advanced PD. Tables 9.1 and 9.2 summarize these disturbances and their management.

Sleep disturbances in PD-D

The main sleep disturbances in PD-D patients include insomnia, rapid eye movement (REM) sleep behaviour disorder (RBD), and excessive daytime sleepiness (EDS).

Insomnia in PD-D

Fragmentation of sleep can have a major impact on quality of life in PD and is a multifactorial problem. Drugs such as selegiline or amantadine can cause insomnia. In advanced disease, 'off'-state-related parkinsonism during the night can also produce insomnia. Nocturia, common in advanced PD, is also a contributing factor. In PD-D patients, nocturnal hallucinations and RBD might also contribute to sleep disturbances.

REM sleep behaviour disorder

RBD is characterized by dream-enacting behaviours (e.g. kicking, talking, swearing, shouting, jumping out of bed) linked to unpleasant dreams (e.g. being attacked, chased, or robbed) and increased electromyographic activity during REM sleep. Infrequently patients may injure themselves or their bed partner. The pathophysiology of RBD is thought to be related to dysfunction of the brainstem REM sleep centres (the locus subcoeruleus, nucleus gigantocellularis, etc.) and their indirect and

Table 9.1 Treatment of sleep disturbances in Parkinson's disease with dementia

	Non-drug strategies	Pharmacological treatment
Insomnia	Sleep hygiene	Quetiapine 25 mg at night
Rapid eye movement sleep behaviour disorder		Clonazepam 0.25–0.5 mg/24 h Melatonin 3–9 mg/24 h
Excessive daytime sleepiness	Sleep hygiene	Methylphenidate, modafinil (could cause nervousness and insomnia)

Table 9.2 Treatment of autonomic dysfunction in Parkinson's disease with dementia

	Non-drug strategies	Pharmacological treatment
Orthostatic hypotension	Water intake Salt intake (at least 8 g) Sleeping with elevation of the head end of the bed	Fludrocortisone 0.1–0.2 mg/day Midodrine 5–10 mg three times a day
Constipation Urinary dysfunction	Fluids, high-fibre diet Water restriction at night	Macrogol Different strategies for overactive bladder, urinary retention, nocturnal polyuria

direct anatomic connections (the amygdala, pallidum, neocortex, etc.) [1]. RBD occurs in about 50% of PD patients. It has been estimated that it can antedate the development of motor symptoms of PD in about 15% of cases [2, 3]. It has not been widely studied whether RBD is more prevalent among PD-D patients than in those without dementia. Marion et al. [4] suggested that RBD worsens with time: a small study in 65 consecutive PD patients showed that the presence of RBD-like symptoms was significantly higher in PD-D (10/13, 77%) than in PD without dementia (14/52, 27%). These studies did not include polysomnographic confirmation of the true presence of unequivocal RBD.

RBD may also predict the development of dementia in PD patients. This is perhaps not surprising considering that idiopathic RBD may also evolve into dementia with Lewy bodies (DLB), a condition pathologically very similar to PD. Some risk factors associated with PD-D such as an akinetic–rigid motor phenotype [5], hallucinations, longer PD duration, male gender, and cholinergic denervation have been also associated with RBD in PD [1, 6–10], whereas other risk factors for PD-D, such as advanced age and depression, have not [7, 8, 11, 12].

In summary, it is not certain from the available data whether RBD is linked to PD-D. Long-term follow-up of PD patients without dementia with and without RBD is necessary to elucidate whether it is associated with a high risk for dementia.

Excessive daytime sleepiness

The causes of EDS in PD are numerous. The most relevant are the effects of dopaminergic medication and the consequences of the disease pathology itself [1]. Other factors that have been found to be associated with excessive sleepiness in PD include dementia, disease severity, disease duration, hallucinations, disruption of the circadian sleep–wake cycle, nocturnal sleep quantity and quality, obstructive sleep apnoea, depression, and genetic susceptibility [1]. The individual contributions of each of these factors, including dementia, have not yet been fully elucidated.

EDS, like RBD, can occur in the early stages of PD, including the pre-motor phase [13]. Studies by Gjerstad et al. [14] and Fabbrini et al. [15] have shown that its prevalence increases with disease duration. However, there are only a few reports that have specifically evaluated the frequency and nature of EDS in PD-D. One such study showed that the frequency of EDS in PD-D (57%) was greater than in PD without dementia (41%) [16]. However, another study showed no differences in scores on the Epworth Sleepiness Scale, as a subjective measure of EDS, between PD and PD-D, although abnormal scale scores were significantly more frequent in PD-D than in PD without dementia [17]. Another study using the Epworth Sleepiness Scale showed that the frequency of PD-D patients reporting EDS increased from 57 to 81% after 2 years of follow-up [16]. In daily clinical practice it is widely recognized that EDS can be a prominent behavioural manifestation occurring in PD-D patients.

Autonomic dysfunction in PD-D

Autonomic disturbances are common in PD, causing significant discomfort to patients and negatively affecting their quality of life [18, 19]. The most common autonomic symptoms (AS) are cardiovascular, gastrointestinal, genitourinary, and thermoregulatory disturbances. Some of these disturbances can occur in the early stages of PD, presenting at the time of diagnosis or even antedating the onset of motor symptoms. Such is the case, for example, for constipation, bladder problems, and erectile dysfunction, and for some cardiovascular abnormalities. Early and pre-motor autonomic dysfunction has been reviewed elsewhere [20, 21].

The prevalence of AS increases with disease progression [22–24]. In his early descriptions James Parkinson indicated the progressive worsening of constipation in advanced PD. Anorectal function was recently found to be more impaired in patients with longer disease duration and higher Hoehn and Yahr stages [25]. There is also a correlation between increasing severity of the disease and increasing bladder problems [26, 27]. In another study, orthostatic hypotension (OH) was found to be related to the duration and severity of the disease and to the use of higher daily doses of levodopa and bromocriptine [28]. Verbaan et al. [29] reported that older, more severely affected, and more heavily medicated subjects had greater autonomic dysfunction.

The presence of autonomic dysfunction in advanced PD has also been documented in the Sidney Multicenter Study of PD [30]. In that study a cohort of newly diagnosed patients were followed longitudinally. At 15-year follow-up symptomatic postural hypotension occurred in 35%, and there were 22 people (41%) who had urinary incontinence. This condition became more frequent with increasing Hoehn and Yahr stage, from 14% in stage 2 to 62% in stage 5 patients. At 20-year follow-up [31] dementia was present in 83% of the survivors. AS were also common: symptomatic postural hypotension in 48% (six required fludrocortisone) and urinary incontinence in 71%. Faecal incontinence occurred in 5 (17%) and constipation requiring daily laxatives was present in 12 (40%). These findings illustrate how common and clinically important AS are in patients with advanced PD. However, it was not specified whether AS were more common or severe in PD-D patients.

Coelho et al. [32] described a cohort of 50 advanced PD patients with a mean age of 74.1 years and mean disease duration of 17.9 years. All of them presented dysautonomic symptoms and 50% of them suffered from dementia. In this study, the most frequent dysautonomic symptoms were constipation (82%) and urinary dysfunction (64%).

PD-D patients generally suffer from severe motor disability due to bradykinesia, freezing of gait, poor balance, and falls. Since AS are frequent in advanced PD and PD-D also develops in these late stages, one can logically expect AS to be prominent in patients with PD-D. This conjecture, however, has not been systematically and comprehensively evaluated, and data on the relative frequency of AS in PD-D as compared with PD patients without dementia are scarce. One recent study assessed the impact of AS on the survival of PD-D and DLB patients. Stubendorff et al. [33] studied data from 16 DLB and 14 PD-D patients followed for 36 months with orthostatic tests performed at baseline and at 12- and 24-week visits. Patients with persistent OH had a significantly shorter survival than those without OH despite equal Mini-Mental State Examination scores and disease duration at baseline.

The assessment of autonomic function in patients with severe parkinsonism and dementia has limitations. Because of severe motor and cognitive impairment, the collaboration of the patient cannot be obtained for some tests or in answering questionnaires, most of which have been validated in patients without dementia. In fact, in many studies on autonomic function in PD, PD-D patients have been specifically excluded.

A few studies have specifically assessed autonomic symptoms in PD patients with cognitive impairment. In the study by Idiaquez et al. [34], 40 PD patients and 30 age-matched controls were assessed for cognitive and behavioural manifestations using standardized neuropsychological tools. They were also assessed for OH, post-prandial hypotension, heart rate responses to deep breathing, and AS using the Scale for Outcomes in Parkinson's Disease for Autonomic Symptoms (SCOPA-AUT). Eleven of the 40 PD patients fulfilled the DSM-IV criteria for dementia. The authors found a higher incidence of cardiovascular symptoms in PD-D patients than in those without dementia. The presence of OH or post-prandial hypotension did not correlate with the severity of cognitive impairment, and there was no correlation between gastrointestinal or urological symptoms and cognitive impairment. The authors suggested that the lack of correlation between AS and cognitive impairment suggests that cognitive and autonomic involvement may progress independently from each other and variably among PD patients.

A clinical study by Peralta et al. [35] provided some evidence that, when tested in an autonomic function laboratory, OH is more frequent in PD-D patients than in PD without dementia, but the difference failed to reach statistical significance. Drop in systolic blood pressure was significantly greater in the PD-D group than in the PD group. In this study 'attention', assessed with the 'Test of Everyday Attention', deteriorated significantly during tilt in the PD-D group, correlating with the blood pressure response and suggesting that OH may exacerbate attentional dysfunction in PD-D patients. Allan et al. [36] assessed autonomic cardiovascular function in 39 patients with Alzheimer's disease (AD), 30 with vascular dementia, 30 with DLB, 40 with PD-D, and 38 elderly controls by Ewing's battery of autonomic function tests and power spectral analysis of variability in heart rate. Autonomic dysfunction occurred in all the common dementias, but was especially prominent in PD-D and DLB. The PD-D patients showed consistent impairment of both parasympathetic and sympathetic function tests in comparison with controls and AD. Patients with advanced PD but without dementia were not studied. Akaogi et al. [37] assessed autonomic function in 12 PD-D, 12 DLB, 12 PD without dementia, and 12 healthy control subjects by sudomotor, skin vasomotor, and cardiovascular reflexes. Impaired cutaneous sudomotor function was present in all patients, but was more prominent in those with PD-D or DLB. The mean skin vasomotor reflex amplitudes in the PD-D and DLB patients were significantly lower than those in the controls but not lower than those reported in the PD patients without dementia.

Graham and Sagar [38] also reported a higher frequency of symptomatic orthostasis in association with cognitive impairment in PD. Hohler et al. [39] assessed the differences in motor and cognitive function in 44 patients with PD with and without OH. Patients with OH (17/44) were found to have significantly lower scores in the Mini-Mental State Examination compared with those without OH, although the disease severity was similar. In another study, Kim et al. [40] evaluated the association of cognitive dysfunction with neurocirculatory abnormalities in early PD. This work included 87 patients with early PD who were classified as having normal cognition (25/87), mild cognitive impairment (48/87), or dementia (14/87). They concluded that even in patients with early PD cognitive impairment was associated with OH and supine hypertension.

This finding is supported by a recent study identifying an association between OH and selective cognitive deficits in PD [41]. Forty-eight PD patients were evaluated with a tilt table test to assess OH, neuropsychological evaluation, and magnetic resonance imaging (MRI). Twenty-three (49%) patients presented OH (13 of them symptomatic) and their cognitive performance was significantly worse in sustained attention and visuospatial and verbal memory when compared with patients without OH. OH was independent of the presence of cerebrovascular damage in MRI.

Pathophysiology of autonomic symptoms

Pathological studies have revealed that α-synuclein pathology, the core pathology associated with PD, can be seen throughout the central and peripheral autonomic nervous system—the hypothalamus, brainstem, pre- and post-ganglionic neurons and plexi [42, 43]—providing an anatomical substrate for the dysautonomic symptoms encountered in PD patients. Both pre- and post-ganglionic neurons and plexi as well as central autonomic structures are thought to become involved early on in the disease process [42, 44, 45]. This explains why AS are common in PD with or without dementia. Involvement of the limbic and cerebral cortices with synuclein pathology [46–49] is the characteristic finding in subjects with PD-D; these lesions may contribute to the worsening of AS since several of these areas, such as the amygdala, anterior cingulate, insular and ventro-medial prefrontal cortices, among others, control the tonic, reflex, and adaptive activities of the sympathetic and parasympathetic nervous systems. Degeneration of neurons in the frontal cortex, for example, may disinhibit the pontine bladder control centre and could play an important role in incontinence in patients with advanced PD who also suffer from dementia [50].

In trying to identify the neural substrate of autonomic dysfunction in PD it becomes difficult to disentangle the role of central versus peripheral lesions. Constipation, for example, could be considered a consequence of lesions in the enteric neurons, but involvement of central structures such as the medullary raphe which projects to spinal nuclei such as Onuf's nucleus may be an important contributing factor [51]. Urinary dysfunction can be ascribed to the involvement of abdomino-pelvic plexi in the neurodegenerative process. On the other hand degeneration in the nigrostriatal dopamine system that causes disinhibition of the micturition reflex may result in detrusor overactivity and explain the worsening of detrusor function with increasing Hoehn and Yahr stages [52–54]. Studies in PD have also revealed significant loss of neurons in the intermediolateral cell column which inhibits detrusor muscle function [55].

Co-morbidities such as prostatic hypertrophy or cerebrovascular pathology must also be considered in the pathophysiology of dysautonomic symptoms. The presence of symptoms such as urinary incontinence or constipation may result, at least in part, from factors such as physical inactivity or from defaecatory dysfunction due to motor impairment; constipation may in part be due to severe immobility and anal sphincter dystonia [56]. Other factors that can cause or contribute to dysautonomia in PD-D include advanced age or the use of numerous medications known to cause autonomic dysfunction. Dopaminergic drugs, for example, frequently cause OH, profuse sweating spells occur in association with levodopa-related on–off fluctuations, and anticholinergic drugs can cause constipation and bladder dysfunction. Cholinesterase inhibitors and atypical antipsychotics can also induce AS. Finally, symptoms such as urinary and faecal incontinence or sexual dysfunction may be due in part to behavioural symptoms such as hallucinations or EDS, which are frequent in PD-D.

Conclusion

Sleep disorders are frequent in PD-D patients and can be an important source of distress for both patients and caregivers. Longitudinal studies have shown that the prevalence of EDS in PD increases over time in parallel with cognitive decline and disease progression. It is not clearly established if RBD represents a risk factor for PD-D, and whether RBD is more common in patients with dementia, although there is some evidence. Sleep disturbances in PD have been attributed to Lewy body pathology in sleep-related extranigral structures (e.g. the brainstem, hypothalamus) and other PD-related lesions. These structures are consistently involved in advanced PD patients, most of whom suffer from dementia. Antiparkinsonian drugs or treatments for hallucinations and agitation can also produce EDS.

Studies on autonomic dysfunction in PD-D patients are scarce. The available information indicates that urinary incontinence, constipation, faecal incontinence, and postural hypotension are common in patients with late-stage PD, a stage of the illness in which dementia frequently develops. However, it is unclear whether dysautonomia is more common in PD-D versus PD patients without dementia in advanced stages. There is hardly any information available on some dysautonomic symptoms (e.g. thermal dysregulation or sexual dysfunction) in patients with PD-D.

The cause of autonomic dysfunction in advanced PD is probably multifactorial and may be difficult to uncover in a given patient. The involvement of peripheral and central autonomic systems plays a central role, but behavioural and motor problems, severe immobility, advanced age, and adverse effects of drugs can all contribute to the presence and severity of AS. In PD-D patients higher autonomic symptoms scores are associated with poorer outcomes in all measures of motor function, activities of daily living, quality of life, and survival. Symptoms of autonomic dysfunction have important treatment implications and need to be addressed in all patients with advanced PD in order to minimize their consequences for the patient and the caregiver.

References

1. Iranzo A, Santamaria J, Tolosa E. The clinical and pathophysiological relevance of REM sleep behavior disorder in neurodegenerative diseases. Sleep Med Rev 2009; **13**: 385–401.

2. Gagnon JF, Bedard MA, Fantini ML, et al. REM sleep behavior disorder and REM sleep without atonia in Parkinson's disease. Neurology 2002; **59**: 585–9.

3. Iranzo A, Tolosa E, Gelpi E, et al. Neurodegenerative disease status and post-mortem pathology in idiopathic rapid-eye-movement sleep behaviour disorder: an observational cohort study. Lancet Neurol 2013; **12**: 443–53.

4. Marion MH, Qurashi M, Marshall G, et al. Is REM sleep behaviour disorder (RBD) a risk factor of dementia in idiopathic Parkinson's disease? J Neurol 2008; **255**: 192–6.

5. Kumru H, Santamaria J, Tolosa E, et al. Relation between subtype of Parkinson's disease and REM sleep behavior disorder. Sleep Med 2007; **8**: 779–83.

6. Sinforiani E, Zangaglia R, Manni R, et al. REM sleep behavior disorder, hallucinations, and cognitive impairment in Parkinson's disease. Mov Disord 2006; **21**: 462–6.

7. De Cock VC, Vidailhet M, Leu S, et al. Restoration of normal motor control in Parkinson's disease during REM sleep. Brain 2007; **130**: 450–6.

8. Wetter TC, Trenkwalder C, Gershanik O, et al. Polysomnographic measures in Parkinson's disease: a comparison between patients with and without REM sleep disturbances. Wien Klin Wochenschr 2001; **113**: 249–53.

9. Iranzo A, Santamaria J, Rye DB, et al. Characteristics of idiopathic REM sleep behavior disorder and that associated with MSA and PD. Neurology 2005; **65**: 247–52.

10. Kotagal V, Albin RL, Muller ML, et al. Symptoms of rapid eye movement sleep behavior disorder are associated with cholinergic denervation in Parkinson disease. Ann Neurol 2012; **71**: 560–8.

11. Postuma RB, Gagnon JF, Vendette M, et al. REM sleep behaviour disorder in Parkinson's disease is associated with specific motor features. J Neurol Neurosurg Psychiatry 2008; **79**: 1117–21.

12. **Postuma RB, Gagnon JF, Vendette M, et al.** Manifestations of Parkinson disease differ in association with REM sleep behavior disorder. Mov Disord 2008; **23**: 1665–72.

13. **Abbott RD, Ross GW, White LR, et al.** Excessive daytime sleepiness and subsequent development of Parkinson disease. Neurology 2005; **65**: 1442–6.

14. **Gjerstad MD, Aarsland D, Larsen JP.** Development of daytime somnolence over time in Parkinson's disease. Neurology 2002; **58**: 1544–6.

15. **Fabbrini G, Barbanti P, Aurilia C, et al.** Excessive daytime somnolence in Parkinson's disease. Follow-up after 1 year of treatment. Neurol Sci 2003; **24**: 178–9.

16. **Boddy F, Rowan EN, Lett D, et al.** Subjectively reported sleep quality and excessive daytime somnolence in Parkinson's disease with and without dementia, dementia with Lewy bodies and Alzheimer's disease. Int J Geriatr Psychiatry 2007; **22**: 529–35.

17. **Compta Y, Santamaria J, Ratti L, et al.** Cerebrospinal hypocretin, daytime sleepiness and sleep architecture in Parkinson's disease dementia. Brain 2009; **132**: 3308–17.

18. **Chaudhuri KR, Healy DG, Schapira AH.** Non-motor symptoms of Parkinson's disease: diagnosis and management. Lancet Neurol 2006; **5**: 235–45.

19. **Martinez-Martin P.** The importance of non-motor disturbances to quality of life in Parkinson's disease. J Neurol Sci 2011; **310**: 12–16.

20. **Tolosa E, Compta Y, Gaig C.** The premotor phase of Parkinson's disease. Parkinsonism Relat Disord 2007; **13**(Suppl.): S2–S7.

21. **Tolosa E, Pont-Sunyer C.** Progress in defining the premotor phase of Parkinson's disease. J Neurol Sci 2011; **310**: 4–8.

22. **Magerkurth C, Schnitzer R, Braune S.** Symptoms of autonomic failure in Parkinson's disease: prevalence and impact on daily life. Clin Auton Res 2005; **15**: 76–82.

23. **Visser M, Marinus J, Stiggelbout AM, et al.** Assessment of autonomic dysfunction in Parkinson's disease: the SCOPA-AUT. Mov Disord 2004; **19**: 1306–12.

24. **Martinez-Martin P, Schapira AH, Stocchi F, et al.** Prevalence of nonmotor symptoms in Parkinson's disease in an international setting; study using nonmotor symptoms questionnaire in 545 patients. Mov Disord 2007; **22**: 1623–9.

25. **Stocchi F, Badiali D, Vacca L, et al.** Anorectal function in multiple system atrophy and Parkinson's disease. Mov Disord 2000; **15**: 71–6.

26. **Sakakibara R, Shinotoh H, Uchiyama T, et al.** Questionnaire-based assessment of pelvic organ dysfunction in Parkinson's disease. Auton Neurosci 2001; **92**: 76–85.

27. **Coelho M, Ferreira JJ.** Late-stage Parkinson disease. Nat Rev Neurol 2012; **8**: 435–42.

28. **Senard JM, Rai S, Lapeyre-Mestre M, et al.** Prevalence of orthostatic hypotension in Parkinson's disease. J Neurol Neurosurg Psychiatry 1997; **63**: 584–9.

29. **Verbaan D, Marinus J, Visser M, et al.** Patient-reported autonomic symptoms in Parkinson disease. Neurology 2007; **69**: 333–41.

30. **Hely MA, Morris JG, Reid WG, et al.** Sydney Multicenter Study of Parkinson's disease: non-L-dopa-responsive problems dominate at 15 years. Mov Disord 2005; **20**: 190–9.

31. **Hely MA, Reid WG, Adena MA, et al.** The Sydney multicenter study of Parkinson's disease: the inevitability of dementia at 20 years. Mov Disord 2008; **23**: 837–44.

32. **Coelho M, Marti MJ, Tolosa E, et al.** Late-stage Parkinson's disease: the Barcelona and Lisbon cohort. J Neurol 2010; **257**: 1524–32.

33. **Stubendorff K, Aarsland D, Minthon L, et al.** The impact of autonomic dysfunction on survival in patients with dementia with Lewy bodies and Parkinson's disease with dementia. PLoS ONE 2012; **7**: e45451.

34. **Idiaquez J, Benarroch EE, Rosales H, et al.** Autonomic and cognitive dysfunction in Parkinson's disease. Clin Auton Res 2007; **17**: 93–8.

35. Peralta C, Stampfer-Kountchev M, Karner E, et al. Orthostatic hypotension and attention in Parkinson's disease with and without dementia. J Neural Transm 2007; **114**: 585–8.

36. Allan LM, Ballard CG, Allen J, et al. Autonomic dysfunction in dementia. J Neurol Neurosurg Psychiatry 2007; **78**: 671–7.

37. Akaogi Y, Asahina M, Yamanaka Y, et al. Sudomotor, skin vasomotor, and cardiovascular reflexes in 3 clinical forms of Lewy body disease. Neurology 2009; **73**: 59–65.

38. Graham JM, Sagar HJ. A data-driven approach to the study of heterogeneity in idiopathic Parkinson's disease: identification of three distinct subtypes. Mov Disord 1999; **14**: 10–20.

39. Hohler AD, Zuzuarregui JR, Katz DI, et al. Differences in motor and cognitive function in patients with Parkinson's disease with and without orthostatic hypotension. Int J Neurosci 2012; **122**: 233–6.

40. Kim JS, Oh YS, Lee KS, et al. Association of cognitive dysfunction with neurocirculatory abnormalities in early Parkinson disease. Neurology 2012; **79**: 1323–31.

41. Pilleri M, Facchini S, Gasparoli E, et al. Cognitive and MRI correlates of orthostatic hypotension in Parkinson's disease. J Neurol 2013; **260**: 253–9.

42. Beach TG, Adler CH, Sue LI, et al. Multi-organ distribution of phosphorylated alpha-synuclein histopathology in subjects with Lewy body disorders. Acta Neuropathol 2010; **119**: 689–702.

43. Gelpi E, Navarro-Otano J, Tolosa E, et al. Multiple organ involvement by alpha-synuclein pathology in Lewy body disorders. Mov Disord 2014; **29**: 1010–18.

44. Braak H, Sastre M, Bohl JR, et al. Parkinson's disease: lesions in dorsal horn layer I, involvement of parasympathetic and sympathetic pre- and postganglionic neurons. Acta Neuropathol 2007; **113**: 421–9.

45. Wakabayashi K, Mori F, Tanji K, et al. Involvement of the peripheral nervous system in synucleinopathies, tauopathies and other neurodegenerative proteinopathies of the brain. Acta Neuropathol 2010; **120**: 1–12.

46. Calopa M, Tolosa E, Ferrer I, al. E. Cortical Lewy bodies in Parkinson's disease with dementia. In: Tolosa E, Schulz B, McKeith IG, et al. (ed.) *Neurodegenerative disorders associated with α-synuclein pathology*. Barcelona: Ars Medica, 2002; pp. 127–34.

47. Apaydin H, Ahlskog JE, Parisi JE, et al. Parkinson disease neuropathology: later-developing dementia and loss of the levodopa response. Arch Neurol 2002; **59**: 102–12.

48. Hurtig HI, Trojanowski JQ, Galvin J, et al. Alpha-synuclein cortical Lewy bodies correlate with dementia in Parkinson's disease. Neurology 2000; **54**: 1916–21.

49. Braak H, Rub U, Jansen Steur EN, et al. Cognitive status correlates with neuropathologic stage in Parkinson disease. Neurology 2005; **64**: 1404–10.

50. Blok BF. Central pathways controlling micturition and urinary continence. Urology 2002; **59**: 13–17.

51. Cersosimo MG, Benarroch EE. Neural control of the gastrointestinal tract: implications for Parkinson disease. Mov Disord 2008; **23**: 1065–75.

52. Winge K, Friberg L, Werdelin L, et al. Relationship between nigrostriatal dopaminergic degeneration, urinary symptoms, and bladder control in Parkinson's disease. Eur J Neurol 2005; **12**: 842–50.

53. Winge K, Fowler CJ. Bladder dysfunction in Parkinsonism: mechanisms, prevalence, symptoms, and management. Mov Disord 2006; **21**: 737–45.

54. Sakakibara R, Uchiyama T, Yamanishi T, et al. Genitourinary dysfunction in Parkinson's disease. Mov Disord 2010; **25**: 2–12.

55. Wakabayashi K, Takahashi H. The intermediolateral nucleus and Clarke's column in Parkinson's disease. Acta Neuropathol 1997; **94**: 287–9.

56. Mathers SE, Kempster PA, Swash M, Lees AJ. Constipation and paradoxical puborectalis contraction in anismus and Parkinson's disease: a dystonic phenomenon? J Neurol Neurosurg Psychiatry 1988; **51**: 1503–7.

Chapter 10

Structural and functional neuroimaging in patients with Parkinson's disease dementia

Gordon W. Duncan, Michael J. Firbank, and John T. O'Brien

Introduction

Structural and functional neuroimaging studies have provided insights into the heterogeneous pathological, anatomical, and neurochemical correlates of cognitive impairment associated with the progression of Parkinson's disease (PD) and the subsequent evolution of Parkinson's disease dementia (PD-D). A key target for clinicians and researchers is to develop robust biomarkers for this common, distressing, and disabling complication of PD. This would permit the early identification of those people at highest risk of PD-D and streamline clinical trials of potentially disease-modifying therapies which are most likely to be effective when initiated early in the disease process, prior to extensive neuronal loss. The absence of such biomarkers has hampered the ability of interventional clinical trials to distinguish between the symptomatic effects and the potential disease-modifying properties of study medications. This chapter will provide an overview of the structural and functional imaging studies of PD and cognitive decline to date.

Structural magnetic resonance imaging

Considerable progress has been made in developing conventional structural magnetic resonance imaging (MRI) into a tool for differentiating Alzheimer's disease (AD) from other causes of dementia, as a biomarker for observational studies of amnestic mild cognitive impairment (MCI) and AD, and, increasingly, as a surrogate outcome measure in trials of therapeutics (see Fig. 10.1). It is a commonly held view that MRI has the potential to fulfil a similar role in PD. MRI is an attractive option as a biomarker: it is safe, well tolerated by patients, non-invasive, and readily available. Crucially, for observational researchers and the pharmaceutical industry, it is not prohibitively costly and is up to ten times cheaper than many other imaging modalities being used in clinical trials.

Early MRI studies of PD and cognitive impairment commonly adopted a region of interest (ROI) approach; however, such methods are time-consuming, laborious, and involve critical issues regarding the choice of anatomical boundary, with potential for influencing intra- and inter-rater reliability. Although there are now fully automated protocols for segmenting individual brain structures such as the cortical lobar regions, hippocampus, basal ganglia, and thalamus, methods which analyse the entire grey matter volume are increasingly being used. Voxel-based morphometry (VBM) provides an automated, largely operator independent, and unbiased

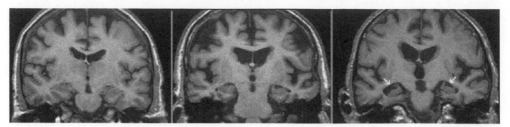

Fig. 10.1 Coronal T$_1$-weighted MRI images of (from left to right) control, PD-D, and AD. Atrophy of the medial temporal structures is most severe in the AD subject (arrows) but mild in the PD subject compared with the control subject of a similar age.

method of assessing differences in the volume of brain tissue between groups of patients. Because the whole of the grey matter may be examined on a voxel-wise basis there is no requirement for an a priori hypothesis, permitting the study of cortical areas which may not have been previously considered relevant and thus ignored by ROI analyses. Corticometry, a measurement of cortical thickness and folding, is a relatively new whole-brain technique and may offer greater sensitivity in detecting early changes to the grey matter than VBM.

Studies using VBM analysis have consistently reported widespread cortical atrophy in patients with established PD-D, with diffuse bilateral loss of grey matter occurring in frontal, parietal, temporal, and occipital areas [1–6]. Studies using cortical thickness analysis have also observed extensive thinning of the frontal, temporal, and parietal cortices in those with PD-D compared with controls [7] and in the temporal lobes relative to PD patients without dementia [8]. Compared with AD, most [1, 6, 9, 10], though not all [8, 11], studies have found less pronounced hippocampal atrophy in PD-D. Atrophy of other limbic structures, including the entorhinal cortex [11, 12], amygdala [13, 14], and anterior cingulate gyrus [4, 10], has also been reported. Atrophy of the caudate nucleus, putamen, and thalamus has been observed in PD-D using both VBM and ROI analyses [1, 4, 15].

Although one study has reported mild posterior atrophy in patients with early PD and intact cognition (PD-NC) [5], significant cortical atrophy in such patients has generally not been observed with VBM [6, 16, 17]. Cortical thinning has been reported in early PD-NC in frontal, temporal, and parietal regions [18]; however, this is not a consistent finding [7]. In studies of PD patients without dementia, with a mean disease duration of over 5 years, VBM studies have demonstrated only mild cortical atrophy relative to control subjects [2, 3, 19, 20]. Mild cortical thinning in frontal, temporal, parietal, and occipital regions has been observed with corticometry [8, 21, 22]. In PD patients without dementia, hippocampal and medial temporal lobe atrophy is not significant when assessed with ROI or VBM techniques [1, 2, 16, 23], although mild loss of grey matter in the amygdala has been reported [24].

PD with mild cognitive impairment (PD-MCI) may represent a transitional state to dementia in patients with PD. The publication in 2012 by the Movement Disorder Society (MDS) of guidance on the diagnosis and classification of PD-MCI aims to harmonize the definition of MCI and standardize methods of testing and classification [25]. Using these criteria, Melzer et al. [6] reported mild loss of grey matter in the temporal, parietal, and frontal cortices and in the hippocampi of PD-MCI patients. In a further study, Mak et al. [26] found loss of grey matter volume in the left insular, left superior frontal, and left middle temporal areas in patients with PD-MCI compared with PD-NC. The predictive value of the VBM approach for determining which patients with PD-MCI will progress to PD-D has been addressed [27]. At the initial scan, patients with PD-MCI who developed PD-D exhibited lower grey matter density in the left frontal area, left insular cortex, and bilateral caudate nucleus compared with patients who did not subsequently develop PD-D. Interestingly, the volume of the substantia innominata was significantly lower in patients who progressed to PD-D. This structure, which is located within the basal forebrain, contains the nucleus basalis of Meynert, one of the major suppliers of cholinergic innervation to the cerebral cortex.

Although not using MDS criteria, Pagonabarraga et al. [8] used corticometry to compare the thickness of grey matter across different cognitive stages of PD. Relative to PD-NC, subjects with PD-MCI displayed grey matter thinning involving the left anterior temporal pole, anterior cingulate cortex, entorhinal cortex, lingual gyrus, and precuneus. On the right, grey matter thinning was seen to involve the cuneus, lateral occipital cortex, inferior temporal cortex, and the fusiform gyrus. Compared with PD-MCI subjects, patients with PD-D displayed even greater atrophy in similar regions.

High-dimensional pattern classification algorithms, such as the regional analysis of volumes examined in normalized space (RAVENS) have been used to predict disease in individual subjects in studies of AD and MCI [28, 29]. An individual's score is generated based upon measures of atrophy of regions such as the hippocampus, posterior cingulate, and peri-hippocampal white matter. Positive scores are indicative of a greater likelihood of dementia and a negative score is more in keeping with healthy control brains. This has been used identify patients who will subsequently progress to PD-D [20, 30]. After 2 years, those PD subjects without dementia with higher baseline SPARE-PDD (spatial pattern of abnormality for recognition of Parkinson's disease with dementia-level cognitive deficits) scores had greater subsequent worsening of global cognitive performance.

Performance in neuropsychological tests has been correlated with atrophy of specific neuroanatomical structures. Atrophy of the prefrontal cortex has been correlated with increased reaction times and hippocampal atrophy has been associated with impairments of verbal memory [31]. Semantic fluency has been correlated with grey matter volume in frontal and temporal areas [32]; visuospatial and visuoperceptual function with occipital grey matter [33]; and impaired decision making with reduced volume of the orbito-frontal cortex [24]. Atrophy of the substantia innominata has been observed across all stages of PD [34, 35], and has been correlated with worsening attention, executive function, and verbal fluency [36].

Visual hallucinations are a prominent feature of PD-D [37, 38]. Patterns of grey matter loss similar to those observed in PD-D are reported in PD subjects without dementia who suffer from visual hallucinations. Compared with those without visual hallucinations, patients who hallucinate display diffuse grey matter loss in the superior parietal lobes (bilaterally), the right medial frontal gyrus, right lingual gyrus, left inferior parietal lobe, and left occipital lobe [39]. After a mean of 29 months' follow-up, the patients with hallucinations had higher rates of conversion to dementia and extensive grey matter loss than those without hallucinations [40].

Few studies have examined longitudinal morphological brain changes in PD. Using the brain boundary shift integral technique, Burton et al. [41] observed significantly higher rates of brain atrophy in those with PD-D (12.2 ml/year; 1.12%) compared with PD patients without dementia (3.4 ml/year; 0.31%) and healthy controls (3.8 ml/year; 0.34%). In PD without dementia rates of atrophy similar to controls have been reported in some, but not all, studies [41–43]. Ventricular dilation may reflect concurrent cerebral atrophy and has been used as a measure of atrophy in studies of AD. Progressive ventricular enlargement of the lateral ventricles in PD-D has been observed [44], and enlargement of the left inferior lateral ventricle and third ventricle is reported in patients with PD-MCI [45, 46].

In routine clinical practice the principal role of MRI is to assist in the differential diagnosis of PD or PD-D from another akinetic–rigid disorder or another dementia syndrome. As discussed, atrophy of structures within the medial temporal lobe is not severe early in the disease course of PD or PD-D when compared with AD; however, with disease progression there is often mild generalized global atrophy. Patients with progressive supranuclear palsy may display prominent midbrain atrophy, while those with multiple system atrophy often show either pontine or cerebellar atrophy. More common, however, is the demonstration of cerebrovascular disease in the form of stroke, lacunar infarcts, microbleeds, or white matter hyperintensities. White matter hyperintensities are a frequent neuroimaging finding in older people and have been associated with both cognitive impairments and mild parkinsonian signs [47–49].

Diffusion tensor imaging

Diffusion tensor imaging (DTI) offers a sensitive technique for assessing changes in white matter by quantifying the magnitude and direction of the motion of water molecules. In doing this DTI provides an in vivo surrogate measure of the integrity of tissue microstructure. The presence of physical barriers constrains the motion of water molecules so that they will preferentially travel in certain directions, termed anisotropy. In the central nervous system such constraints include microtubules, axon walls, and myelin sheaths. Three eigenvalues (λ_1, λ_2, and λ_3) quantify the diffusivities along the three principal axes of the diffusion tensor; the direction of this motion is given as the corresponding eigenvectors (ε_1, ε_2, and ε_3). Mean diffusivity (MD) is the average of the eigenvalues. The degree of this preferential movement is quantified with the fractional anisotropy (FA) metric and values vary between 0 and 1, where 0 indicates isotropic diffusion and 1 is highly constrained diffusion. Voxels which display high FA contain highly organized structures such as axons where the direction of diffusion is limited, causing the direction of travel of the water molecules to occur maximally along the white matter tract. With axonal degeneration and tract disruption the measured FA is reduced [50]. Normal ageing is accompanied by minor changes in both FA and MD, but more extensive changes are present in neurodegenerative and cerebrovascular disease.

Earlier studies typically adopted the ROI approach, often focusing on the substantia nigra and its projections [51, 52]. A more recent technique is tract-based spatial statistics (TBSS) which interrogates the integrity of the major white matter tracts throughout the brain without the limitations of the operator-dependent ROI approach [53] and may offer a more sensitive measure of white matter integrity in patients with PD with regard to cognition [54]. Significant reductions in FA and increases in MD are a feature of PD-D. Applying TBSS in patients with PD-D, Hattori et al. [2] reported reduced FA in the superior longitudinal fasciculus, the anterior limb of the internal capsule, and the inferior longitudinal fasciculus relative to controls. Compared with subjects with PD, patients with PD-D displayed significantly reduced FA in the superior longitudinal fasciculus, inferior longitudinal fasciculus, inferior fronto-occipital fasciculus, uncinate fasciculus, cingulum, and the corpus callosum. Subjects with PD-MCI displayed widespread reductions in FA in similar regions when compared with healthy controls, but this was not significant when compared with PD-NC patients. In addition to extensive reductions in white matter FA, Melzer et al. [55] observed significant increases in MD in patients with PD-D relative to PD-NC and control subjects. Subjects with PD-MCI displayed reduced FA and increased MD compared with PD-NC patients and controls.

Using a ROI analysis in a purely executively impaired cohort of subjects with PD, Matsui et al. [56] reported significantly reduced FA in the left parietal lobe compared with those with PD-NC. Subjects with PD-D displayed reductions in FA in the bilateral posterior cingulate bundles compared with PD-NC patients; however, both groups had lower FA in frontal, temporal, and occipital white matter than controls [57].

In summary, loss of grey matter occurs in the context of advancing disease. Measures of grey matter loss may not be sensitive to changes that occur early in the disease process when the pathological processes are limited to the brainstem; however, with disease progression there appears to be progressive loss of grey matter. Changes in the FA and MD of white matter microstructure appear early in the disease process and may offer a more sensitive measure of early axonal degeneration. The value of structural MRI analysis techniques for identifying those patients at highest risk of PD-D requires further study.

Functional activity imaging

Imaging studies of brain activation have mainly been undertaken with functional MRI (fMRI), in which subjects perform specific tasks in the MR scanner, and the MR signal is compared between tasks or with a baseline. Changes in oxygen consumption, blood flow, and blood volume result in a decrease in the concentration of deoxyhaemoglobin. This leads to a localized change in the magnetic field which is detectable using a T_2^*-weighted sequence. This blood-oxygen-level-dependent (BOLD) signal provides a surrogate measure of focal brain activity, but the precise relationships between changes in the BOLD signal and patterns of neuronal activation are not yet fully understood [58].

In PD subjects without dementia, fMRI has been used to examine the specific neuroanatomical substrates for memory [59], attentional functions [60], and executive functions [61]. Using working memory or executive function tasks, abnormal basal ganglia and prefrontal task-related activity has been observed. Lewis et al. [61] had PD patients perform a working memory task; those with impaired executive function had reduced fronto-striatal activity compared with those with normal executive function. Using a card-sorting test of executive function, Monchi et al. [62], concluded that the caudate is involved in set-shifting (adjusting to new rules) and that activity in the prefrontal areas, which co-activated with the caudate in controls, is reduced along with caudate activity in tasks involving set-shifting; those frontal and parietal areas not related to caudate activity showed hyperactivation in PD. In PD subjects with no impairment of executive performance, cortical hyperactivation may also occur, possibly as a result of compensatory activity [63, 64].

Functional MRI studies have examined the relationship between dopaminergic medication and cognitive function. Use of levodopa has been found to modulate task-related activation in frontal and occipital regions, associated with an improved response to executive tasks but with slightly worse performance on a motor sequence learning task [65–68]. Some of the variation in attentional and executive function may be partly mediated through the Val158Met polymorphism in the catechol O-methyltransferase gene which influences dopaminergic availability [60]. In patients with PD and visual hallucinations, reduced activation to visual stimuli in occipital, parietal, and temporal regions [69, 70] and also increased activation in the superior and inferior frontal gyrus and caudate has been observed [71].

The study of resting-state networks has attracted recent interest. The BOLD signal shows low-frequency oscillations, with correlated activity being seen across distributed networks of brain regions while the subject lies in the scanner with no specific task to perform. These networks can be identified using techniques such as independent component analysis. The default-mode network (DMN) is characterized by basal activity which increases at rest or passive visual fixation and becomes less active during a cognitive task. It has attracted particular interest in studies of dementia because it includes the posterior cingulate and hippocampus. In the absence of significant structural abnormalities, reduced DMN functional connectivity has been observed in the right medial temporal lobe and bilateral inferior parietal cortices in PD-NC subjects. These changes correlated with performance on tests of memory and visuospatial function, respectively, and were independent of the severity of motor symptoms, disease duration, or levodopa therapy [72]. Dysfunction of the DMN has also been observed in patients in the hypodopaminergic state [73] and it is postulated that dopaminergic therapy may modulate the DMN, with patterns of DMN activation being similar to those of healthy controls when in the 'on' state [74].

Perfusion and metabolism

The techniques of single-photon emission computed tomography (SPECT) and positron emission tomography (PET) have traditionally been used to study cerebral perfusion and metabolism. Recently there has been interest in the application of advanced MRI techniques such as arterial spin labelling (ASL-MRI) and magnetic resonance spectroscopy. Unlike PET and SPECT these techniques are non-invasive and do not require intravenously injected radioactive ligands to form brain images, thus making them attractive for longitudinal studies.

Glucose metabolism has been measured using ^{18}F-fluorodeoxyglucose (FDG)-PET. Perfusion imaging using SPECT is achieved with a variety of ligands: ^{99m}Tc-hexamethylpropyleneamine oxime (HMPAO), N-isopropyl-p-^{123}I-iodoamphetamine (IMP), and ^{99m}Tc-ethylcysteinate dimer (ECD). Using blood samples the FDG uptake signal can be quantified in absolute units, but is often analysed relative to a reference region, with either a whole brain average or cerebellar uptake being chosen. Perfusion, likewise, is nearly always semi-quantitative. The choice of reference region is also important; a potential disadvantage of using average whole brain (or grey matter) values as a reference is that if there is a large area of hypoperfusion unaffected areas will appear relatively hyperperfused (and the affected area will seem relatively less hypoperfused). The choice of a reference region is not completely standard, the cerebellum has been shown to be a good choice in AD since it is relatively unaffected [75]. However, cerebellar activity may be increased in PD, and Borghammer et al. [76] have suggested using the white matter region as a reference, but this has not yet been widely adopted.

FDG-PET has shown widespread reductions in glucose metabolism, including in the midline frontal and parietal regions, lateral frontal, lateral parieto-temporal, and occipital cortex, in those with PD-D [77–79]. Using FDG and principal components analysis, Huang et al. [80] identified specific patterns of relative regional metabolism which accounted for the variability in FDG scans across PD subjects. They then identified one of these component patterns where FDG uptake correlated with cognitive function in PD. This consisted of relatively reduced metabolism in the midline frontal, precuneus, inferior parietal, and prefrontal regions, with increased metabolism in the cerebellum and pons. The same authors also demonstrated that this pattern of altered regional metabolism was associated with PD-MCI [81] and that longitudinal changes in it were associated with decreasing cognitive ability [82]. Bohnen et al. [83] have further demonstrated reduced metabolism in the occipital cortex and posterior cingulate cortex in those with PD without dementia at baseline who then went on to develop PD-D.

SPECT studies of perfusion in PD-D report similar results to those using FDG-PET, with reduced perfusion in the midline and lateral parietal regions [84–88]; moreover, posterior parietal perfusion has been found to correlate with cognitive ability [89] (see Fig. 10.2) These changes are very similar to those seen in dementia with Lewy bodies (DLB) [77, 88, 90].

ASL-MRI provides a surrogate measure of cerebral blood flow and perfusion. The magnetic state of the protons in the cerebral circulation provides contrast; as the blood flows towards the brain the magnetization of the protons is inverted and when the blood reaches the brain tissue the change in magnetization is detected. In studies of AD, ASL-MRI has demonstrated patterns

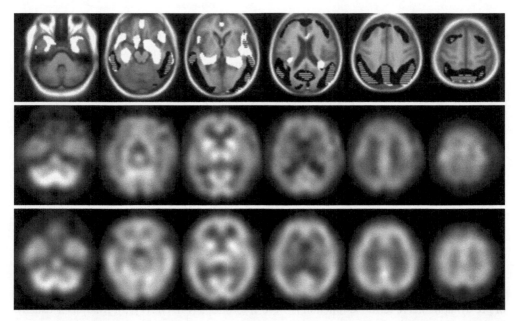

Fig. 10.2 SPECT perfusion in AD and PD-D. Top row (adapted from data in Firbank *et al* 2003): over-laid on an axial MRI are averaged perfusion deficits—PD-D in black; AD in white; both AD and PDD in horizontal shading. Second row: perfusion image from a typical subject with PDD. Third row: normal perfusion image.

Reprinted from NeuroImage, 20, Firbank MJ, Colloby SJ, Burn DJ, McKeith IG, O'Brien JT., Regional cerebral blood flow in Parkinson's disease with and without dementia, 1309–19, ©(2003), with permission from Elsevier.

of temporo-parietal hypoperfusion comparable with those observed with FDG-PET [91]. In sub-jects with PD-D, hypoperfusion has been observed in the precuneus, cuneus, and middle frontal gyri when compared with healthy controls [92, 93], and there is preservation of perfusion in the globus pallidus, putamen, anterior cingulate, and pre- and post-central gyri [93].

Magnetic resonance spectroscopy provides an in vivo surrogate measure of specific aspects of cerebral metabolism. Proton magnetic resonance spectroscopy (^{1}H-MRS) detects the small signal changes of protons from molecules of particular metabolites found within the brain on the basis that the resonance frequency is altered by the surrounding chemical milieu. These key 'biomolecules' include: *N*-acetyl aspartate (NAA), considered to be a marker of neuronal dens-ity and integrity reflecting cell metabolism and mitochondrial activity; creatine (Cr), a molecule found in all types of neuronal cell and used as a concentration reference because of its steady state; myo-inositol, principally found in glial cells acting as a major osmosregulator within these cells; and choline, a precursor of acetylcholine which is increased in membrane breakdown and found in glycerophosphorylcholine as a breakdown product of membrane phosphatidylcholine. Either multislice or single-voxel spectroscopy is performed and a large size is often chosen for the single voxel owing to the small concentrations of the measured molecules of interest [94]. A few small studies have demonstrated that ^{1}H-MRS may be able to identify metabolic changes in the cerebral structures implicated in PD-related cognitive decline.

An observation that supports the concept of significant 'posterior' cortical dysfunction driving the evolution of PD-D [95] is the lower NAA/Cr ratios in the hippocampus [96] and occipital cortices of patients with PD-D relative to subjects with PD-NC and healthy controls [97]. In comparison with those with AD, subjects with PD-D had reduced glutamate and NAA/Cr was reduced relative to controls [98]. A further study observed reduced NAA concentrations in the right dorsolateral prefrontal cortex compared with PD-NC [96] which correlated with performance on frontal subcortical tasks. In subjects with seemingly normal cognition, reduced NAA/Cr has also been observed in the posterior cingulate gyrus [99].

In summary, PD-D patients have markedly reduced perfusion and metabolism throughout the brain, particularly in the parietal and frontal regions. The degree of reduction in perfusion appears to be linked to cognitive decline, and patients with specific cognitive impairments also demonstrate metabolic changes. Currently the data from ^{1}H-MRS and ASL-MRI are too limited to inform any role as possible biomarkers for cognitive decline in PD and further research is required to characterize the changes in cerebral blood flow and metabolism detectable with MRI and how these compare with changes observed with PET and SPECT.

Dopaminergic imaging

Degeneration in the dopaminergic system in PD has been investigated with PET and SPECT imaging measures of pre- and post-synaptic function and integrity. A widely used PET measure of pre-synaptic nerve terminal function is ^{18}F-6-fluorodopa (F-DOPA) [73]. Analysis is usually by the graphical method of Patlak and Blasberg [100], which calculates the k_i or tracer influx constant using a reference region, usually the occipital lobe. Reduced F-DOPA tracer uptake has been demonstrated in the whole striatum in PD, particularly in the putamen, relative to healthy controls. Decreased F-DOPA uptake in both the putamen and caudate has been correlated with measures of motor severity, although generally the putamen shows a stronger correlation [101–103]. The caudate and ventral striatum may play a more significant role in cognition than the putamen, and uptake of F-DOPA by the caudate has been correlated with measures of executive function and memory [102, 103].

Ito et al. [104] used F-DOPA to compare PD-D patients with controls and those with PD. They observed that patients with PD-D had reduced striatal F-DOPA uptake compared with control and PD subjects. However, in a study by Klein et al. [105], although the authors observed reduced F-DOPA uptake in the striatum of those with PD, PD-D, and DLB relative to control subjects the differences between the groups were not significant. Increased cortical uptake of F-DOPA in the anterior cingulate and medial frontal cortex has been observed in unmedicated PD subjects, possibly as a compensatory mechanism; however, decreased cortical uptake has also been found [102]. Cropley et al. [106] reported a greater calculated F-DOPA influx constant in white versus grey matter, contrary to the expected distribution, and the authors postulated that the Patlak method may be unreliable for this tracer for cortical areas due to differences in perfusion in the reference occipital region. A further PET measure of pre-synaptic dopaminergic uptake is achieved using the vesicular monoamine transporter type 2 (VMAT2) ligand ^{11}C-dihyrdotertabenazine which binds to VMAT2 terminals within the striatum. Reduced pre-synaptic tracer uptake has been reported in the striatum in both PD and PD-D [107].

PET has also been used to investigate post-synaptic dopamine receptors. Cropley et al. [106] found no difference between PD and controls with a D1 receptor ligand ^{11}C-NNC 112. Using ^{11}C-raclopride, a marker of D2 receptor availability, decreased binding potential (indicative of greater endogenous dopamine) was found in a working memory task relative to a visuomotor task in controls and PD, with a small region of the caudate having greater task-related decreases in controls compared with PD subjects.

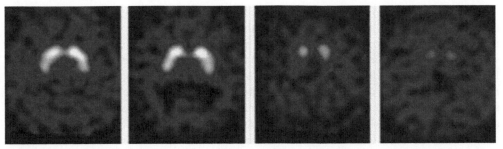

Fig. 10.3 Typical FP-CIT (dopamine transporter) images: from left to right control, AD, PD, and PD-D.

SPECT studies of PD-D and DLB show that uptake of the pre-synaptic dopamine transporter ligand [^{123}I]-2β-carbomethoxy-3β-(4-iodophenyl)-N-(3-fluoropropyl)-N-nortropane ([^{123}I]-FP-CIT) is virtually absent in the putamen and reduced in the caudate (Fig. 10.3). The presence of abnormal [^{123}I]-FP-CIT uptake has excellent diagnostic accuracy for differentiating DLB and PD-D from AD, with a sensitivity and specificity of approximately 80 and 90%, respectively [108]. Adding to the evidence from PET and fMRI studies implicating dopaminergic loss and caudate dysfunction in cognitive impairment in PD, relative to PD-NC, where the putamen is affected more than the caudate, PD-D subjects show a relatively uniform reduction in FP-CIT uptake throughout the striatum [109, 110].

In summary, in PD and PD-D profound deficits in the basal ganglia dopaminergic system can be demonstrated with PET and SPECT; however, these are generally not significant across the different stages of cognitive decline in patients with PD.

Cholinergic imaging

Autopsy and neuroimaging studies confirm that cholinergic dysfunction plays a major role in the evolution of cognitive impairment and dementia in PD. This is supported by the observation that medications with anticholinergic properties can impair performance on tests of attention and executive function when used in patients with PD [111]. Furthermore, clinical trials report modest but consistent improvements in cognitive impairment, in particular in attentional and executive dysfunction in PD-D patients following the initiation of cholinesterase inhibitor therapy [112, 113]. Degeneration of cholinergic neurons within the pedunculopontine nucleus and nucleus basalis of Meynert occurs early in PD resulting in the reduced cholinergic innervation of cortical and subcortical nuclei [114–117]. SPECT and PET radiotracers have been used to investigate the integrity of the cholinergic system in PD.

In the pre-synaptic neuron, vesicle-associated acetylcholine transporters (VAChT) translocate acetylcholine from the neuronal cytoplasm into intracellular vesicles. These may be labelled in vivo with the SPECT radioligand [^{123}I]-iodobenzovesamicol ([^{123}I]-IBVM) providing a measure of integrity of the pre-synaptic terminal. Kuhl et al. [118] observed significantly reduced retention of VAChT in the occipital cortex and posterior cingulate in those with PD-D, but only mild reductions in the parietal cortex and occipital cortex were present in PD subjects without dementia. Imaging of cholinergic muscarinic receptors with SPECT using (R,R) ^{123}I-iodo-quinuclidinyl-benzilate (QNB) [119] and nicotinic receptors with ^{125}I-5-iodo-3-[2(S)-2-azetidinylmethoxy] pyridine (5IA-85380) has revealed decreases in the frontal and temporal lobes in PD-D and DLB, and a relative increase in uptake of both ligands in the occipital lobe, with the uptake of the nicotinic ligand being higher in DLB subjects with recent hallucinations [120].

PET radiotracers may be used to measure the activity of the enzyme acetylcholinesterase (AChE) which is found within the synapse, both at the pre-synaptic terminals of cholinergic neurons and anchored to post-synaptic neuronal membranes. Lipophilic acetylcholine analogues such as methyl-4-piperidyl acetate (MP4A) and N-^{11}C-methyl-4-piperidinyl propionate (^{11}C-PMP) have been used. Using both F-DOPA and MP4A, Hilker et al. [107] observed moderately reduced MP4A binding in PD subjects without dementia relative to those with PD-D, in whom severe widespread reductions were seen. Cortical binding of MP4A in some regions showed a significant association with striatal F-DOPA in both PD and PD-D, although there were no significant differences between PD and PD-D in striatal F-DOPA. These reductions in cortical AChE activity are also present in DLB to a similar extent as seen in PD-D. Furthermore, reduced cortical AChE activity in the medial occipital lobe has been reported early in the disease and preceding dementia [121]. The cholinergic deficit in PD-D and DLB may actually be more profound than that seen in AD; using ^{11}C-PMP Bohnen et al. [122] reported moderate reductions in PD, and marked reductions in PD-D (about 20%) relative to controls [123] and AD [122]. Levels of PMP were reduced by about 10% in AD subjects in all regions apart from the inferior temporal lobe, where the reduction was greater (about 20%) and comparable to that of PD-D. Reductions in the PMP uptake correlated well with poor performance on executive and spatial tasks, which are typically impaired in PD-D, but not with verbal memory tasks or motor impairment [123].

Amyloid imaging

The binding of the PET tracer N-methyl-^{11}C-2-(4'-methylaminophenyl)-6-hydroxybenzothiazole (Pittsburgh Compound B, ^{11}C-PIB) to fibrillary amyloid-beta provides an in vivo surrogate measure of the aggregation of amyloid protein. Increased binding of ^{11}C-PIB relative to the cerebellum throughout the cortex has been found in AD [124], particularly in the posterior cingulate, frontal, lateral temporal, and parietal regions. Although increased uptake is a sensitive indicator of AD, 10–20% of subjects without any cognitive impairment also show increased ^{11}C-PIB uptake [125, 126]. Studies of PD and PD-D generally demonstrate lower levels of cortical uptake when compared with AD patients and no significant increases in PD relative to controls; however, a subgroup of cases of PD-D may have increased uptake but to a lesser extent than that seen in DLB or AD [127–129].

Cardiac scintigraphy imaging

There is loss of sympathetic innervation in the heart in patients with PD [130]. This has been demonstrated with cardiac scintigraphy using ^{123}I-metaiodobenzylguanidine ([^{123}I]-MIBG), an analogue of noradrenaline, with the ratio of uptake in the heart to the mediastinum calculated to quantify the images. This ratio has been found to be reduced in PD and also in DLB and PD-D in comparison with both AD and healthy subjects [131]. Studies have found a diagnostic accuracy of approximately 90% for differentiating PD from other causes of neurodegenerative parkinsonism, with a sensitivity and specificity of 83% [132]. However, since decreased uptake is present in those with cardiovascular disease, caution must be exercised in the interpretation of MIBG scans in such patients [131].

Conclusion

Because the pathological, anatomical, and neurochemical mechanisms underlying the evolution of cognitive decline in PD are heterogeneous, it is unlikely that any single neuroimaging modality will be a reliable biomarker for all patients. Structural imaging studies with MRI have demonstrated that the evolution of dementia in PD is underpinned by significant and progressive loss of grey matter and disruption of the integrity of the white matter tracts. Functional imaging techniques show that such changes are accompanied by significant disturbances not only in perfusion and metabolism but also within the dopaminergic and cholinergic neurotransmitter systems, and these changes become more pronounced with disease progression.

Future research should focus on the development of harmonized protocols for image acquisition and processing to facilitate large multicentre studies, the development of radiotracers for α-synuclein and tau aggregation, and standardized neuropsychological testing schedules. Longitudinal studies should be of sufficient size and duration to track the significance of early cognitive changes and be able to correlate these to atrophic changes as they develop and include, where possible, pathological evaluation post-mortem.

References

1. **Burton EJ, McKeith IG, Burn DJ, et al**. Cerebral atrophy in Parkinson's disease with and without dementia: a comparison with Alzheimer's disease, dementia with Lewy bodies and controls. Brain 2004; **127**: 791–800.

2. **Hattori T, Orimo S, Aoki S, et al**. Cognitive status correlates with white matter alteration in Parkinson's disease. Hum Brain Mapp 2012; **33**: 727–39.

3. **Nagano-Saito A, Washimi Y, Arahata Y, et al**. Cerebral atrophy and its relation to cognitive impairment in Parkinson's disease. Neurology 2005; **64**: 224–9.

4. **Summerfield C, Junque C, Tolosa E, et al**. Structural brain changes in Parkinson disease with dementia: a voxel-based morphometry study. Arch Neurol 2005; **62**: 281–5.

5. **Song SK, Lee JE, Park HJ, et al**. The pattern of cortical atrophy in patients with Parkinson's disease according to cognitive status. Mov Disord 2011; **26**: 289–96.

6. **Melzer TR, Watts R, MacAskill MR, et al**. Grey matter atrophy in cognitively impaired Parkinson's disease. J Neurol Neurosurg Psychiatry 2012; **83**: 188–94.

7. **Zarei M, Ibarretxe-Bilbao N, Compta Y, et al**. Cortical thinning is associated with disease stages and dementia in Parkinson's disease. J Neurol Neurosurg Psychiatry 2013; **84**: 875–81.

8. **Pagonabarraga J, Corcuera-Solano I, Vives-Gilabert Y, et al**. Pattern of regional cortical thinning associated with cognitive deterioration in Parkinson's disease. PLoS ONE 2013; **8**: e54980.

9. **Tam CW, Burton EJ, McKeith IG, et al**. Temporal lobe atrophy on MRI in Parkinson disease with dementia: a comparison with Alzheimer disease and dementia with Lewy bodies. Neurology 2005; **64**: 861–5.

10. **Beyer MK, Janvin CC, Larsen JP, et al**. A magnetic resonance imaging study of patients with Parkinson's disease with mild cognitive impairment and dementia using voxel-based morphometry. J Neurol Neurosurg Psychiatry 2007; **78**: 254–9.

11. **Goldman JG, Stebbins GT, Bernard B, et al**. Entorhinal cortex atrophy differentiates Parkinson's disease patients with and without dementia. Mov Disord 2012; **27**: 727–34.

12. **Kenny ER, Burton EJ, O'Brien JT**. A volumetric magnetic resonance imaging study of entorhinal cortex volume in dementia with Lewy bodies. A comparison with Alzheimer's disease and Parkinson's disease with and without dementia. Dement Geriatr Cogn Disord 2008; **26**: 218–25.

13. **Junque C, Ramirez-Ruiz B, Tolosa E, et al**. Amygdalar and hippocampal MRI volumetric reductions in Parkinson's disease with dementia. Mov Disord 2005; **20**: 540–4.

14. **Bouchard TP, Malykhin N, Martin WR, et al**. Age and dementia-associated atrophy predominates in the hippocampal head and amygdala in Parkinson's disease. Neurobiol Aging 2008; **29**: 1027–39.

15. **Almeida OP, Burton EJ, McKeith I, et al**. MRI study of caudate nucleus volume in Parkinson's disease with and without dementia with Lewy bodies and Alzheimer's disease. Dement Geriatr Cogn Disord 2003; **16**: 57–63.

16. **Dalaker TO, Zivadinov R, Larsen JP, et al**. Gray matter correlations of cognition in incident Parkinson's disease. Mov Disord 2010; **25**: 629–33.

17. **Agosta F, Canu E, Stojkovic T, et al.** The topography of brain damage at different stages of Parkinson's disease. Hum Brain Mapp 2013; **34**: 2798–807.

18. **Lyoo CH, Ryu YH, Lee MS.** Topographical distribution of cerebral cortical thinning in patients with mild Parkinson's disease without dementia. Mov Disord 2010; **25**: 496–9.

19. **Martin WR, Wieler M, Gee M, et al.** Temporal lobe changes in early, untreated Parkinson's disease. Mov Disord 2009; **24**: 1949–54.

20. **Weintraub D, Doshi J, Koka D, et al.** Neurodegeneration across stages of cognitive decline in Parkinson disease. Arch Neurol 2011; **68**: 1562–8.

21. **Tinaz S, Courtney MG, Stern CE.** Focal cortical and subcortical atrophy in early Parkinson's disease. Mov Disord 2011; **26**: 436–41.

22. **Pereira JB, Ibarretxe-Bilbao N, Marti MJ, et al.** Assessment of cortical degeneration in patients with Parkinson's disease by voxel-based morphometry, cortical folding, and cortical thickness. Hum Brain Mapp 2012; **33**: 2521–34.

23. **Jubault T, Gagnon JF, Karama S, et al.** Patterns of cortical thickness and surface area in early Parkinson's disease. NeuroImage 2011; **55**: 462–7.

24. **Ibarretxe-Bilbao N, Junque C, Tolosa E, et al.** Neuroanatomical correlates of impaired decision-making and facial emotion recognition in early Parkinson's disease. Eur J Neurosci 2009; **30**: 1162–71.

25. **Litvan I, Goldman JG, Troster AI, et al.** Diagnostic criteria for mild cognitive impairment in Parkinson's disease: Movement Disorder Society Task Force guidelines. Mov Disord 2012; **27**: 349–56.

26. **Mak E, Zhou J, Tan LC, et al.** Cognitive deficits in mild Parkinson's disease are associated with distinct areas of grey matter atrophy. J Neurol Neurosurg Psychiatry 2013; **85**: 576–80.

27. **Lee JE, Cho KH, Song SK, et al.** Exploratory analysis of neuropsychological and neuroanatomical correlates of progressive mild cognitive impairment in Parkinson's disease. J Neurol Neurosurg Psychiatry 2014; **85**: 7–16.

28. **Davatzikos C, Xu F, An Y, et al.** Longitudinal progression of Alzheimer's-like patterns of atrophy in normal older adults: the SPARE-AD index. Brain 2009; **132**: 2026–35.

29. **Fan Y, Batmanghelich N, Clark CM, et al.** Spatial patterns of brain atrophy in MCI patients, identified via high-dimensional pattern classification, predict subsequent cognitive decline. NeuroImage 2008; **39**: 1731–43.

30. **Weintraub D, Dietz N, Duda JE, et al.** Alzheimer's disease pattern of brain atrophy predicts cognitive decline in Parkinson's disease. Brain 2012; **135**: 170–80.

31. **Bruck A, Kurki T, Kaasinen V, et al.** Hippocampal and prefrontal atrophy in patients with early non-demented Parkinson's disease is related to cognitive impairment. J Neurol Neurosurg Psychiatry 2004; **75**: 1467–9.

32. **Pereira JB, Junque C, Marti MJ, et al.** Structural brain correlates of verbal fluency in Parkinson's disease. NeuroReport 2009; **20**: 741–4.

33. **Pereira JB, Junque C, Marti MJ, et al.** Neuroanatomical substrate of visuospatial and visuoperceptual impairment in Parkinson's disease. Mov Disord 2009; **24**: 1193–9.

34. **Hanyu H, Asano T, Sakurai H, et al.** MR analysis of the substantia innominata in normal aging, Alzheimer disease, and other types of dementia. Am J Neuroradiol 2002; **23**: 27–32.

35. **Oikawa H, Sasaki M, Ehara S, et al.** Substantia innominata: MR findings in Parkinson's disease. Neuroradiology 2004; **46**: 817–21.

36. **Choi SH, Jung TM, Lee JE, et al.** Volumetric analysis of the substantia innominata in patients with Parkinson's disease according to cognitive status. Neurobiol Aging 2012; **33**: 1265–72.

37. **Aarsland D, Bronnick K, Ehrt U, et al.** Neuropsychiatric symptoms in patients with Parkinson's disease and dementia: frequency, profile and associated care giver stress. J Neurol Neurosurg Psychiatry 2007; **78**: 36–42.

38. **Aarsland D, Larsen JP, Cummins JL, et al.** Prevalence and clinical correlates of psychotic symptoms in Parkinson disease: a community-based study. Arch Neurol 1999; **56**: 595–601.

39. **Ramirez-Ruiz B, Marti MJ, Tolosa E, et al.** Cerebral atrophy in Parkinson's disease patients with visual hallucinations. Eur J Neurol 2007; **14**: 750–6.

40. **Ibarretxe-Bilbao N, Ramirez-Ruiz B, Junque C, et al.** Differential progression of brain atrophy in Parkinson's disease with and without visual hallucinations. J Neurol Neurosurg Psychiatry 2010; **81**: 650–7.

41. **Burton EJ, McKeith IG, Burn DJ, et al.** Brain atrophy rates in Parkinson's disease with and without dementia using serial magnetic resonance imaging. Mov Disord 2005; **20**: 1571–6.

42. **Hu MT, White SJ, Chaudhuri KR, et al.** Correlating rates of cerebral atrophy in Parkinson's disease with measures of cognitive decline. J Neural Transm 2001; **108**: 571–80.

43. **Ramirez-Ruiz B, Marti MJ, Tolosa E, et al.** Longitudinal evaluation of cerebral morphological changes in Parkinson's disease with and without dementia. J Neurol 2005; **252**: 1345–52.

44. **Camicioli R, Sabino J, Gee M, et al.** Ventricular dilatation and brain atrophy in patients with Parkinson's disease with incipient dementia. Mov Disord 2011; **26**: 1443–50.

45. **Lewis MM, Smith AB, Styner M, et al.** Asymmetrical lateral ventricular enlargement in Parkinson's disease. Eur J Neurol 2009; **16**: 475–81.

46. **Dalaker TO, Zivadinov R, Ramasamy DP, et al.** Ventricular enlargement and mild cognitive impairment in early Parkinson's disease. Mov Disord 2011; **26**: 297–301.

47. **de Leeuw FE, de Groot JC, Achten E, et al.** Prevalence of cerebral white matter lesions in elderly people: a population based magnetic resonance imaging study. The Rotterdam Scan Study. J Neurol Neurosurg Psychiatry 2001; **70**: 9–14.

48. **de Groot JC, de Leeuw FE, Oudkerk M, et al.** Cerebral white matter lesions and cognitive function: the Rotterdam Scan Study. Ann Neurol 2000; **47**: 145–51.

49. **de Laat KF, Tuladhar AM, van Norden AG, et al.** Loss of white matter integrity is associated with gait disorders in cerebral small vessel disease. Brain 2011; **134**: 73–83.

50. **Nucifora PG, Verma R, Lee SK, et al.** Diffusion-tensor MR imaging and tractography: exploring brain microstructure and connectivity. Radiology 2007; **245**: 367–84.

51. **Yoshikawa K, Nakata Y, Yamada K, et al.** Early pathological changes in the parkinsonian brain demonstrated by diffusion tensor MRI. J Neurol Neurosurg Psychiatry 2004; **75**: 481–4.

52. **Chan LL, Rumpel H, Yap K, et al.** Case control study of diffusion tensor imaging in Parkinson's disease. J Neurol Neurosurg Psychiatry 2007; **78**: 1383–6.

53. **Smith SM, Jenkinson M, Johansen-Berg H, et al.** Tract-based spatial statistics: voxelwise analysis of multi-subject diffusion data. NeuroImage 2006; **31**: 1487–505.

54. **Rae CL, Correia MM, Altena E, et al.** White matter pathology in Parkinson's disease: the effect of imaging protocol differences and relevance to executive function. NeuroImage 2012; **62**: 1675–84.

55. **Melzer TR, Watts R, MacAskill MR, et al.** White matter microstructure deteriorates across cognitive stages in Parkinson disease. Neurology 2013; **80**: 1841–9.

56. **Matsui H, Nishinaka K, Oda M, et al.** Wisconsin Card Sorting Test in Parkinson's disease: diffusion tensor imaging. Acta Neurol Scand 2007; **116**: 108–12.

57. **Matsui H, Nishinaka K, Oda M, et al.** Dementia in Parkinson's disease: diffusion tensor imaging. Acta Neurol Scand 2007; **116**: 177–81.

58. **Jezzard P, Matthews PM, Smith SM (ed.)** *Functional MRI: an introduction to methods.* Oxford: Oxford University Press, 2003.

59. **Ibarretxe-Bilbao N, Zarei M, Junque C, et al.** Dysfunctions of cerebral networks precede recognition memory deficits in early Parkinson's disease. NeuroImage 2011; **57**: 589–97.

60. **Williams-Gray CH, Hampshire A, Barker RA, et al.** Attentional control in Parkinson's disease is dependent on COMT val 158 met genotype. Brain 2008; **131**: 397–408.

61. **Lewis SJ, Dove A, Robbins TW, et al.** Cognitive impairments in early Parkinson's disease are accompanied by reductions in activity in frontostriatal neural circuitry. J Neurosci 2003; **23**: 6351–6.

62. **Monchi O, Petrides M, Mejia-Constain B, et al.** Cortical activity in Parkinson's disease during executive processing depends on striatal involvement. Brain 2007; **130**: 233–44.

63. Tinaz S, Schendan HE, Stern CE. Fronto-striatal deficit in Parkinson's disease during semantic event sequencing. Neurobiol Aging 2008; **29**: 397–407.

64. Marie RM, Lozza C, Chavoix C, et al. Functional imaging of working memory in Parkinson's disease: compensations and deficits. J Neuroimaging 2007; **17**: 277–85.

65. Feigin A, Ghilardi MF, Carbon M, et al. Effects of levodopa on motor sequence learning in Parkinson's disease. Neurology 2003; **60**: 1744–9.

66. Mattay VS, Tessitore A, Callicott JH, et al. Dopaminergic modulation of cortical function in patients with Parkinson's disease. Ann Neurol 2002; **51**: 156–64.

67. Tessitore A, Hariri AR, Fera F, et al. Dopamine modulates the response of the human amygdala: a study in Parkinson's disease. J Neurosci 2002; **22**: 9099–103.

68. Rowe JB, Hughes L, Ghosh BC, et al. Parkinson's disease and dopaminergic therapy—differential effects on movement, reward and cognition. Brain 2008; **131**: 2094–105.

69. Stebbins GT, Goetz CG, Carrillo MC, et al. Altered cortical visual processing in PD with hallucinations: an fMRI study. Neurology 2004; **63**: 1409–16.

70. Howard R, David A, Woodruff P, et al. Seeing visual hallucinations with functional magnetic resonance imaging. Dement Geriatr Cogn Disord 1997; **8**: 73–7.

71. Meppelink AM, de Jong BM, Renken R, et al. Impaired visual processing preceding image recognition in Parkinson's disease patients with visual hallucinations. Brain 2009; **132**: 2980–93.

72. Tessitore A, Esposito F, Vitale C, et al. Default-mode network connectivity in cognitively unimpaired patients with Parkinson disease. Neurology 2012; **79**: 2226–32.

73. van Eimeren T, Monchi O, Ballanger B, et al. Dysfunction of the default mode network in Parkinson disease: a functional magnetic resonance imaging study. Arch Neurol 2009; **66**: 877–83.

74. Nagano-Saito A, Liu J, Doyon J, et al. Dopamine modulates default mode network deactivation in elderly individuals during the Tower of London task. Neurosci Lett 2009; **458**: 1–5.

75. Soonawala D, Amin T, Ebmeier KP, et al. Statistical parametric mapping of (99m)Tc-HMPAO-SPECT images for the diagnosis of Alzheimer's disease: normalizing to cerebellar tracer uptake. NeuroImage 2002; **17**: 1193–202.

76. Borghammer P, Jonsdottir KY, Cumming P, et al. Normalization in PET group comparison studies—the importance of a valid reference region. NeuroImage 2008; **40**: 529–40.

77. Yong SW, Yoon JK, An YS, et al. A comparison of cerebral glucose metabolism in Parkinson's disease, Parkinson's disease dementia and dementia with Lewy bodies. Eur J Neurol 2007; **14**: 1357–62.

78. Jokinen P, Scheinin N, Aalto S, et al. [(11)C]PIB-, [(18)F]FDG-PET and MRI imaging in patients with Parkinson's disease with and without dementia. Parkinsonism Relat Disord 2010; **16**: 666–70.

79. Vander Borght T, Minoshima S, Giordani B, et al. Cerebral metabolic differences in Parkinson's and Alzheimer's diseases matched for dementia severity. J Nucl Med 1997; **38**: 797–802.

80. Huang C, Mattis P, Tang C, et al. Metabolic brain networks associated with cognitive function in Parkinson's disease. NeuroImage 2007; **34**: 714–23.

81. Huang C, Mattis P, Perrine K, et al. Metabolic abnormalities associated with mild cognitive impairment in Parkinson disease. Neurology 2008; **70**: 1470–7.

82. Huang C, Tang C, Feigin A, et al. Changes in network activity with the progression of Parkinson's disease. Brain 2007; **130**: 1834–46.

83. Bohnen NI, Koeppe RA, Minoshima S, et al. Cerebral glucose metabolic features of Parkinson disease and incident dementia: longitudinal study. J Nucl Med 2011; **52**: 848–55.

84. Waragai M, Yamada T, Matsuda H. Evaluation of brain perfusion SPECT using an easy Z-score imaging system (eZIS) as an adjunct to early-diagnosis of neurodegenerative diseases. J Neurol Sci 2007; **260**: 57–64.

85. Matsui H, Udaka F, Miyoshi T, et al. N-isopropyl-p-^{123}I iodoamphetamine single photon emission computed tomography study of Parkinson's disease with dementia. Intern Med 2005; **44**: 1046–50.

86. **Osaki Y, Morita Y, Fukumoto M, et al.** Three-dimensional stereotactic surface projection SPECT analysis in Parkinson's disease with and without dementia. Mov Disord 2005; **20**: 999–1005.

87. **Derejko M, Slawek J, Wieczorek D, et al.** Regional cerebral blood flow in Parkinson's disease as an indicator of cognitive impairment. Nucl Med Commun 2006; **27**: 945–51.

88. **Firbank MJ, Colloby SJ, Burn DJ, et al.** Regional cerebral blood flow in Parkinson's disease with and without dementia. NeuroImage 2003; **20**: 1309–19.

89. **Van Laere K, Santens P, Bosman T, et al.** Statistical parametric mapping of (99m)Tc-ECD SPECT in idiopathic Parkinson's disease and multiple system atrophy with predominant parkinsonian features: correlation with clinical parameters. J Nucl Med 2004; **45**: 933–42.

90. **Mito Y, Yoshida K, Yabe I, et al.** Brain 3D-SSP SPECT analysis in dementia with Lewy bodies, Parkinson's disease with and without dementia, and Alzheimer's disease. Clin Neurol Neurosurg 2005; **107**: 396–403.

91. **Chen Y, Wolk DA, Reddin JS, et al.** Voxel-level comparison of arterial spin-labeled perfusion MRI and FDG-PET in Alzheimer disease. Neurology 2011; **77**: 1977–85.

92. **Kamagata K, Motoi Y, Hori M, et al.** Posterior hypoperfusion in Parkinson's disease with and without dementia measured with arterial spin labeling MRI. J Magn Reson Imaging 2011; **33**: 803–7.

93. **Melzer TR, Watts R, MacAskill MR, et al.** Arterial spin labelling reveals an abnormal cerebral perfusion pattern in Parkinson's disease. Brain 2011; **134**: 845–55.

94. **Soares DP, Law M.** Magnetic resonance spectroscopy of the brain: review of metabolites and clinical applications. Clin Radiol 2009; **64**: 12–21.

95. **Williams-Gray CH, Evans JR, Goris A, et al.** The distinct cognitive syndromes of Parkinson's disease: 5 year follow-up of the CamPaIGN cohort. Brain 2009; **132**: 2958–69.

96. **Pagonabarraga J, Gomez-Anson B, Rotger R, et al.** Spectroscopic changes associated with mild cognitive impairment and dementia in Parkinson's disease. Dement Geriatr Cogn Disord 2012; **34**: 312–18.

97. **Summerfield C, Gomez-Anson B, Tolosa E, et al.** Dementia in Parkinson disease: a proton magnetic resonance spectroscopy study. Arch Neurol 2002; **59**: 1415–20.

98. **Griffith HR, den Hollander JA, Okonkwo OC, et al.** Brain metabolism differs in Alzheimer's disease and Parkinson's disease dementia. Alzheimers Dement 2008; **4**: 421–7.

99. **Griffith HR, den Hollander JA, Okonkwo OC, et al.** Brain N-acetylaspartate is reduced in Parkinson disease with dementia. Alzheimer Dis Assoc Disord 2008; **22**: 54–60.

100. **Patlak CS, Blasberg RG.** Graphical evaluation of blood-to-brain transfer constants from multiple-time uptake data. Generalizations. J Cereb Blood Flow Metab 1985; **5**: 584–90.

101. **Broussolle E, Dentresangle C, Landais P, et al.** The relation of putamen and caudate nucleus 18F-Dopa uptake to motor and cognitive performances in Parkinson's disease. J Neurol Sci 1999; **166**: 141–51.

102. **Rinne JO, Portin R, Ruottinen H, et al.** Cognitive impairment and the brain dopaminergic system in Parkinson disease: [18F]fluorodopa positron emission tomographic study. Arch Neurol 2000; **57**: 470–5.

103. **van Beilen M, Portman AT, Kiers HA, et al.** Striatal FDOPA uptake and cognition in advanced non-demented Parkinson's disease: a clinical and FDOPA-PET study. Parkinsonism Relat Disord 2008; **14**: 224–8.

104. **Ito K, Nagano-Saito A, Kato T, et al.** Striatal and extrastriatal dysfunction in Parkinson's disease with dementia: a 6-[^{18}F]fluoro-L-dopa PET study. Brain 2002; **125**: 1358–65.

105. **Bruck A, Aalto S, Nurmi E, et al.** Cortical 6-[^{18}F]fluoro-L-dopa uptake and frontal cognitive functions in early Parkinson's disease. Neurobiol Aging 2005; **26**: 891–8.

106. **Cropley VL, Fujita M, Bara-Jimenez W, et al.** Pre- and post-synaptic dopamine imaging and its relation with frontostriatal cognitive function in Parkinson disease: PET studies with [^{11}C]NNC 112 and [^{18}F]FDOPA. Psychiatry Res 2008; **163**: 171–82.

107. Hilker R, Thomas AV, Klein JC, et al. Dementia in Parkinson disease: functional imaging of cholinergic and dopaminergic pathways. Neurology 2005; **65**: 1716–22.

108. McKeith I, O'Brien J, Walker Z, et al. Sensitivity and specificity of dopamine transporter imaging with (^{123})I-FP-CIT SPECT in dementia with Lewy bodies: a phase III, multicentre study. Lancet Neurol 2007; **6**: 305–13.

109. O'Brien JT, Colloby S, Fenwick J, et al. Dopamine transporter loss visualized with FP-CIT SPECT in the differential diagnosis of dementia with Lewy bodies. Arch Neurol 2004; **61**: 919–25.

110. Walker Z, Costa DC, Walker RW, et al. Striatal dopamine transporter in dementia with Lewy bodies and Parkinson disease: a comparison. Neurology 2004; **62**: 1568–72.

111. Ehrt U, Broich K, Larsen JP, et al. Use of drugs with anticholinergic effect and impact on cognition in Parkinson's disease: a cohort study. J Neurol Neurosurg Psychiatry 2010; **81**: 160–5.

112. Dubois B, Tolosa E, Katzenschlager R, et al. Donepezil in Parkinson's disease dementia: a randomized, double-blind efficacy and safety study. Mov Disord 2012; **27**: 1230–8.

113. Emre M, Aarsland D, Albanese A, et al. Rivastigmine for dementia associated with Parkinson's disease. N Engl J Med 2004; **351**: 2509–18.

114. Perry E, Walker M, Grace J, et al. Acetylcholine in mind: a neurotransmitter correlate of consciousness? Trends Neurosci 1999; **22**: 273–80.

115. Braak H, Ghebremedhin E, Rub U, et al. Stages in the development of Parkinson's disease-related pathology. Cell Tissue Res 2004; **318**: 121–34.

116. Pahapill PA, Lozano AM. The pedunculopontine nucleus and Parkinson's disease. Brain 2000; **123**: 1767–83.

117. Tiraboschi P, Hansen LA, Alford M, et al. Cholinergic dysfunction in diseases with Lewy bodies. Neurology 2000; **54**: 407–11.

118. Kuhl DE, Minoshima S, Fessler JA, et al. In vivo mapping of cholinergic terminals in normal aging, Alzheimer's disease, and Parkinson's disease. Ann Neurol 1996; **40**: 399–410.

119. Colloby SJ, Pakrasi S, Firbank MJ, et al. In vivo SPECT imaging of muscarinic acetylcholine receptors using (R,R) ^{123}I-QNB in dementia with Lewy bodies and Parkinson's disease dementia. NeuroImage 2006; **33**: 423–9.

120. O'Brien JT, Colloby SJ, Pakrasi S, et al. Nicotinic alpha4beta2 receptor binding in dementia with Lewy bodies using ^{123}I-5IA-85380 SPECT demonstrates a link between occipital changes and visual hallucinations. NeuroImage 2008; **40**: 1056–63.

121. Shimada H, Hirano S, Shinotoh H, et al. Mapping of brain acetylcholinesterase alterations in Lewy body disease by PET. Neurology 2009; **73**: 273–8.

122. Bohnen NI, Kaufer DI, Ivanco LS, et al. Cortical cholinergic function is more severely affected in parkinsonian dementia than in Alzheimer disease: an in vivo positron emission tomographic study. Arch Neurol 2003; **60**: 1745–8.

123. Bohnen NI, Kaufer DI, Hendrickson R, et al. Cognitive correlates of cortical cholinergic denervation in Parkinson's disease and parkinsonian dementia. J Neurol 2006;**253**:242–7.

124. Klunk WE, Engler H, Nordberg A, et al. Imaging brain amyloid in Alzheimer's disease with Pittsburgh Compound-B. Ann Neurol 2004; **55**: 306–19.

125. Mintun MA, Larossa GN, Sheline YI, et al. [^{11}C]PIB in a nondemented population: potential antecedent marker of Alzheimer disease. Neurology 2006; **67**: 446–52.

126. Gomperts SN, Rentz DM, Moran E, et al. Imaging amyloid deposition in Lewy body diseases. Neurology 2008; **71**: 903–10.

127. Edison P, Rowe CC, Rinne JO, et al. Amyloid load in Parkinson's disease dementia and Lewy body dementia measured with [^{11}C]PIB positron emission tomography. J Neurol Neurosurg Psychiatry 2008; **79**: 1331–8.

128. Maetzler W, Reimold M, Liepelt I, et al. [^{11}C]PIB binding in Parkinson's disease dementia. NeuroImage 2008; **39**: 1027–33.

129. **Donaghy P, Thomas AJ, O'Brien JT**. Amyloid PET imaging in Lewy body disorders. Am J Geriatr Psychiatry 2013; doi: 10.1016/j.jagp.2013.03.001

130. **Goldstein DS**. Dysautonomia in Parkinson's disease: neurocardiological abnormalities. Lancet Neurol 2003; **2**: 669–76.

131. **Treglia G, Cason E**. Diagnostic performance of myocardial innervation imaging using MIBG scintigraphy in differential diagnosis between dementia with Lewy bodies and other dementias: a systematic review and a meta-analysis. J Neuroimaging 2012; **22**: 111–17.

132. **Orimo S, Suzuki M, Inaba A, et al**. ^{123}I-MIBG myocardial scintigraphy for differentiating Parkinson's disease from other neurodegenerative parkinsonism: a systematic review and meta-analysis. Parkinsonism Relat Disord 2012; **18**: 494–500.

Chapter 11

Biomarkers for cognitive impairment and dementia in Parkinson's disease

Guido Alves, Kenn Freddy Pedersen,
and Jan Petter Larsen

Introduction

Cognitive impairment is one of the most frequent and disabling non-motor features in Parkinson's disease (PD). Long-term observational studies indicate that up to 80% of PD patients develop dementia (PD-D) [1, 2]. PD-D evolves gradually, and many PD patients report mild cognitive impairment (PD-MCI) years before the onset of PD-D; this signals increased risk for progression to PD-D within 3–4 years, in both early [3] and advanced [4] disease stages.

While impaired episodic memory is the characteristic cognitive feature in patients with incipient Alzheimer's disease (AD) [5], cognitive impairment in PD is more heterogeneous. Several large-scale studies in patients with newly diagnosed PD have revealed mild deficits in various cognitive domains, including attention and executive, memory, and visuospatial function, while language is less affected [6–8]. However, the profile of cognitive deficits in PD varies from patient to patient and may change over the course of the disease [9]. It has been proposed that cognitive deficits with a posterior-cortical basis rather than frontal-executive dysfunction predict subsequent development of dementia [10], yet this view is challenged by several longitudinal studies that also find executive and attentional deficits to herald an increased risk of PD-D [3, 11, 12].

Substantial inter-individual variability is also observed in the onset and progression of cognitive deficits, and the time from onset of motor symptoms to dementia varies considerably between individuals. Longitudinal studies indicate that about 20% of patients with PD develop dementia within 5 years of diagnosis [10], whereas another 20% are still without dementia after 20 years [1].

Biological heterogeneity

The clinical heterogeneity in PD probably reflects variability in the underlying neuropathological and biochemical changes. While loss of dopaminergic neurons in substantia nigra and aggregation of α-synuclein (αSyn) with the formation of Lewy bodies are the pathological hallmarks of PD, the disease is now recognized as a widespread, multisystem brain disorder that may cause multiple transmitter deficits from its very earliest stages. In addition, vascular lesions and AD-type changes, such as amyloid-beta (Aβ) and tau pathologies, are found post mortem in a number of patients with PD-D [13]. These pathologies have been proposed to influence the spread of αSyn and the rate of cognitive decline in PD [13]. The large inter-individual variability in risk and time to PD-D may further be explained by individual differences in the capacity of the brain to tolerate ('cognitive reserve') [14] or counteract these pathologies, for example through activation of the innate immune system or degradation of pathological protein aggregates [15]. Finally, clinical, biochemical and neuropathological heterogeneity in PD may be genetically determined, and several genetic polymorphisms that modify the risk of PD-D have been proposed.

The need for biomarkers

There has been an extensive search for biomarkers that could help to identify patients at risk for developing dementia at an early stage of disease. Such biomarkers would be valuable for better patient management and more efficient recruitment to clinical trials. Biomarkers, if measured repeatedly, could also serve to track cognitive decline and monitor the response to treatment. Finally, biomarkers may provide important insights into the molecular mechanisms driving PD-associated cognitive decline, which could fuel the development of novel preventive agents.

According to the Biomarkers Definitions Working Group, a biomarker is 'a characteristic that is objectively measured and evaluated as an indicator of normal biological processes, pathogenic processes, or pharmacological response to a therapeutic intervention' [16]. The ideal biomarker should reflect 'a fundamental feature of neuropathology, be validated in neuropathologically-confirmed cases, be reliable, reproducible', safe, and easy to measure (non-invasive) at low cost [17]. Importantly, to be useful in clinical practice, a new biomarker should add value to already existing biomarkers and available clinical measures.

Potential sources of biomarkers include different bodily fluids such as cerebrospinal fluid, blood, saliva, or urine. Such biomarkers may be classified as 'wet' biomarkers, in contrast to the 'dry' markers derived from different neuroimaging modalities, such as magnetic resonance imaging (MRI), single-photon emission computed tomography (SPECT), positron emission tomography (PET), or neurophysiological examinations (e.g. an electroencephalogram, EEG). While the dry markers and genetic risk factors are covered in detail in other chapters and will be discussed only briefly here, our main focus will be on the wet biomarkers of cognitive impairment and dementia in PD.

Cerebrospinal fluid markers

Cerebrospinal fluid (CSF) is produced mainly in the choroid plexi of the lateral ventricles from where it circulates through the inner ventricles to the subarachnoid space surrounding the brain and spinal cord. Because of its close proximity to the brain, CSF is considered to be an excellent source of possible biomarkers of neurodegenerative diseases. Not surprisingly, most studies exploring wet cognitive biomarkers in PD have focused on CSF. While untargeted strategies such as proteomics [18, 19] have so far been little applied in the search for such markers, the vast majority of studies have used targeted approaches with a priori defined candidate markers. Most of these candidates were explored because of their key role in the pathogenesis of PD and PD-D, as evidenced by clinico-pathological or genetic association studies.

α-Synuclein

αSyn is a small (14 kDa) protein that is expressed in different tissues, but most abundantly in the brain [20] where it primarily localizes to pre-synaptic terminals and is thought to be involved in vesicular trafficking and release; however, its detailed physiological functions are not fully understood [20]. αSyn has been considered as an attractive candidate biomarker ever since linkage studies revealed that mutations and multiplications in *SNCA*, the gene encoding αSyn, cause rare familial forms of young-onset PD [21]. These *SNCA* mutations alter the function of the protein and promote its oligomerization, fibrillization, and aggregation into Lewy bodies and

Lewy neurites [20], which mainly contain αSyn that has been post-translationally modified (e.g. phosphorylated) [22]. The interest in αSyn as a diagnostic biomarker has been further fuelled by genome-wide association studies demonstrating strong associations between the *SNCA* locus and sporadic PD with a more typical age at disease onset [23]. Finally, most clinico-pathological studies find a higher burden of Lewy bodies and αSyn to be strongly correlated with PD-D [13], indicating that αSyn in CSF could be a promising biomarker for cognitive impairment in PD.

The vast majority of CSF studies so far have focused on the potential of αSyn to discriminate PD from other neurodegenerative disorders or the healthy state [24]. Most studies have measured the content of total αSyn using (different) enzyme-linked immunosorbent assay (ELISA) techniques, whereas a few groups have also investigated other forms, such as oligomeric or phosphorylated αSyn [24]. A meta-analysis from 2013 of 18 independent CSF studies showed that total αSyn levels are reduced in PD compared with controls [25]. However, these reductions were mild in the majority of studies, with considerable overlap between diagnostic groups and thus insufficient diagnostic accuracy [24]. Less overlap has been observed for oligomeric αSyn and its ratio to total αSyn, with higher levels in PD patients than controls [26]. Most studies report no or only weak correlations of CSF αSyn levels with clinical measures of motor impairment or disease stage [24]. These observations, together with findings of lowered total αSyn CSF levels in drug-naïve, incident patients [27], may indicate that slight alterations in CSF αSyn occur early (before motor onset) but with no or only small changes during the symptomatic phase of PD. Longitudinal studies with repeated CSF measurements would be needed to clarify this issue.

Despite strong pathological evidence pointing towards a significant role of αSyn in the pathogenesis of PD-D, relatively few studies have investigated the association of CSF αSyn with neuropsychological measures or cognitive state (e.g. PD-MCI and PD-D). At least two cross-sectional CSF studies observed no differences in total αSyn levels between dementia with Lewy bodies (DLB), PD-D, and PD without dementia [28, 29]. Two other studies investigated patients with de novo PD, and found no association between total αSyn levels in CSF and neuropsychological measures or presence/absence of PD-MCI [27, 30]. One of these studies, however, reported lowered total αSyn concentrations in the CSF of patients who presented with the postural instability and gait disturbance (PIGD) subtype [27]. This finding is of interest, since this motor phenotype has previously been reported to indicate an increased risk for PD-D compared with the more benign tremor-dominant variant [31, 32]. No longitudinal studies investigating the association between αSyn, including oligomeric or post-translationally modified forms, and subsequent cognitive decline and PD-D risk have been published to date.

Amyloid-beta

Aβ peptides are derived by cleavage of the amyloid precursor protein (APP) and are the main constituents of the neuritic plaques that are characteristic of AD [5]. Amyloid plaques are particularly rich in Aβ peptides with a length of 42 amino acids (Aβ42), which are prone to aggregate [5]. Aβ42 is abundant in CSF and low levels of Aβ42 in the CSF are inversely correlated with plaque pathology post mortem [33] and in vivo [34], as assessed by amyloid PET. It is well established that reductions in Aβ42 can be seen in the CSF many years before related cognitive symptoms emerge [35], and CSF Aβ42, along with Aβ brain imaging, has recently been incorporated in diagnostic research guidelines to define the pre-clinical stages of AD [36].

In AD, the concentration of Aβ42 in the CSF is usually decreased by about 50% compared with the levels in normal controls [5]. Still, reductions in CSF Aβ42 are not entirely specific to AD as altered levels can be found in other diseases in which aggregation and deposition of Aβ is observed, such as Lewy body disorders. These include DLB (development of dementia within 1 year of motor onset) and PD with or without dementia. Across this spectrum, Aβ pathology is most frequently observed in DLB, followed by patients with PD-D and PD without dementia [37–39]. A number of studies show a similar pattern in CSF, with the most extensive reductions in Aβ42 found in DLB, followed by moderate reductions in PD-D, and mostly mild changes in PD without dementia [40–46], including patients with incident PD [27, 30, 47], compared with normal controls.

Although the burden of cortical Lewy bodies is a strong correlate of PD-D, some autopsy studies report that a combination of Lewy body and AD pathologies is a more robust correlate of PD-D than any single pathology alone [48]. In addition, several clinico-pathological studies indicate that concomitant Aβ pathology may accelerate the spread of Lewy body pathology and the rate of cognitive decline in PD, resulting in a shorter time to PD-D [38, 39, 49]. Therefore, an increasing number of studies have focused on more detailed assessments of PD patients without dementia (Table 11.1). In some studies significant, but usually modest, correlations between CSF Aβ42 and executive function [42], verbal [47] or visual [30] memory, or processing speed [50] were observed, whereas others [27] found no correlations with neuropsychological measures. The association between CSF Aβ and PD-MCI has been little studied, although one recent study in de novo PD reported lower levels of CSF Aβ42 and Aβ40 in PD-MCI compared with PD patients with normal cognition [30]. Another study in de novo PD patients [47] also reported significant reductions in CSF Aβ40 and Aβ38 compared with normal controls, which may reflect production of Aβ rather than deposition [51]. Significant correlations were also found between Aβ levels, ventricular enlargement [52], and PIGD subtype [53], both known risk factors for PD-D. The association between lowered CSF Aβ concentrations and PIGD subtype was replicated in another study in incident PD [27]. Overall, these cross-sectional observations from de novo PD patients link early reductions in CSF Aβ to a clinical profile that heralds an increased risk for PD-D.

There is limited, but so far consistent, evidence from longitudinal studies to support the prognostic value of CSF Aβ42 in PD (Table 11.1). One study with 1–3 years of follow-up found significantly more rapid cognitive decline, as measured by the Mattis Dementia Rating Scale (DRS-2), in patients with low baseline levels of CSF Aβ42, independent of age, disease duration, and baseline cognitive status [54]. Another small study found significantly decreased baseline CSF Aβ42 levels in PD patients without dementia who converted to PD-D during 18 months of follow-up, compared with those who remained without dementia [55]. These findings were replicated and extended in a 5-year longitudinal study that followed a larger cohort of patients with incident PD and quantified CSF Aβ42 at diagnosis using two different detection methods at two different laboratories. Regardless of the detection method, low Aβ42 levels predicted early onset PD-D at high sensitivity (≥85%), independent of age and cognitive status at baseline [56]. Additional longitudinal studies in large cohorts and with long-term follow-up are, however, required to further validate these findings.

Tau

Tau is a 68-kDa microtubule-associated protein important for cell stability and axonal transport in neurons [5]. Tau exists in several isoforms and may be phosphorylated at numerous sites. Tangles characteristic of AD are composed of hyperphosphorylated tau [5]. Concentrations of total tau (t-tau) as well as phosphorylated tau (p-tau) can be measured in CSF. Levels of t-tau in CSF are increased about three-fold in AD compared with normal controls [5]. However, similar elevations in CSF t-tau concentrations may be seen after stroke and traumatic brain injury [57], and even

Table 11.1 Cross-sectional and longitudinal studies assessing the associations of CSF biomarkers with neuropsychological performance or dementia risk in PD patients

Authors	*n*	Setting	αSyn	Aβ42	Tau/p-tau	Comments
Cross-sectional studies:						
Compta et al. [42]	20	Clinic-based	NA	Phonemic fluency	0/0	Increased t-tau and p-tau values associated with impaired verbal learning and naming in PD-D
Alves et al. [47]	109	Population-based, de novo	NA	Verbal memory	0/0	Verbal memory also correlated with Aβ40 and Aβ38 levels
Leverenz et al. [50]	22	Clinic-based	NA	Processing speed	0/0	Correlation lost after adjustment for age
Kang et al. [27]	63	Clinic-based, de novo	0	0	0/0	First results from Parkinson's Progression Markers Initiative
Yarnall et al. [30]	67	Clinic-based, incident	0	Visual memory	0/0	Aβ42 correlated with Montreal Cognitive Assessment Score; lower Aβ42 and Aβ40 in PD-MCI than PD with normal cognition
Longitudinal studies:						
Siderowf et al. [54]	45	Clinic-based, 19 months' follow-up	NA	↑ cognitive decline (DRS-2)	0/0	Largest effect size for decline in attention subscale of DRS-2; no association between CSF markers and baseline DRS-2 scores; low baseline Aβ42 levels in APOE e4 carriers
Compta et al. [55]	27	Clinic-based, 18 months' follow-up	NA	↑ PD-D risk	0/0	Low baseline Aβ42 predicted limbic and posterior-cortical neuropsychological decline as well as frontal, limbic and posterior-cortical thinning on MRI

Table 11.1 (continued) Cross-sectional and longitudinal studies assessing the associations of CSF biomarkers with neuropsychological performance or dementia risk in PD patients

Authors	n	Setting	αSyn	Aβ42	Tau/p-tau	Comments
Alves et al. [56]	104	Population-based, incident cohort, 60 months' follow-up	NA	↑ PDD risk	0/0	Baseline Aβ42 levels measured by two analytic methods and at two different laboratories; low Aβ42 levels predicted PD-D at high sensitivity (≥85%) and independently of age and cognitive status at baseline; no association of baseline Aβ40 or Aβ38 levels with PD-D risk

PD-D, Parkinson's disease dementia; PD-MCI, Parkinson's disease with mild cognitive impairment; NA, not assessed; 0, no significant correlation with cognitive measures (cross-sectional studies) or association with PD-D risk (longitudinal studies); DRS-2, Mattis Dementia Rating Scale.

higher values are found in rapidly progressing neurodegenerative disorders such as Creutzfeld–Jakob disease [58]. Hence, t-tau is considered as a rather non-specific CSF marker of neuronal cell loss. Increased CSF p-tau levels, in contrast, appear to be more closely related to tangle pathology and are therefore a more specific marker for AD.

Neuronal loss and tangle pathology may be found in the brains of patients with PD-D and DLB but are usually less extensive and severe than in AD [13]. In agreement with this, CSF tau proteins have been shown to be valuable in distinguishing AD from the synucleinopathies, particularly in combination with other CSF markers [29, 45, 59].

In PD, the association of CSF tau protein levels with cognition has been investigated extensively, mainly by cross-sectional studies. Most of these studies show normal or even decreased levels of CSF tau in patients without dementia, including individuals with de novo PD and PD-MCI [27, 30, 47]. Results are more inconsistent in patients with PD-D, although several groups reported mild to moderately increased t-tau levels in PD-D relative to PD without dementia and normal controls [40–42]. In PD-D, but not in PD without dementia, CSF levels of t-tau and p-tau have been shown to correlate with neuropsychological deficits indicating dysfunction of the posterior cortex [42]. Combined, these findings could indicate that tau levels—at least in some patients—may increase with progressive cognitive decline in PD; however, these changes appear to occur later than those observed for CSF Aβ. Indeed, while Aβ42 predicted PD-D in the few longitudinal studies conducted so far this was not the case for tau proteins [54–56]. Longitudinal studies with repeated CSF measures would be valuable to clarify the trajectories of CSF tau proteins in relation to cognitive changes in PD.

Other CSF biomarker candidates

There are a number of other candidates that might be of interest as cognitive biomarkers in PD. Genetic and molecular studies point towards several partly interrelated pathways that may directly or indirectly drive the abnormal protein accumulation and neurodegeneration observed in PD, such as impaired protein degradation, mitochondrial dysfunction, oxidative stress, and neuroinflammation [15]. Given the central pathogenic role of αSyn, and probably Aβ, pathology in cognitive impairment related to PD, CSF markers that reflect these pathways appear particularly promising and have been increasingly explored. However, few studies have investigated these markers with specific focus on their relation to cognitive impairment in PD.

Markers of protein degradation

Impaired protein degradation by the ubiquitin–proteosome system, the autophagy–lysosomal pathway, and possibly other proteolytic systems, is considered to contribute to the pathological cascade leading to accumulation of αSyn in PD [13, 60]. Indeed, differences between PD patients and controls in activity levels of several lysosomal enzymes in the CSF have been reported in cross-sectional studies [61, 62]. However, associations with cognitive measures or state were not explored. Another study found significantly reduced levels of neurosin, an enzyme proposed to be involved in the cleavage of extracellular αSyn [63], in patients with synucleinopathies compared with controls and AD, with the lowest levels observed in subjects with DLB [28]. However, no differences were seen between PD-D patients versus PD without dementia, questioning its utility as cognitive marker in PD.

Markers of Aβ production and clearance

CSF markers that reflect the production or clearance of Aβ have been extensively studied in AD. Some have had promising results, such as the β-site APP cleaving enzyme-1 (BACE1) [64] and neprilysin [65], an Aβ-degrading protein found at pre-synaptic terminals. Lowered levels of activity of neprilysin in the CSF of patients with DLB and PD-D compared with PD without dementia and normal controls have been reported in one cross-sectional study [66], but no longitudinal studies have yet been published. Visinin-like protein-1 (VILIP-1), a marker of neuronal injury, has also been shown to predict the rate of cognitive decline in cognitively normal individuals and those with very mild and mild AD [67, 68], but has not been investigated in PD.

Oxidative stress markers

Mitochondrial dysfunction and oxidative stress have been implicated in the pathogenesis of PD. DJ-1 is a multifunctional protein that is involved in mitochondrial regulation and protection against oxidative stress. Studies of DJ-1 in the CSF are inconsistent, showing either reduced [69] or elevated [70] levels in PD compared with controls, and have not explored possible associations with cognitive impairment in PD. CSF levels of 8-hydroxy-2′-deoxyguanosine (8-OHdG), a marker of oxidative stress, have been reported by several groups to be elevated in PD. One of these also reported an inverse correlation of this marker with Mini-Mental State Examination scores in PD-D but no significant differences in levels of 8-OHdG in the CSF of PD-D, DLB, and AD patients [71].

Neuroinflammatory markers

Neuroinflammatory changes including microglial activation are thought to play an important role in many neurodegenerative diseases, including PD [72]. Microglial activation has potential beneficial effects by clearing aggregates of pathological protein and remodelling synapses, but may also damage neurons through the release of cytokines, proteases, and nitric oxide [72, 73]. Hence, inter-individual differences in microglial activation may have an impact on the spread of pathology [73], and therefore the rate of cognitive decline and risk for dementia in PD. Cross-sectional correlations of several inflammatory CSF markers, such as tumour necrosis factor-alpha (TNF-α)

[74] and brain-derived neurotrophic factor (BDNF) [50], with cognition have been described in PD but await further replication and exploration in longitudinal studies.

Markers in other bodily fluids

In addition to markers in CSF, several other bodily fluids may provide potential markers for cognitive impairment and dementia in PD. These include plasma, serum, saliva, and urine. Examination of these fluids may be more practical, less expensive, or less stressful for patients. However, these fluids are more prone to be confounded by factors introduced by other organ systems and may therefore be considered as less attractive than CSF for the identification of cognitive biomarkers in PD. The number of studies examining these bodily fluids is still limited, yet some interesting candidates have been identified.

For example, lowered serum levels of uric acid, a potent antioxidant, have been associated with increased risk for PD in the general population and more rapid clinical decline in patients with symptomatic PD [75]. One group also reported potential associations of serum and urine levels of uric acid with neuropsychological impairment in a small PD cohort [76, 77]. Another, probably even more promising, observation comes from a longitudinal study that examined 102 plasma proteins and their association with cognitive performance in PD, as measured by DRS-2. Baseline cognitive performance correlated with concentrations of 11 plasma proteins, of which epidermal growth factor (EGF) was identified as the strongest candidate. Importantly, low levels of EGF also predicted an eight-fold greater risk for progression to dementia during follow-up [78]. This finding has been replicated in part in a more recent study that found serum EGF levels in early PD to correlate with frontal and temporal cognitive functioning and to predict cognitive performance after 2 years of follow-up [79]. However, additional longitudinal studies are needed to further validate these findings.

Genetic risk markers

Several epidemiological studies have shown an increased risk of PD-D or AD in first-degree relatives of patients with PD [80, 81], suggesting a possible role for genetic factors in PD-D. Indeed, research has revealed several genetic polymorphisms that have been proposed to influence cognitive function or dementia risk in PD.

Apolipoprotein E (APOE)

The co-manifestation of AD and PD in families has led to the hypothesis of shared susceptibility genes, such as the apolipoprotein E (*APOE*) gene [82]. The *APOE* gene is located on chromosome 19q13.2 and has three major alleles designated ε2, ε3, and ε4. The ε4 variant is associated with an increased risk and possibly lower age at onset of AD [83]. In PD, evidence for an association between the ε4 variant and dementia risk is less clear. Longitudinal studies show inconstant findings on the impact of ε4 carrier status on the rate of cognitive decline [84–86]. However, a large meta-analysis conducted in 2009 found a modest overrepresentation of ε4 carriers in PD-D versus PD without dementia [85]. In keeping with this, studies in autopsy-confirmed cases suggest that the ε4 allele increases the risk of dementia across the spectrum of Lewy body diseases, including PD-D [87, 88].

Microtubule-associated protein tau (MAPT)

The *MAPT* gene encodes tau and is located on chromosome 17q21.1. It has two major haplotypes, H1 and H2. The H1/H1 genotype has been associated with increased risk for several neurodegenerative disorders, including PD [89]. Furthermore, two studies found the H1/H1 genotype to be strongly associated with increased risk for PD-D [90, 91], and a synergistic interaction between the H1/H1 genotype and a specific SNCA polymorphism on PD-D risk was reported in one of these studies [90]. However, no association between H1/H1 genotype and PD-D was found in a large clinico-pathological study [88].

Glucocerebrosidase (GBA)

The *GBA* gene is located on chromosome 1q21 and encodes the lysosomal enzyme beta-glucocerebrosidase. Homozygous mutations in *GBA* cause the lysosomal storage disorder Gaucher's disease. During recent years, heterozygous *GBA* mutations have emerged as the most common genetic risk factor for PD [92, 93], affecting 4–7% of patients with the disease. Moreover, *GBA*-linked PD has also been associated with increased risk and earlier onset of dementia compared with PD patients without *GBA* mutations [93, 94]. A recent autopsy study reported glucocerebrosidase deficits to be associated with increased levels of αSyn even in sporadic PD without *GBA* mutations [95]. This supports the notion that in the general PD population dysfunctional lysosomal pathways may contribute to increased deposition and cortical spreading of αSyn, which has been linked to PD-D [13].

Cathecol-O-methyltransferase (COMT)

The *COMT* gene is located on chromosome 22q11.21 and encodes an enzyme that is involved in the catabolism of monoamines, including dopamine. In PD, the *COMT* Val158Met functional polymorphism has been proposed to be associated with frontal-executive deficits but not with incidence of dementia [10]. Similar findings have been described by another group [86], while a third study observed no direct effect of *COMT* Val158Met genotype on attention or executive function in PD [96].

Neuroimaging markers

Although a detailed discussion of neuroimaging and neurophysiological markers is beyond the scope of this chapter, we want to point out that increasing evidence supports the potential usefulness of structural MRI [97], SPECT [98], PET [99], or quantitative EEG [100] in predicting cognitive decline and dementia in PD (see Chapter 10). These techniques are considered attractive because they are not very invasive and can be combined with neuropsychological measures or wet biomarkers in order to optimize prognostic accuracy. Indeed, one recent longitudinal study demonstrated that baseline abnormalities in three different modalities (CSF Aβ42, volumetric MRI, neuropsychological impairment) combined separated perfectly PD patients who did or did not develop PD-D during 18 months of follow-up [55]. Despite the small cohort and short follow-up, these findings are encouraging for future research and support the notion that combining biomarkers from different modalities is superior to single measures in predicting PD-D.

Conclusion

This review shows that considerable efforts have been made to identify cognitive biomarkers in PD. A range of biochemical markers are now available that are thought to reflect key mechanisms in the pathogenesis of PD-D. However, although several promising markers have been identified, findings have not been replicated or are inconsistent for the vast majority of candidates. This lack of consistency may be due to a number of reasons from bench to bedside, including variability in pre-analytical or analytical procedures, patient characteristics, range and choice of cognitive tests, and definitions of PD-MCI and PD-D. This hampers the comparability of studies, and also the possibility for collaboration between different study sites. The harmonization of laboratory and clinical procedures will be important for the translation from biomarker discovery to validation and eventually use in clinical routine.

In addition to variability in pre-clinical and clinical procedures, the scarcity of prospective longitudinal studies for the majority of explored markers represents another major limitation in the search for clinically useful cognitive biomarkers in PD. Indeed, because current evidence on cognitive biomarkers is dominated by cross-sectional studies, the predictive value of most markers is unknown.

The slowly progressive nature of the disease and the substantial biological and clinical heterogeneity per se make the search for biomarkers in PD challenging. For example, some patients develop dementia within a couple of years of diagnosis whereas others remain cognitively normal for more than two decades. For these reasons, large-scale studies that follow patients over a long period of time, ideally from diagnosis to death, are needed. In such studies, repeated assessment of biomarkers is desirable, not only in the search for markers that may help to track cognitive decline but also because changes in biomarkers over time might be a more powerful predictor of subsequent progression to dementia. However, such studies are difficult to perform at single centres and demand collaboration between multiple study sites and possibly countries. One important example of such a multicentre international cooperation is the Parkinson's Progression Markers Initiative [27].

Finally, the genetics, neuropathology, and biochemistry underlying cognitive changes in PD are complex and therefore best covered by combined assessments of multiple biomarkers from different modalities. These could be further combined with genetic, demographic, and clinical risk factors in order to identify those patients at highest risk for PD-D as early as possible during the course of their disease (Fig. 11.1). This would not only be important for patient management and efficient recruitment to clinical trials testing therapies to prevent PD-D, but also for timely initiation of such treatments once they become available in the future.

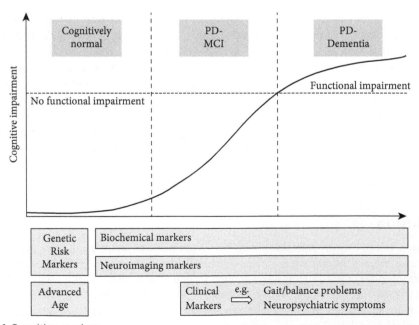

Fig. 11.1 Cognition markers.

References

1. **Hely MA, Reid WG, Adena MA, et al.** The Sydney multicenter study of Parkinson's disease: the inevitability of dementia at 20 years. Mov Disord 2008; **23**: 837–44.

2. **Aarsland D, Andersen K, Larsen JP, et al.** Prevalence and characteristics of dementia in Parkinson disease: an 8-year prospective study. Arch Neurol 2003; **60**: 387–92.

3. **Pedersen KF, Larsen JP, Tysnes OB, et al.** Prognosis of Mild Cognitive Impairment in Early Parkinson Disease: The Norwegian ParkWest Study. J Am Med Assoc Neurol 2013; **70**: 580–6.

4. **Janvin CC, Larsen JP, Aarsland D, et al.** Subtypes of mild cognitive impairment in Parkinson's disease: progression to dementia. Mov Disord 2006; **21**: 1343–9.

5. **Blennow K, de Leon MJ, Zetterberg H.** Alzheimer's disease. Lancet 2006; **368**: 387–403.

6. **Aarsland D, Bronnick K, Larsen JP, et al.** Cognitive impairment in incident, untreated Parkinson disease: the Norwegian ParkWest study. Neurology 2009; **72**: 1121–6.

7. **Elgh E, Domellof M, Linder J, et al.** Cognitive function in early Parkinson's disease: a population-based study. Eur J Neurol 2009; **16**: 1278–84.

8. **Muslimovic D, Post B, Speelman JD, et al.** Cognitive profile of patients with newly diagnosed Parkinson disease. Neurology 2005; **65**: 1239–45.

9. **Kehagia AA, Barker RA, Robbins TW.** Neuropsychological and clinical heterogeneity of cognitive impairment and dementia in patients with Parkinson's disease. Lancet Neurol 2010; **9**: 1200–13.

10. **Williams-Gray CH, Evans JR, Goris A, et al.** The distinct cognitive syndromes of Parkinson's disease: 5 year follow-up of the CamPaIGN cohort. Brain 2009; **132**: 2958–69.

11. **Levy G, Jacobs DM, Tang MX, et al.** Memory and executive function impairment predict dementia in Parkinson's disease. Mov Disord 2002; **17**: 1221–6.

12. **Woods SP, Troster AI.** Prodromal frontal/executive dysfunction predicts incident dementia in Parkinson's disease. J Int Neuropsychol Soc 2003; **9**: 17–24.

13. **Irwin DJ, Lee VM, Trojanowski JQ.** Parkinson's disease dementia: convergence of alpha-synuclein, tau and amyloid-beta pathologies. Nat Rev Neurosci 2013; **14**: 626–36.

14. **Hindle JV, Martyr A, Clare L.** Cognitive reserve in Parkinson's disease: a systematic review and meta-analysis. Parkinsonism Relat Disord 2014; **20**: 1–7.

15. **Schapira AH, Jenner P.** Etiology and pathogenesis of Parkinson's disease. Mov Disord 2011; **26**: 1049–55.

16. **Biomarkers Definitions Working Group.** Biomarkers and surrogate endpoints: preferred definitions and conceptual framework. Clin Pharmacol Therapeut 2001; **69**: 89–95.

17. Consensus report of the Working Group on: 'Molecular and biochemical markers of Alzheimer's disease'. The Ronald and Nancy Reagan Research Institute of the Alzheimer's Association and the National Institute on Aging Working Group. Neurobiol Aging 1998; **19**: 109–16.

18. **Jesse S, Lehnert S, Jahn O, et al.** Differential sialylation of serpin A1 in the early diagnosis of Parkinson's disease dementia. PLoS ONE 2012; **7**: e48783.

19. **Lehnert S, Jesse S, Rist W, et al.** iTRAQ and multiple reaction monitoring as proteomic tools for biomarker search in cerebrospinal fluid of patients with Parkinson's disease dementia. Exp Neurol 2012; **234**: 499–505.

20. **George S, Rey NL, Reichenbach N, et al.** Alpha-synuclein: the long distance runner. Brain Pathol 2013; **23**: 350–7.

21. **Polymeropoulos MH, Lavedan C, Leroy E, et al.** Mutation in the alpha-synuclein gene identified in families with Parkinson's disease. Science 1997; **276**: 2045–7.

22. **Fujiwara H, Hasegawa M, Dohmae N, et al.** Alpha-synuclein is phosphorylated in synucleinopathy lesions. Nat Cell Biol 2002; **4**: 160–4.

23. **Edwards TL, Scott WK, Almonte C, et al.** Genome-wide association study confirms SNPs in SNCA and the MAPT region as common risk factors for Parkinson disease. Ann Hum Genet 2010; **74**: 97–109.

24. Parnetti L, Castrioto A, Chiasserini D, et al. Cerebrospinal fluid biomarkers in Parkinson disease. Nat Rev Neurol 2013; **9**: 131–40.

25. Zetterberg H, Petzold M, Magdalinou N. Cerebrospinal fluid alpha-synuclein levels in Parkinson's disease—changed or unchanged? Eur J Neurol 2014; **21**: 365–7.

26. Tokuda T, Qureshi MM, Ardah MT, et al. Detection of elevated levels of alpha-synuclein oligomers in CSF from patients with Parkinson disease. Neurology 2010; **75**: 1766–72.

27. Kang JH, Irwin DJ, Chen-Plotkin AS, et al. Association of cerebrospinal fluid beta-amyloid 1–42, t-tau, p-tau181, and alpha-synuclein levels with clinical features of drug-naive patients with early Parkinson disease. J Am Med Assoc Neurol 2013; **70**: 1277–87.

28. Wennstrom M, Surova Y, Hall S, et al. Low CSF levels of both alpha-synuclein and the alpha-synuclein cleaving enzyme neurosin in patients with synucleinopathy. PLoS ONE 2013; **8**: e53250.

29. Hall S, Ohrfelt A, Constantinescu R, et al. Accuracy of a panel of 5 cerebrospinal fluid biomarkers in the differential diagnosis of patients with dementia and/or parkinsonian disorders. Arch Neurol 2012; **69**: 1445–52.

30. Yarnall AJ, Breen DP, Duncan GW, et al. Characterizing mild cognitive impairment in incident Parkinson disease: the ICICLE-PD Study. Neurology 2014; **82**: 308–16.

31. Alves G, Larsen JP, Emre M, et al. Changes in motor subtype and risk for incident dementia in Parkinson's disease. Mov Disord 2006; **21**: 1123–30.

32. Burn DJ, Rowan EN, Allan LM, et al. Motor subtype and cognitive decline in Parkinson's disease, Parkinson's disease with dementia, and dementia with Lewy bodies. J Neurol Neurosurg Psychiatry 2006; **77**: 585–9.

33. Strozyk D, Blennow K, White LR, et al. CSF Abeta 42 levels correlate with amyloid-neuropathology in a population-based autopsy study. Neurology 2003; **60**: 652–6.

34. Fagan AM, Mintun MA, Mach RH, et al. Inverse relation between in vivo amyloid imaging load and cerebrospinal fluid Abeta42 in humans. Ann Neurol 2006; **59**: 512–19.

35. Jack CR, Jr, Knopman DS, Jagust WJ, et al. Tracking pathophysiological processes in Alzheimer's disease: an updated hypothetical model of dynamic biomarkers. Lancet Neurol 2013; **12**: 207–16.

36. Sperling RA, Aisen PS, Beckett LA, et al. Toward defining the preclinical stages of Alzheimer's disease: recommendations from the National Institute on Aging–Alzheimer's Association workgroups on diagnostic guidelines for Alzheimer's disease. Alzheimers Dement 2011; **7**: 280–92.

37. Jellinger KA, Attems J. Prevalence and impact of vascular and Alzheimer pathologies in Lewy body disease. Acta Neuropathol 2008; **115**: 427–36.

38. Ballard C, Ziabreva I, Perry R, et al. Differences in neuropathologic characteristics across the Lewy body dementia spectrum. Neurology 2006; **67**: 1931–4.

39. Halliday G, Hely M, Reid W, et al. The progression of pathology in longitudinally followed patients with Parkinson's disease. Acta Neuropathol 2008; **115**: 409–15.

40. Mollenhauer B, Trenkwalder C, von Ahsen N, et al. Beta-amlyoid 1–42 and tau-protein in cerebrospinal fluid of patients with Parkinson's disease dementia. Dement Geriatr Cogn Disord 2006; **22**: 200–8.

41. Parnetti L, Tiraboschi P, Lanari A, et al. Cerebrospinal fluid biomarkers in Parkinson's disease with dementia and dementia with Lewy bodies. Biol Psychiatry 2008; **64**: 850–5.

42. Compta Y, Marti MJ, Ibarretxe-Bilbao N, et al. Cerebrospinal tau, phospho-tau, and beta-amyloid and neuropsychological functions in Parkinson's disease. Mov Disord 2009; **24**: 2203–10.

43. Montine TJ, Shi M, Quinn JF, et al. CSF Abeta(42) and tau in Parkinson's disease with cognitive impairment. Mov Disord 2010; **25**: 2682–5.

44. Mulugeta E, Londos E, Ballard C, et al. CSF amyloid beta38 as a novel diagnostic marker for dementia with Lewy bodies. J Neurol Neurosurg Psychiatry 2011; **82**: 160–4.

45. Parnetti L, Chiasserini D, Bellomo G, et al. Cerebrospinal fluid tau/alpha-synuclein ratio in Parkinson's disease and degenerative dementias. Mov Disord 2011; **26**: 1428–35.

46. Andersson M, Zetterberg H, Minthon L, et al. The cognitive profile and CSF biomarkers in dementia with Lewy bodies and Parkinson's disease dementia. Int J Geriatr Psychiatry 2011; **26**: 100–5.

47. Alves G, Bronnick K, Aarsland D, et al. CSF amyloid-beta and tau proteins, and cognitive performance, in early and untreated Parkinson's disease: the Norwegian ParkWest study. J Neurol Neurosurg Psychiatry 2010; **81**: 1080–6.

48. Compta Y, Parkkinen L, O'Sullivan SS, et al. Lewy- and Alzheimer-type pathologies in Parkinson's disease dementia: which is more important? Brain 2011; **134**: 1493–505.

49. Pletnikova O, West N, Lee MK, et al. Abeta deposition is associated with enhanced cortical alpha-synuclein lesions in Lewy body diseases. Neurobiol Aging 2005; **26**: 1183–92.

50. Leverenz JB, Watson GS, Shofer J, et al. Cerebrospinal fluid biomarkers and cognitive performance in non-demented patients with Parkinson's disease. Parkinsonism Relat Disord 2011; **17**: 61–4.

51. Andreasson U, Portelius E, Andersson ME, et al. Aspects of β-amyloid as a biomarker for Alzheimer's disease. Biomark Med 2007; **1**: 59–78.

52. Beyer MK, Alves G, Hwang KS, et al. Cerebrospinal fluid Abeta levels correlate with structural brain changes in Parkinson's disease. Mov Disord 2013; **28**: 302–10.

53. Alves G, Pedersen KF, Bloem BR, et al. Cerebrospinal fluid amyloid-beta and phenotypic heterogeneity in de novo Parkinson's disease. J Neurol Neurosurg Psychiatry 2013; **84**: 537–43.

54. Siderowf A, Xie SX, Hurtig H, et al. CSF amyloid β 1–42 predicts cognitive decline in Parkinson disease. Neurology 2010; **75**: 1055–61.

55. Compta Y, Pereira JB, Rios J, et al. Combined dementia-risk biomarkers in Parkinson's disease: a prospective longitudinal study. Parkinsonism Relat Disord 2013; **19**: 717–24.

56. Alves G, Lange J, Blennow K, et al. Cerebrospinal fluid Aβ42 predicts early onset dementia in Parkinson disease. Neurology 2014; **82**: 1784–90.

57. Ost M, Nylen K, Csajbok L, et al. Initial CSF total tau correlates with 1-year outcome in patients with traumatic brain injury. Neurology 2006; **67**: 1600–4.

58. Van Everbroeck B, Quoilin S, Boons J, et al. A prospective study of CSF markers in 250 patients with possible Creutzfeldt–Jakob disease. J Neurol Neurosurg Psychiatry 2003; **74**: 1210–14.

59. Mollenhauer B, Locascio JJ, Schulz-Schaeffer W, et al. Alpha-synuclein and tau concentrations in cerebrospinal fluid of patients presenting with parkinsonism: a cohort study. Lancet Neurol 2011; **10**: 230–40.

60. Xilouri M, Brekk OR, Stefanis L. Alpha-synuclein and protein degradation systems: a reciprocal relationship. Mol Neurobiol 2013; **47**: 537–51.

61. Balducci C, Pierguidi L, Persichetti E, et al. Lysosomal hydrolases in cerebrospinal fluid from subjects with Parkinson's disease. Mov Disord 2007; **22**: 1481–4.

62. van Dijk KD, Persichetti E, Chiasserini D, et al. Changes in endolysosomal enzyme activities in cerebrospinal fluid of patients with Parkinson's disease. Mov Disord 2013; **28**: 747–54.

63. Tatebe H, Watanabe Y, Kasai T, et al. Extracellular neurosin degrades alpha-synuclein in cultured cells. Neurosci Res 2010; **67**: 341–6.

64. Zetterberg H, Andreasson U, Hansson O, et al. Elevated cerebrospinal fluid BACE1 activity in incipient Alzheimer disease. Arch Neurol 2008; **65**: 1102–7.

65. Maruyama M, Higuchi M, Takaki Y, et al. Cerebrospinal fluid neprilysin is reduced in prodromal Alzheimer's disease. Ann Neurol 2005; **57**: 832–42.

66. Maetzler W, Stoycheva V, Schmid B, et al. Neprilysin activity in cerebrospinal fluid is associated with dementia and amyloid-beta42 levels in Lewy body disease. J Alzheimers Dis 2010; **22**: 933–8.

67. Tarawneh R, D'Angelo G, Macy E, et al. Visinin-like protein-1: diagnostic and prognostic biomarker in Alzheimer disease. Ann Neurol 2011; **70**: 274–85.

68. Tarawneh R, Lee JM, Ladenson JH, et al. CSF VILIP-1 predicts rates of cognitive decline in early Alzheimer disease. Neurology 2012; **78**: 709–19.

69. Hong Z, Shi M, Chung KA, et al. DJ-1 and alpha-synuclein in human cerebrospinal fluid as biomarkers of Parkinson's disease. Brain 2010; **133**: 713–26.

70. Waragai M, Wei J, Fujita M, et al. Increased level of DJ-1 in the cerebrospinal fluids of sporadic Parkinson's disease. Biochem Biophys Res Commun 2006; **345**: 967–72.

71. Gmitterova K, Heinemann U, Gawinecka J, et al. 8-OHdG in cerebrospinal fluid as a marker of oxidative stress in various neurodegenerative diseases. Neurodegener Dis 2009; **6**: 263–9.

72. Phani S, Loike JD, Przedborski S. Neurodegeneration and inflammation in Parkinson's disease. Parkinsonism Relat Disord 2012; **18**: S207–S209.

73. Halliday GM, Stevens CH. Glia: initiators and progressors of pathology in Parkinson's disease. Mov Disord 2011; **26**: 6–17.

74. Menza M, Dobkin RD, Marin H, et al. The role of inflammatory cytokines in cognition and other non-motor symptoms of Parkinson's disease. Psychosomatics 2010; **51**: 474–9.

75. Cipriani S, Chen X, Schwarzschild MA. Urate: a novel biomarker of Parkinson's disease risk, diagnosis and prognosis. Biomark Med 2010; **4**: 701–12.

76. Annanmaki T, Pessala-Driver A, Hokkanen L, et al. Uric acid associates with cognition in Parkinson's disease. Parkinsonism Relat Disord 2008; **14**: 576–8.

77. Annanmaki T, Pohja M, Parviainen T, et al. Uric acid and cognition in Parkinson's disease: a follow-up study. Parkinsonism Relat Disord 2011; **17**: 333–7.

78. Chen-Plotkin AS, Hu WT, Siderowf A, et al. Plasma epidermal growth factor levels predict cognitive decline in Parkinson disease. Ann Neurol 2011; **69**: 655–63.

79. Pellecchia MT, Santangelo G, Picillo M, et al. Serum epidermal growth factor predicts cognitive functions in early, drug-naive Parkinson's disease patients. J Neurol 2013; **260**: 438–44.

80. Marder K, Tang MX, Alfaro B, et al. Risk of Alzheimer's disease in relatives of Parkinson's disease patients with and without dementia. Neurology 1999; **52**: 719–24.

81. Kurz MW, Larsen JP, Kvaloy JT, et al. Associations between family history of Parkinson's disease and dementia and risk of dementia in Parkinson's disease: a community-based, longitudinal study. Mov Disord 2006; **21**: 2170–4.

82. Pankratz N, Byder L, Halter C, et al. Presence of an APOE4 allele results in significantly earlier onset of Parkinson's disease and a higher risk with dementia. Mov Disord 2006; **21**: 45–9.

83. Farrer LA, Cupples LA, Haines JL, et al. Effects of age, sex, and ethnicity on the association between apolipoprotein E genotype and Alzheimer disease. A meta-analysis. APOE and Alzheimer Disease Meta Analysis Consortium. J Am Med Assoc 1997; **278**: 1349–56.

84. Kurz MW, Dekomien G, Nilsen OB, et al. APOE alleles in Parkinson disease and their relationship to cognitive decline: a population-based, longitudinal study. J Geriatr Psychiatry Neurol 2009; **22**: 166–70.

85. Williams-Gray CH, Goris A, Saiki M, et al. Apolipoprotein E genotype as a risk factor for susceptibility to and dementia in Parkinson's disease. J Neurol 2009; **256**: 493–8.

86. Morley JF, Xie SX, Hurtig HI, et al. Genetic influences on cognitive decline in Parkinson's disease. Mov Disord 2012; **27**: 512–18.

87. Tsuang D, Leverenz JB, Lopez OL, et al. APOE epsilon4 increases risk for dementia in pure synucleinopathies. J Am Med Assoc Neurol 2013; **70**: 223–8.

88. Irwin DJ, White MT, Toledo JB, et al. Neuropathologic substrates of Parkinson disease dementia. Ann Neurol 2012; **72**: 587–98.

89. Zabetian CP, Hutter CM, Factor SA, et al. Association analysis of MAPT H1 haplotype and subhaplotypes in Parkinson's disease. Ann Neurol 2007; **62**: 137–44.

90. Goris A, Williams-Gray CH, Clark GR, et al. Tau and alpha-synuclein in susceptibility to, and dementia in, Parkinson's disease. Ann Neurol 2007; **62**: 145–53.

91. Williams-Gray CH, Mason SL, Evans JR, et al. The CamPaIGN study of Parkinson's disease: 10-year outlook in an incident population-based cohort. J Neurol Neurosurg Psychiatry 2013; **84**: 1258–64.

92. **Sidransky E, Nalls MA, Aasly JO, et al.** Multicenter analysis of glucocerebrosidase mutations in Parkinson's disease. N Engl J Med 2009; **361**: 1651–61.

93. **Neumann J, Bras J, Deas E, et al.** Glucocerebrosidase mutations in clinical and pathologically proven Parkinson's disease. Brain 2009; **132**: 1783–94.

94. **Winder-Rhodes SE, Evans JR, Ban M, et al.** Glucocerebrosidase mutations influence the natural history of Parkinson's disease in a community-based incident cohort. Brain 2013; **136**: 392–9.

95. **Murphy KE, Gysbers AM, Abbott SK, et al.** Reduced glucocerebrosidase is associated with increased alpha-synuclein in sporadic Parkinson's disease. Brain 2014; **137**: 834–48.

96. **Hoogland J, de Bie RM, Williams-Gray CH, et al.** Catechol-O-methyltransferase val158met and cognitive function in Parkinson's disease. Mov Disord 2010; **25**: 2550–4.

97. **Weintraub D, Dietz N, Duda JE, et al.** Alzheimer's disease pattern of brain atrophy predicts cognitive decline in Parkinson's disease. Brain 2012; **135**(Pt 1): 170–80.

98. **Nobili F, Arnaldi D, Campus C, et al.** Brain perfusion correlates of cognitive and nigrostriatal functions in de novo Parkinson's disease. Eur J Nucl Med Molec Imaging 2011; **38**: 2209–18.

99. **Bohnen NI, Koeppe RA, Minoshima S, et al.** Cerebral glucose metabolic features of Parkinson disease and incident dementia: longitudinal study. J Nucl Med 2011; **52**: 848–55.

100. **Klassen BT, Hentz JG, Shill HA, et al.** Quantitative EEG as a predictive biomarker for Parkinson disease dementia. Neurology 2011; **77**: 118–24.

Chapter 12

Electrophysiological and other auxiliary investigations in patients with Parkinson's disease dementia

Yasuyuki Okuma and Yoshikuni Mizuno

Introduction

Patients with Parkinson's disease (PD) often show cognitive deficits. Impairments have been documented in almost all areas of cognition, including general intellectual functions, visuospatial functions, attention, memory, and executive functions [1–4]. Various electrophysiological investigations have been used to study these cognitive dysfunctions in patients with PD. In this chapter, the results of electrophysiological investigations in PD patients with and without dementia are reviewed. In addition, data on ^{123}I-metaiodobenzylguanidine ($[^{123}$I]-MIBG) myocardial scintigraphy, which has been found to be very useful for differentiating Lewy body diseases such as PD and dementia with Lewy bodies (DLB) from Alzheimer's disease (AD) [5, 6], are also reviewed.

Electrophysiological methods

Electroencephalography (EEG)

Early studies showed that EEG findings are abnormal in around 30–40% of PD patients. The slowing of the alpha rhythm and a generalized or focal increase in slow-wave activities are the common findings, particularly in patients with dementia [7–13]. Tanaka et al. [14] conducted EEG power spectral analyses and their results agreed with the previous findings that delta and theta power increased in PD patients with dementia (PD-D), but they did not see a decreased alpha power compared with controls. Recently, Kamei and colleagues [15–18] made an extensive quantitative EEG (qEEG) study by employing multiple logistic regression analysis, as well as estimating the distribution of frequency changes, in a large number of PD patients without brain ischaemia. They showed diffuse slowing except for the frontal pole in the qEEG compared with age-matched healthy controls [15] and a decreased spectral ratio at all electrode locations with progression of the disease [16]. They also studied qEEG alterations in PD patients with executive dysfunction (ExD) and cognitive impairment; they found an increase in slow-wave activity in frontal and frontal-pole locations in ExD [17] and at all brain areas in patients with dementia [18]. Klassen et al. [19] reported qEEG findings such as decreased frequency of background rhythm and relative power in the theta band being predictive biomarkers for incident PD-D. The underlying pathophysiology of EEG changes in PD is difficult to elucidate. Both subcortical and cortical involvement may account for the EEG slowing, Soikkeli et al. [12] suggested that deficits in cholinergic transmission could in part explain the slowing in EEG, particularly in PD-D patients.

To explore whether EEG abnormalities can discriminate between DLB, AD, and PD-D in the early stages, Bonanni et al. [20] studied EEG in 50 DLB, 50 AD, and 40 PD-D patients with earliest stage of dementia (MMSE 20 ≤) at first visit. Dominant mean frequencies were 8.3 Hz for the AD group and 7.4 Hz for DLB. The variability of the dominant frequency also differed between the AD (1.1 Hz) and DLB groups (1.8 Hz). By comparison, fewer than half of the patients with PD-D exhibited the EEG abnormalities seen in those with DLB. The authors concluded that if revised consensus criteria for DLB diagnosis [21] are properly applied, EEG may be helpful for discriminating between AD and DLB in the early stages of dementia. The difference in qEEG findings between PD-D and AD was also investigated by Fonseca et al. [22]. Differences in beta coherence were found between AD and PD-D, with an increase in PD-D and a decrease in AD, along with a greater increase in the slow-wave absolute powers (delta and theta) in PD-D. These neurophysiological differences are likely to be related to distinct mechanisms involved in the pathogenesis of dementia in AD and PD-D.

Evoked potentials

Auditory evoked potentials (AEPs)

There are several reports regarding AEPs in PD. Gawel et al. [23] described prolongation of wave V latency, whereas Prasher and Bannister [24] reported normal AEP findings. This difference may be due to the selection of patients. Tachibana et al. [25] showed normal latencies in PD patients without dementia. By contrast, PD-D patients revealed a significant prolongation of wave I–V (particularly wave III–V) inter-peak latencies compared with patients without dementia and healthy subjects. These results show that auditory brainstem pathways are involved in PD-D and could be explained by the more widespread involvement of the brainstem pathways by the disease process and/or other concomitant pathologies in such patients. Green and colleagues [26, 27] reported that the P1 (50 ms) of the middle-latency AEP was lacking in 39% of AD and 58% of PD-D patients and suggested that abnormalities of P1 in patients with dementia may be due to cholinergic dysfunction.

Visual evoked potentials (VEPs)

There have been contradictory results concerning the changes in VEPs in patients with PD. Bodis-Wollner and Yahr [28] reported that the average latency was prolonged but became less prolonged on levodopa therapy, suggesting that the extrapyramidal connections of the visual cortex and the retinal dopaminergic neurons can be affected in PD. Dinner et al. [29] and Nightingale et al. [30] did not find prolonged VEP latencies. Calzetti et al. [31] compared VEP and electroretinogram data and concluded that changes in VEPs are not entirely dependent on alterations at the retinal level. Okuda et al. [32] found that prolonged P100 latency was found only in PD-D patients and speculated that dysfunction in the central visual system plays a role in the abnormal pattern of VEPs in PD. In conclusion, the disturbance of both retinal and nigrostriatal dopaminergic systems may contribute to the delayed VEP latency.

Somatosensory evoked potentials (SEPs)

Short-latency SEPs were reported to be normal when recorded from the parietal region regardless of cognitive function [24, 33, 34], although Potolicchio and O'Doherty [35] found that inter-wave latencies were prolonged in some patients. In contrast to parietal SEPs, Rossini et al. [34] described reduced frontal N30 amplitude in PD patients. They suggested that dysfunctions of the thalamo-basal ganglia–frontal cortex circuit or supplementary motor cortex might play a role in the reduction of frontal N30 amplitude.

Event-related potentials (ERPs)

P300 (P3, target P3) The P3 ERP can be elicited whenever one stimulus is discriminated from another [36]. The subject is instructed to respond to the infrequent (oddball) or target stimulus and not to respond to the frequently presented or standard stimulus. Goodin et al. [37] showed that the peak latency of P3 becomes longer with increasing age. In addition, P3 latency was found to be longer in patients with dementia than the normal values for a given age [37, 38]. P3 is sensitive to cognitive changes associated with ageing and mental dysfunction associated with various diseases, including PD.

There have been a number of studies examining P3 in PD patients. The results of P3 latencies in PD patients without dementia are contradictory, whereas P3 latency in PD-D patients is found to be consistently prolonged. Table 12.1 summarizes the studies on auditory oddball P3 latency and amplitude in PD patients without dementia [14, 39–49]. Interestingly, the effects of levodopa therapy are variable. Amabile et al. [42] reported that the basal P3 latency was delayed but became normalized after levodopa therapy. Starkstein et al. [43] examined PD patients with severe motor fluctuation and reported a significant improvement of the P3 latency of the ERP in the 'on' phase. In contrast, Prasher and Findley [44] showed that P3 was normal before treatment but that after treatment P3 latency was significantly prolonged with the reduction of reaction time. Dopamine replacement is followed by a significantly reduced motor processing time despite the increased cognitive processing time. They suggest that dopaminergic overstimulation of other regions may adversely affect cognitive processing. Yamada and Hirayama [50] also observed a similar effect and speculated that it may be due to a hyperarousal state provoked by levodopa. Regarding the relationship between P3 latency and neuropsychological testing, Hansch et al. [39] reported that the Symbol Digit Modalities Test, but not the Mini-Mental State Examination (MMSE), showed correlation with P3 latency. O'Brien et al. [51] showed that P3 latency was correlated with MMSE score and other psychological measures, indicating that cognitive decline influences P3 latency.

Table 12.1 Auditory oddball P300 latency and amplitude in PD patients without dementia

Study	Medication	Latency	Amplitude
Hansch et al. (1982) [39]	+	↑	N
Goodin and Aminoff (1987) [41]	+	N	N
Amabile et al. (1990) [42]	+	N	N
	−	↑	N
Prasher and Findlay (1991) [44]	+	↑	N
	−	N	N
Ebmeier et al. (1992) [45]	+	N	N
Vieregge et al. (1994) [46]	+	N	N
Green et al. (1996) [47]	+	N	↑
Lagopoulos et al. (1998) [48]	+/−	N	N
Iijima et al. (2000) [49]	+	↑	N
Tanaka et al. (2000) [14]	+	N	↑

Medication: +, on levodopa treatment; −, off levodopa treatment.

N, normal; ↑, prolonged (latency) or increased (amplitude).

ERPs during the performance of visual discrimination tasks have also been studied. Tachibana et al. [52] reported that P3 latency was normal in PD without dementia, but was significantly prolonged in PD-D patients. However, they observed that during semantic discrimination tasks, P3 latency was significantly prolonged even in PD patients without dementia compared with the controls [53]. Wang et al. [54, 55] used the same methods as those of Tachibana et al., and showed that P3 latency was only delayed in PD patients without dementia when long inter-stimulus intervals (5100 ms) were used. Some of these discrepancies may appear to be task specific, depending on both stimulus modality and response requirements. Bodis-Wollner et al. [56] studied auditory and visual ERPs in PD patients without dementia and found that visual P3 was prolonged but auditory P3 was not. To study the mechanisms of visual hallucinations, Kurita et al. [57] compared visual (a visual discrimination paradigm) and auditory ERP latencies among PD-D patients with (PD-DH) and without visual hallucinations, DLB patients, and AD patients. The mean visual P3 latencies in the PD-DH and DLB groups were significantly longer than that in the AD group, while the mean auditory P3 latencies in all groups were comparable, suggesting that visual cognitive functions are selectively impaired in DLB and PD-DH patients. Somatosensory ERPs are less well studied. Ito [58] showed that P3 latency was significantly prolonged compared with that in controls in PD-D, AD, and vascular dementia.

P3 amplitude has mostly been reported to be normal with the auditory oddball paradigm, but some investigators have shown an increased amplitude in PD patients without dementia. Green et al. [47] showed an enlarged P3 amplitude in unmedicated patients with mild PD, and speculated that it reflects abnormality in the use of attentional resources to compensate for brain dysfunction. Tanaka et al. [14] reported increased P3 amplitude and resting EEG total power in PD without dementia, but both decreased with increasing severity of dementia. Future prospective studies will determine whether increased P3 and EEG amplitude in intellectually normal PD patients is a predictor of later intellectual changes. Iijima et al. [49] reported that topographical mapping (TM) of P300 demonstrated abnormal distribution in four of 20 PD patients without dementia, and three of them showed frontal shift. Its significance is difficult to determine, since their P300 latencies were normal. P3 latency has been considered to be the index of the time for controlled information processing, whereas P3 TM and amplitude are indices of selective attention to stimulation and allocation of information resources. Wang et al. [54] used a visual oddball and an S1–S2 paradigm to evoke ERPs in PD patients without dementia and showed decreased P3 amplitude in the S1–S2 paradigm but not in the usual oddball paradigm.

Non-target P3 (P3a, novelty P3, no-go P3) Two types of P3 have been reported in normal subjects— one is a parietal maximal P3 component designated P3b and the other is a fronto-central or sometimes parietal maximal P3 component named P3a [60, 61]. P3a is elicited by unexpected neutral stimuli under conditions of passive attention. Tachibana et al. [60] studied actively and passively evoked P3 components (P3a and P3b) using visual discrimination tasks. P3a and P3b were identified as responses to infrequent target stimuli and infrequent non-target stimuli. Although P3b latency was prolonged in PD-D patients, P3a latency was normal. In AD, however, both P3a and P3b latencies were prolonged. They suggested that the automatic processing stage associated with P3a may be less impaired than the attention-controlled processing reflected by P3b in PD-D patients [60].

Hozumi et al. [62] studied auditory ERP topography in 15 PD patients without dementia using two kinds of novelty tones (10% each) added to target tones (20%). Patients had shorter P3a latencies to the novel stimuli and a more frontal distribution on the P3 map. These findings suggest that decreased mental switching causes a lack of novelty P3 habituation in PD and that this is related to learning disabilities due to dysfunction of the frontal-basal ganglia circuits.

No-go ERPs are known to reflect the process of inhibition of motor responses. Iijima et al. [59] studied push/wait paradigm no-go P3 using two Japanese Kanji words: 'push' as the go stimulus and 'wait' as the no-go stimulus. The latency of go P3 did not differ significantly between PD and controls, but the no-go P3 had a longer latency in PD patients without dementia than in controls. They concluded that the process of inhibition of motor response declines earlier than does the production process, and no-go P3 might be a useful tool for evaluating inhibitory cognitive function in PD.

N100, P200, N200 (N1, P2, N2) Although Goodin and Aminoff [41] reported that N1 latency was prolonged in PD-D compared with PD without dementia and control subjects, subsequent reports showed normal N1 and P2 latencies even in PD-D patients [52, 63]. Ebmeier et al. [45] reported increased P2 and N2 latencies in PD patients without dementia; in particular increased peak latencies of N2 were moderately associated with parkinsonian motor impairment and lower score in Benton Multiple Choice Visual Retention Test. The original N2 response can be divided into two components, NA and N2, and they reflect stages of processing associated with pattern recognition and stimulus classification, respectively [64]. Tachibana et al. [52] also obtained NA and N2 components by subtraction methods and applied these to PD patients without dementia. They found that N2 latency was significantly longer than that of controls, although NA latency was normal. These results suggest that the automatic processing stage associated with NA may be less impaired than the attention-controlled processing reflected by N2 in patients with PD [52]. Wang et al. [54] also found delayed N2 latency with the visual S1–S2 paradigm.

Mismatch negativity (MMN) (N2a) MMN reflects the automatic aspect of attention and it is elicited by deviant stimuli when compared with standard stimuli. Vieregge et al. [46] studied MMN during a two-channel selective auditory attention task. They measured MMN by subtracting the average of ignored standard tones from the average of the ignored deviant tones. MMN did not differ between PD patients and controls, indicating that there is no gross pre-attentive deficit in PD. Karayanidis et al. [65] also found that MMN in PD showed little further disruption with ageing.

Processing negativity (PN) Selective attention refers to the ability to focus on one channel of information in the presence of other distracting channels [66]. The auditory ERPs evoked by the attended tones are negatively shifted in relation to those of unattended tones. The shift often begins before the peak of the N1 wave and may last for several hundred milliseconds. This is called processing negativity (PN) and is attributed to subjects' maintenance of a vivid internal template of the attended stimulus. Wright et al. [66] found PN to be significantly smaller in PD patients than in controls, providing evidence for an impairment of auditory selective attention in PD patients.

Contingent negative variation (CNV) Changes in attention and response preparation are reflected by CNV. Analysis of components in the cue–target interval permits an assessment of cue processing and response preparation that occurs prior to an anticipated target stimulus. Wright et al. [66] showed greatly reduced CNV for a PD group during a task involving covert orientation of visual attention. Oishi et al. [67] examined CNV and movement-related cortical potentials using an S1 (click)–S2 (flash)–key press paradigm. The amplitude of early CNV was smaller in the PD group than in the control group. However, the amplitude increased significantly after levodopa infusion, indicating that the small amplitude of the early CNV is related to decreased levels of dopaminergic activity [67, 68].

MIBG myocardial scintigraphy

MIBG is a physiological analogue of noradrenaline (norepinephrine), and [^{123}I]-MIBG myocardial scintigraphy is used to evaluate post-ganglionic cardiac sympathetic innervation [69]. This method was briefly mentioned in Chapter 10 and will be described in more detail here. Recent studies have shown that reduction of myocardial MIBG uptake is associated with Lewy body diseases such as PD and DLB regardless of the presence of autonomic failure [70–72]. In PD, cardiac uptake tends to decrease as the disease progresses, and it decreases more in DLB than in PD [70, 73, 74]. MIBG myocardial scintigraphy is particularly useful for differentiating PD from atypical parkinsonism, for example progressive supranuclear palsy and multiple system atrophy [70, 75–77]. It has also been reported to be useful in differentiating DLB from AD; MIBG uptake is markedly reduced in DLB, whereas it is normal in AD [5, 6] (Fig. 12.1). MIBG myocardial scintigraphy is a sensitive tool for discriminating DLB from AD even in patients without parkinsonism [78]. MIBG myocardial scintigraphy is more useful than medial occipital hypoperfusion measurement using single-photon emission computed tomography in diagnosing DLB [79]. Wada-Isoe et al. [80] found that MIBG scintigraphy is superior to cerebrospinal fluid markers such as amyloid-beta 42 and p-tau in differentiating AD from DLB. The same group found that the presence of visual hallucinations independently predicted decreased cardiac MIBG uptake [81]. Since its importance has been increasingly recognized, the low MIBG uptake has been included as a supportive feature in the revised criteria for the clinical diagnosis of DLB [20].

Conclusion

EEG abnormalities in patients with PD consist of slowing of the background activities, particularly in PD-D patients. P3 latency is prolonged in patients with PD-D, but conflicting results are obtained in PD patients without dementia. The conflicting results may be due to both patient selection and methodological differences. P3 amplitude is largely normal or even increased in PD patients without dementia, but it decreases as dementia emerges. N1, P2, and NA components and MMN are normal, whereas N2, CNV, and PN are abnormal. These results suggest that the automatic processing stage may be less affected than attention-controlled processing and that

(A)   (B)

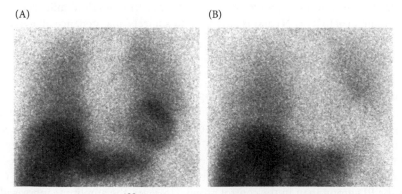

Fig. 12.1 Examples of myocardial ^{123}I-MIBG uptake in a patient with Alzheimer's disease (AD) (A) and dementia with Lewy bodies (DLB) (B). The myocardial uptake of MIBG is normal in AD, but cardiac accumulation is markedly reduced in DLB.

both the speed of cognitive processing and the amount of processed information decrease as cognitive dysfunction develops in PD. MIBG myocardial scintigraphy is a sensitive tool for discriminating DLB and PD-D from AD.

References

1. **Raskin SA, Borod JC, Tweedy J.** Neuropsychological aspects of Parkinson's disease. Neuropsychol Rev 1990; **1**: 185–221.

2. **Biggins CA, Boyd JL, Harrop FM, et al.** A controlled, longitudinal study of dementia in Parkinson's disease. J Neurol Neurosurg Psychiatry 1992; **55**: 566–71.

3. **Bayles KA, Tomoeda CK, Wood JA, et al.** Change in cognitive function in idiopathic Parkinson's disease. Arch Neurol 1996; **53**: 1140–6.

4. **Jacobs DM, Marder K, Cote LJ, et al.** Neuropsychological characteristics of preclinical dementia in Parkinson's disease. Neurology 1995; **45**: 1691–6.

5. **Watanabe H, Iida T, Katayama T, et al.** Cardiac ^{123}I-meta-iodobenzylguanidine (MIBG) uptake in dementia with Lewy bodies: comparison with Alzheimer's disease. J Neurol Neurosurg Psychiatry 2001; **70**: 781–3.

6. **Yoshita M, Taki J, Yamada M.** A clinical role for [123 I] MIBG myocardial scintigraphy in the distinction between dementia of the Alzheimer's type and dementia with Lewy bodies. J Neurol Neurosurg Psychiatry 2001; **71**: 583–8.

7. **Sirakov AA, Mezan IS.** EEG findings in parkinsonism. Electroencephalogr Clin Neurophysiol 1963; **15**: 321–2.

8. **Yeager CL, Alberts WW, Delattre LD.** Effect of stereotaxic surgery upon electroencephalographic status of parkinsonian patients. Neurology 1966; **16**: 904–10.

9. **Neufeld MY, Inzelberg R, Korczyn AD.** EEG in demented and non-demented parkinsonian patients. Acta Neurol Scand 1988; **78**: 1–5.

10. **de Weed AW, Perquin WVM, Jonkman EJ.** Role of the EEG in the prediction of dementia in Parkinson's disease. Dementia 1990; **1**: 115–18.

11. **Neufeld MY, Blumen S, Aitkin I, et al.** EEG frequency analysis in demented and nondemented Parkinsonian patients. Dementia 1994; **5**: 23–8.

12. **Soikkeli R, Partanen J, Soininen H, et al.** Slowing of EEG in Parkinson's disease. Electroencephalogr Clin Neurophysiol 1991; **79**: 159–65.

13. **Domitrz I, Friedman A.** Electroencephalography of demented and non-demented Parkinson's disease patients. Parkinsonism Relat Disord 1999; **5**: 37–41.

14. **Tanaka H, Koenig T, Pascual-Marqui RD, et al.** Event-related potential and EEG measures in Parkinson's disease without and with dementia. Dement Geriatr Cogn Disord 2000; **11**: 39–45.

15. **Serizawa K, Kamei S, Morita A, et al.** Comparison of quantitative EEGs between Parkinson disease and age-adjusted normal controls. J Clin Neurophysiol 2008; **25**: 361–6.

16. **Morita A, Kamei S, Serizawa K, et al.** The relationship between slowing EEGs and the progression of Parkinson's disease. J Clin Neurophysiol 2009; **26**: 426–9.

17. **Kamei S, Morita A, Serizawa K, et al.** Quantitative EEG analysis of executive dysfunction in Parkinson's disease. J Clin Neurophysiol 2010; **27**: 193–7.

18. **Morita A, Kamei S, Mizutani T.** Relationship between slowing of the EEG and cognitive impairment in Parkinson's disease. J Clin Neurophysiol 2011; **28**: 384–7.

19. **Klassen BT, Hentz JG, Shill HA, et al.** Quantitative EEG as a predictive biomarker for Parkinson disease dementia. Neurology 2011; **77**: 118–24.

20. **Bonanni L, Thomas A, Tiraboschi P, et al.** EEG comparisons in early Alzheimer's disease, dementia with Lewy disease and Parkinson's disease with dementia patients with a 2-year follow-up. Brain 2008; **131**: 690–705.

21. McKeith IG, Dickson DW, Lowe J, et al. Diagnosis and management of dementia with Lewy bodies: third report of the DLB Consortium. Neurology 2005; **65**: 1863–72.

22. Fonseca LC, Tedrus GM, Carvas PN, et al. Comparison of quantitative EEG between patients with Alzheimer's disease and those with Parkinson's disease dementia. Clin Neurophysiol 2013; **124**: 1970–4.

23. Gawel MJ, Das P, Vincent S, et al. Visual and auditory evoked responses in patients with Parkinson's disease. J Neurol Neurosurg Psychiatry 1981; **44**: 227–32.

24. Prasher D, Bannister R. Brain stem auditory evoked potentials in patients with multiple system atrophy with progressive autonomic failure (Shy–Drager syndrome). J Neurol Neurosurg Psychiatry 1986; **49**: 278–89.

25. Tachibana H, Takeda M, Sugita M. Short-latency somatosensory and brainstem auditory evoked potentials in patients with Parkinson's disease. Int J Neurosci 1989; **44**: 321–6.

26. Green JB, Flagg L, Freed DM, et al. The middle latency auditory evoked potential may be abnormal in dementia. Neurology 1992; **42**: 1034–6.

27. Buchwald JS, Erwin S, Read D, et al. Midlatency auditory evoked responses: differential abnormality of P1 in Alzheimer's disease. Electroenchephalogr Clin Neurophysiol 1989; **74**: 378–84.

28. Bodis-Wollner I, Yahr MD. Measurements of visual evoked potentials in Parkinson's disease. Brain 1978; **101**: 661–71.

29. Dinner DS, Luders H, Hanson M, et al. Pattern evoked potentials (PEPs) in Parkinson's disease. Neurology 1985; **35**: 610–13.

30. Nightingale S, Mitchell KW, Howe JW. Visual evoked cortical potentials and pattern electroretinograms in Parkinson's disease and control subjects. J Neurol Neurosurg Psychiatry 1986; **49**: 1280–7.

31. Calzetti S, Franchi A, Taratufolo G, et al. Simultaneous VEP and PERG investigations in early Parkinson's disease. J Neurol Neurosurg Psychiatry 1990; **53**: 114–17.

32. Okuda B, Tachibana H, Kawabata M, et al. Correlation of visual evoked potentials with dementia in Parkinson's disease. Jpn J Geriat 1992; **29**: 475–9.

33. Koller WC. Sensory symptoms in Parkinson's disease. Neurology 1984; **34**: 957–9.

34. Rossini PM, Babiloni F, Bernardi G, et al. Abnormalities of short-latency somatosensory evoked potentials in parkinsonian patients. Electroencephalogr Clin Neurophysiol 1989; **74**: 277–89.

35. Potolicchio SJ, Jr, O'Doherty DS. Somatosensory evoked potentials in subcortical and cortical lesions. In: Nodar RH, Barber C (ed.), *Evoked potentials II. Second International Evoked Potentials Symposium.* London: Butterworth, 1984; pp. 423–31.

36. Polich J. P300 in clinical applications: meaning, method, and management. Am J EEG Technol 1991; **31**: 201–31.

37. Goodin DS, Squires KC, Starr A. Long latency event-related components of the auditory evoked potential in dementia. Brain 1978; **101**: 635–48.

38. Goodin DS, Squires K, Henderson B, et al. Age-related variations in evoked potentials to auditory stimuli in normal human subjects. Electroencephalogr Clin Neurophysiol 1978; **44**: 447–58.

39. Hansch EC, Syndulko K, Cohen SN, et al. Cognition in Parkinson disease: an event-related potential perspective. Ann Neurol 1982; **11**: 599–607.

40. Goodin DS, Aminoff MJ. Electrophysiological differences between subtypes of dementia. Brain 1986; **109**: 1103–13.

41. Goodin DS, Aminoff MJ. Electrophysiological differences between demented and nondemented patients with Parkinson's disease. Ann Neurol 1987; **21**: 90–4.

42. Amabile G, Fattapposta F, Pierelli F. Evoked potentials in Parkinson's disease: sensory and cognitive aspects. A review. J Psychophysiol 1990; **4**: 115–22.

43. Starkstein SE, Esteguy M, Berthier ML, et al. Evoked potentials, reaction time and cognitive performance in on and off phases of Parkinson's disease. J Neurol Neurosurg Psychiatry 1989; **52**: 338–40.

44. Prasher D, Findley L. Dopaminergic induced changes in cognitive and motor processing in Parkinson's disease: an electrophysiological investigation. J Neurol Neurosurg Psychiatry 1991; **54**: 603–9.

45. **Ebmeier KP, Potter DD, Cochrane RHB, et al**. Event related potentials, reaction time, and cognitive performance in idiopathic Parkinson's disease. Biol Psychol 1992; **33**: 73–89.

46. **Vieregge P, Verleger R, Wascher E, et al**. Auditory selective attention is impaired in Parkinson's disease–event-related evidence from EEG potentials. Cogn Brain Res 1994; **2**: 117–29.

47. **Green J, Woodard JL, Sirockman BE, et al**. Event-related potential P3 change in mild Parkinson's disease. Mov Disord 1996; **11**: 33–42.

48. **Lagopoulos J, Clouston P, Barhamali H, et al**. Late components of the event-related potentials and their topography in Parkinson's disease. Mov Disord 1998; **2**: 262–7.

49. **Iijima M, Osawa M, Ushijima R, et al**. Nogo event-related potentials in Parkinson's disease. Electoroencephalogr Clin Neurophysiol 1999; **49**(Suppl.): 199–203.

50. **Yamada T, Hirayama K**. Effect of L-dopa on P300 component—study in patients with juvenile parkinsonism having wearing off phenomena. Clin Neurol 1987; **27**: 53–7.

51. **O'Donnell BF, Squires NK**. Evoked potentials changes and neuropsychological performance in Parkinson's disease. Biol Psychol 1987; **24**: 23–7.

52. **Tachibana H, Aragane K, Miyata Y, et al**. Electrophysiological analysis of cognitive slowing in Parkinson's disease. J Neurol Sci 1997; **149**: 47–56.

53. **Tachibana H, Aragane K, Kawabata K, et al**. P3 latency change in aging and Parkinson's disease. Arch Neurol 1997; **54**: 296–302.

54. **Wang L, Kuroiwa Y, Kamitani T**. Visual event-related potential changes at two different tasks in nondemented Parkinson's disease. J Neurol Sci 1999; **164**: 139–47.

55. **Wang L, Kuroiwa Y, Kamitani T, et al**. Effect of interstimulus interval on visual P300 in Parkinson's disease. J Neurol Neurosurg Psychiatry 1999; **67**: 497–503.

56. **Bodis-Wollner I, Borod JC, Cicero B, et al**. Modality dependent changes in event-related potentials correlate with specific cognitive functions in nondemented patients with Parkinson's disease. J Neural Transm 1995; **9**: 197–209.

57. **Kurita A, Murakami M, Takagi S, et al**. Visual hallucinations and altered visual information processing in Parkinson disease and dementia with Lewy bodies. Mov Disord 2010; **25**: 167–71.

58. **Ito J**. Somatosensory event-related potentials (ERPs) in patients with different types of dementia. J Neurol Sci 1994; **121**: 139–46.

59. **Iijima M, Osawa M, Iwata M, et al**. Topographic mapping of P300 and frontal cognitive function in Parkinson's disease. Behav Neurol 2000; **12**: 143–8.

60. **Tachibana H, Toda K, Sugita M**. Actively and passively evoked P3 latency of event-related potentials in Parkinson's disease. J Neurol Sci 1992; **111**: 134–42.

61. **Squires NK, Squires KC, Hillyard SA**. Two varieties of long-latency positive waves evoked by unpredictable auditory stimuli. Electroencephalogr Clin Neurophysiol 1975; **38**: 387–401.

62. **Hozumi A, Hirata K, Tanaka H, et al**. Perseveration for novel stimuli in Parkinson's disease: an evaluation based on event-related potentials topography. Mov Disord, 2000; **15**: 835–42.

63. **Filipovic S, Kostic VS, Sternic N, et al**. Auditory event-related potentials in different types of dementia. Eur Neurol 1990; **30**: 189–93.

64. **Ritter W, Simson R, Vaughan HG**. Event-related potentials correlates of two stages of information processing in physical and semantic discrimination tasks. Psychophysiology 1983; **20**: 168–79.

65. **Karayanidis F, Andrews S, Ward PB, Michie PT**. ERP indices of auditory selective attention in aging and Parkinson's disease. Psychophysiology 1995; **32**: 335–50.

66. **Wright MJ, Geffen GM, Geffen LB**. Event-related potentials associated with covert orientation of visual attention in Parkinson's disease. Neuropsychologia 1993; **31**: 1283–97.

67. **Oishi M, Mochizuki Y, Du C, et al**. Contingent negative variation and movement-related cortical potentials in parkinsonism. Electroencephalogr Clin Neurophysiol 1995; **95**: 346–9.

68. **Amabile G, Fattapposta F, Pozzessere G, et al**. Parkinson disease: electrophysiological (CNV) analysis related to pharmacological treatment. Electroencephalogr Clin Neurophysiol 1986; **64** 521–4.

69. Wieland DM, Brown LE, Rogers WL, et al. Myocardial imaging with a radioiodinated norepinephrine storage analog. J Nucl Med 1981; **22**: 22–31.

70. Orimo S, Ozawa E, Nakade S, et al. ^{123}I-metaiodobenzylguanidine myocardial scintigraphy in Parkinson's disease. J Neurol Neurosurg Psychiatry 1999; **67**: 189–94.

71. Braune S, Reinhardt M, Schnitzer R, et al. Cardiac uptake of MIBG separates Parkinson's disease from multiple system atrophy. Neurology 1999; **53**: 1020–5.

72. Taki J, Nakajima K, Hwang E-H, et al. Peripheral sympathetic dysfunction in patients with Parkinson's disease without autonomic failure is heart selective and disease specific. Eur J Nucl Med 2000; **27**: 566–73.

73. Saiki S, Hirose G, Sakai K, et al. Cardiac ^{123}I-MIBG scintigraphy can assess the disease severity and phenotype of PD. J Neurol Sci, 2004; **220**: 105–11.

74. Suzuki M, Kurita A, Hashimoto M, et al. Impaired myocardial ^{123}I-metaiodobenzylguanidine uptake in Lewy body disease: comparison between dementia with Lewy bodies and Parkinson's disease. J Neurol Sci 2006; **240**: 15–19.

75. Yoshita M. Differentiation of idiopathic Parkinson's disease from striatonigral degeneration and progressive supranuclear palsy using iodine-123 meta-iodobenzylguanidine myocardial scintigraphy. J Neurol Sci 1998; **155**: 60–7.

76. Druschky A, Hilz MJ, Platsch G, et al. Differentiation of Parkinson's disease and multiple system atrophy in early disease stages by means of I-123-MIBG-SPECT. J Neurol Sci 2000; **175**: 3–12.

77. Nagayama H, Hamamoto M, Ueda M, et al. Reliability of MIBG myocardial scintigraphy in the diagnosis of Parkinson's disease. J Neurol Neurosurg Psychiatry 2005; **76**: 249–51.

78. Yoshita M, Taki J, Yokoyama K, et al. Value of [123]I -MIBG radioactivity in the differential diagnosis of DLB from AD. Neurology 2006; **66**: 1850–4.

79. Hanyu H, Shimizu S, Hirao K, et al. Comparative value of brain perfusion SPECT and [^{123}I]-MIBG myocardial scintigraphy in distinguishing between dementia with Lewy bodies and Alzheimer's disease. Eur J Nucl Med Mol Imaging 2006; **33**: 248–53.

80. Wada-Isoe K, Kitayama M, Nakaso K, et al. Diagnostic markers for diagnosing dementia with Lewy bodies: CSF and MIBG cardiac scintigraphy study. J Neurol Sci 2007; **260**: 33–7.

81. Kitayama M, Wada-Isoe K, Irizawa Y, et al. Association of visual hallucinations with reduction of MIBG cardiac uptake in Parkinson's disease. J Neurol Sci 2008; **264**: 22–6.

Chapter 13

The genetic basis of dementia in Parkinson's disease

Rita Guerreiro and Andrew Singleton

Introduction

Parkinson's disease (PD) is a heterogeneous disease both genetically and clinically. It is hoped that we will eventually be able to dissect out the role of genetics in the clinical heterogeneity of PD. The occurrence of dementia in PD (PD-D) has been a particular target of genotype–phenotype research. In the last 10 years genetics has played a major role in helping us to understand the pathobiological underpinnings of PD. However, the role of genetics in PD-D is still poorly understood. In this chapter we examine the evidence for a genetic component of PD-D, first by reviewing studies of familial PD-D and reporting on the genes and mutations involved, then by discussing the role of genetic risk factors such as apolipoprotein E (*APOE*), the best-known genetic risk factor for Alzheimer's disease (AD). Finally, we examine the expected next steps in genetics research that are likely to yield insight into the basis of PD-D, in light of the new technologies that have become available.

Finding genes that underlie disease

Disease genetics is a discipline that aims to detect a signal in the background of an extremely large amount of noise, the proverbial 'needle in a haystack'. We can be most sure of the results, and most confident of success, when a systematic genome-wide approach is taken to define a risk or causative locus; this approach does not rely on a perceived understanding of the processes underlying the disease to nominate genes of interest for interrogation. As a consequence, some of the most successful genetic approaches in PD have been those centred on, or founded on evidence from, family-based studies, where genome-wide linkage (a method that surveys the whole genome to define segregation between DNA segments and disease) and positional cloning (analysis of those segments for mutations) are used.

Family-based genetic work has led to the identification of several genes containing mutations that cause PD, and some of the patients with these mutations progress to, or even present with, dementia. Because dementia is a relatively common occurrence in the ageing population, a critical question is whether the co-occurring dementia observed in these PD families is related to the underlying PD aetiology or just a random coincidence. This is not necessarily an easy question to answer; although one can compare age-matched incidence rates between the population and patients within families that harbour particular mutations, the number of people in the latter group affected by these mutations is relatively low (with some exceptions discussed later). With this in mind, we will now discuss the incidence of dementia in monogenic forms of PD. Mutation in three genes (*PARK2*, *PINK1*, and *PARK7*) cause autosomal recessive forms of early onset

PD [1–3]. Patients with PD caused by mutations in these genes are rarely reported to show signs of dementia. For this reason, herein we will discuss the autosomal dominant forms of PD with a focus on *SNCA* and *LRRK2*-associated PD, for which dementia has been shown to be an important phenotypic factor.

Gene mutations known to cause dominant PD associated with dementia

In 2011, vacuolar protein sorting 35 (*VPS35*) was the first PD gene identified using a direct next-generation sequencing strategy [4, 5]. Only one mutation (p.D620N) has been shown to be unequivocally pathogenic, with a frequency ranging from 0.1 to 1% in familial cases with autosomal dominant PD [6]. From the clinical descriptions of the 35 unrelated PD cases reported in the literature, dementia seems to be a very rare event in this type of PD, with only one Asian patient reported to have mild cognitive impairment [6, 7]. Dementia is also an uncommon event in *LRRK2*-associated PD, but is much more common when *SNCA* mutation is the cause of disease.

SNCA (previously PARK1, PARK4; encoding the protein α-synuclein)

The first key advance that occurred in the genetics of PD was closely related with PD-D. A study of a large kindred with early onset, Lewy body-positive autosomal dominant PD [8] identified a missense mutation (p.A53T) in the gene encoding α-synuclein [9].

Although mutations in *SNCA* are very rare in patients with PD, they did provide the first clue that this protein is involved in the molecular pathway leading to the disease. The advantage of studying a rare familial form of the disease for understanding the more common, apparently sporadic forms became evident when Lewy bodies and Lewy neurites present in sporadic PD were found to contain aggregates of α-synuclein [10]. This work neatly demonstrated a link between familial and sporadic disease and placed α-synuclein at the centre of scientific research into PD. Five missense mutations have been identified in α-synuclein to date (p.A30P, p.E46K, p.H50Q, p.G51D, and p.A53T) [9, 11–14]. Furthermore, several families have now been described where the cause of PD lies in the genetic burden of α-synuclein: patients presenting with one or two extra copies of this gene (locus duplication and triplication, respectively) [15]. PD-D and dementia with Lewy bodies (DLB) were explicitly described as the presenting diseases in the family carrying the p.E46K mutation. However, it is clear that dementia occurs as a common feature of families linked to α-synuclein mutation, both missense and copy number mutations (see Table 13.1).

It is also worth noting that within those families where disease is caused by multiplication of the α-synuclein locus, the genetic load appears to be correlated with both the severity of disease and the presence/absence of dementia. Thus, patients who carry two additional copies of α-synuclein tend to present in their 30s and the disease progresses to include severe dementia, whereas patients who carry only one additional copy of α-synuclein tend to get the disease a decade or so later and dementia is not as frequent a feature (although it does still occur) [15–17]. The prevalence of dementia in these families argues strongly that this is truly a facet of the disease process and not simply coincidental. This notion is supported by neuropathological examination of patients who carry these mutations, which reveals a widespread and severe α-synuclein pathology involving neocortical as well as archi-cortical systems [18]. Table 13.1 summarizes the main features of PD families where a genetic mutation in *SNCA* has been associated with the disease [11–17, 19–44].

Table 13.1 Main features of Parkinson's disease families where a genetic mutation in *SNCA* has been associated with the disease

	SNCA mutation						
	p.A30P	**p.E46K**	**p.H50Q**	**p.G51D**	**p.A53T**	**Duplication**	**Triplication**
No. of cases (families)	4 cases; 1 family	5 cases; 1 family	3 cases; 2 families	8 cases (2 families; 1 case apparently sporadic)	70 cases; 22 families	36 cases; 10 families, sporadic cases, 2 unaffected carriers reported	25 triplications and 2 homozygous duplications
Age at onset (years)	60 ± 11	60 ± 7	62 ± 8	36 ± 12	47 ± 12	50 ± 11	40 ± 14
Dementia	2 of 4 (50%)	4 of 5 (80%)	All	3 of 6 (50%)	9 of 23 (39%)	12 of 24 (50%)	All (*n* = 13)
AAO dementia	At ages 52 and 76	2 within 4 years, 1 after 14 years	2 within 3 years, third case after 9 years	2 and 9 years after onset; not known for the third case	51 ±13 years (*n* = 57)	57 ± 11 years (*n* = 11)	39 ± 4 years
References	[11, 19]	[12]	[13, 20]	[14, 21, 22]	[9, 23–27]	[16, 28–39]	[15, 17, 40–43]

AAO dementia, age at onset of dementia.

Kasten, M. and C. Klein, Mov Disord, The many faces of alpha-synuclein mutations, 28, 6, 697–701 ©2007.

LRRK2 (PARK8; encoding the protein Lrrk2/dardarin)

The leucine-rich repeat kinase 2 gene (*LRRK2*), located on chromosome 12 (12q12), encodes the protein dardarin. This contains both GTPase and kinase domains, as well as two protein–protein interaction domains (leucine-rich and WD40 repeats) [45]. In 2004, mutations in this gene were associated with the development of PD in several kindreds [46, 47]. Since then, pathogenic *LRRK2* substitutions have become recognized as one of the most important causes of both familial and sporadic forms of PD [48–50].

While the majority of patients with *LRRK2*-linked disease present with a phenotype that is clinically indistinguishable from typical PD, there are several case reports of patients who present with clinically and neuropathologically atypical forms of the disease [47]. Two members of family A (one of the families in which mutations in *LRRK2* were first described as being associated with PD) [47] presented with dementia in the absence of parkinsonian symptoms and carried the p.Y1699C amino acid change [51]. A novel mutation (p.L1165P) was also found in a PD patient who developed severe neuropsychological symptoms and dementia [52], although in this instance the pathogenicity of the mutation has not been proven. In 2012, Meeus et al. [53] screened the major AD and PD genes in a cohort of DLB and PD-D cases from Belgium. They identified a female PD-D patient with an onset of parkinsonism at 70 years and progressive cognitive decline that led to dementia with important functional impairment [Mini-Mental State Examination (MMSE) score 14/30 at age 86] who carried the p.R1441C *LRRK2* mutation.

The most common *LRRK2* mutation in White populations is the p.G2019S variant, which affects a key residue in the kinase domain of this large and complex protein. This variant appears to underlie disease in about 1% of patients with sporadic PD and 4% of patients with hereditary PD, and its frequency varies greatly with geographical or ethnic origin, being highest in the Middle East and higher in southern than in northern Europe [54].

Overall, the prevalence of cognitive dysfunction and dementia among *LRRK2* p.G2019S patients is low [54–56]. Four studies assessing cognitive dysfunction in *LRRK2* p.G2019S PD cases in different populations have found no significant differences between p.G2019S carriers and non-carriers [57–60]. However, a larger study performed in a worldwide series showed a significantly lower prevalence of cognitive impairment in *LRRK2*-related PD than in idiopathic PD: only 23% of patients with *LRRK2* p.G2019S were found to have evidence of cognitive impairment (MMSE score ≤24) compared with 70% of patients with idiopathic PD [54]. This finding clearly argues against the speculation that genetic variability at the *LRRK2* locus could underlie both AD and PD, given the previous association of the chromosome 12q12 locus with late-onset AD [61].

Dementias with parkinsonism

The clinical expression of mutations in genes proven to be associated with different dementias is variable. Some of these mutations may give rise to parkinsonian syndromes and thus these genes may be of potential importance in the development of PD-D. For example, mutations of *PSEN1* and *PSEN2* cause a familial form of young-onset AD. In *PSEN1* the p.G217D mutation was found in a Japanese family affected by a disease characterized by dementia, parkinsonism, a stooped posture, and an antiflexion gait with an onset in the fourth decade of life. Neuropathologically, the disease was characterized by the presence of 'cotton wool' plaques, senile plaques, severe amyloid angiopathy, neurofibrillary tangles, neuronal rarefaction, and gliosis [62]. In *PSEN2*, the p.A85V mutation was found in an Italian family in which the proband was diagnosed with DLB. All the other affected members exhibited a clinical phenotype typical of AD. Neuropathologically, the proband presented with unusually abundant and widespread cortical Lewy bodies in addition to the hallmark lesions of AD [63]. To clarify the role of mutations in the major dementia (*APP, PSEN1, PSEN2, MAPT, GRN, TARDBP*) and PD (*SNCA, LRRK2, PARK2, PINK1, PARK7, GBA*) genes in DLB and PD-D, Meeus et al. [53] performed sequencing and dosage analyses in 99 DLB and 75 PD-D patients from Belgium. They identified 14 known or novel variants in these genes, but most were associated with a diagnosis of DLB, with only three variants (*PSEN2* p.V191E, *LRRK2* p.R1441C, and *PARK2* p.P37L) being found in PD-D or probable PD-D cases. From these three, only the *LRRK2* p.R1441C mutation was considered as definitely pathogenic. Interestingly, the sequencing of *GBA* revealed five rare and two common heterozygous variants in the studied cohort. The five rare mutations were found in seven patients, six of whom had a diagnosis of PD-D and only one of DLB. One of these mutations was a novel frameshift mutation (p.Q256SfX9), predicted to create a premature stop codon, in a familial early onset PD-D patient whose father also suffered from early onset PD. Even though this study analysed a small series of patients, the results suggest that rare variants in dementia genes have a more pronounced role in the genetics of DLB, while variants in PD genes seem to be more frequently associated with PD-D.

Synucleinopathies

DLB is a disorder mainly characterized by dementia and parkinsonism, but with other distinguishing features. The question of whether PD-D and DLB are different entities or different demonstrations of the same pathological spectrum has been extensively discussed (including elsewhere in this book); however, it is important to stress that even fully penetrant, autosomal dominant mutations may lead to different clinical phenotypes across the spectrum of PD-D, DLB, and beyond. Families with mutations in *SNCA* emphasize this premise: (1) the family described by Zarranz et al. [12] includes individuals carrying the same mutation (p.E46K) but with PD-D and DLB phenotypes within the same cohort; (2) multiplications of the *SNCA* locus may lead to either PD-D or DLB [15, 16, 30]. Neuropathological examination of brain tissue from dominantly inherited forms of AD and from Down's syndrome patients frequently reveals Lewy body pathology. Mutations in *LRRK2* may lead to α-synuclein, tau, or ubiquitin pathology with or without Lewy bodies. Clearly there are multiple genetic factors that can trigger the formation of Lewy bodies, irrespective of the disease phenotype, and this implicitly links the underlying molecular aetiology of these diseases to that of PD.

Multiple system atrophy (MSA) is the second most common parkinsonian syndrome after idiopathic PD, presenting clinically with various combinations of parkinsonism, cerebellar ataxia, and autonomic failure. Even though cognitive dysfunction appears to be minimal, the majority of patients have frontal system impairment and some develop dementia late in the course of the disease. Pathologically, it is characterized by glial cytoplasmic inclusions mainly composed of α-synuclein. MSA is usually a sporadic disease, but the fact that several MSA patients have relatives with PD led to the study of various genes. Clearly, from the point of view of molecular pathology, the most plausible gene responsible for the pathogenesis of MSA is *SNCA*. Several genetic analyses of *SNCA* in MSA cases have been conducted, but they have largely failed to identify any pathogenic mutations, particularly when only pathologically confirmed cases were screened [64, 65]. More recently, an individual with a *SNCA* multiplication mutation was reported with a clinical syndrome reminiscent of MSA [31]. Common genetic variability at this locus may also confer risk for MSA in White populations [66–68].

Tauopathies

The tauopathies are a heterogeneous group of neurodegenerative diseases that share the presence of aberrant tau aggregates [69]. Tau is a microtubule-associated protein that binds to tubulin and works to stabilize microtubules and promote microtubule assembly [70]. The microtubule-associated protein tau gene (*MAPT*) is located in an atypical genomic region of chromosome 17 and produces six isoforms of the tau protein by alternative splicing of exons 2, 3, and 10 [71]. The interaction of tau with the microtubules occurs through three (3R) or four (4R) imperfect repeat sequences in the carboxyl terminal of the protein. One of these four domains is encoded by exon 10; hence, the alternative splicing of this exon determines the number of microtubule-binding domains. In the adult human brain, 3R and 4R tau are present in approximately equal quantities [72].

Several pathogenic mutations in *MAPT* have been associated with different clinical phenotypes. These mutations appear clustered between exons 9 and 13 of the gene and may be roughly divided into two categories, depending on the pathogenic mechanism involved: protein function mutations and splicing regulation mutations. The first group of mutations impairs the ability of tau to interact with microtubules or to promote microtubule assembly; the second corresponds to mutations located in exon 10 (with the exception of those occurring in codon 301) and in flanking intronic regions that affect the alternative splicing of this exon and consequently increase the 4R/3R tau ratio. 4R tau appears to aggregate more readily than 3R tau, thus overproduction of 4R tau may lead to an excess of free 4R and consequently promote tau aggregation [73].

The most frequent phenotype associated with *MAPT* mutations is frontotemporal dementia with parkinsonism linked to chromosome 17 (FTDP-17). This is a familial disorder mainly characterized by behavioural and cognitive disturbances with progression to dementia followed by parkinsonism. The clinical spectrum associated with *MAPT* mutations is, however, extensive. The same mutation may cause different clinical expressions in different families and even within the same family. This is the case with the most frequent *MAPT* mutation, p.P301L, that has been associated with cases resembling Pick's disease, corticobasal degeneration, and progressive supranuclear palsy [74, 75]. Whereas it can be clearly argued that FTDP-17 and PD-D are undoubtedly distinct entities, recent evidence implicating genetic variability in *MAPT* to lifetime risk for PD suggests that expression of this protein is a critical factor in PD, despite the general lack of tau pathology in this disease.

Genetic risk factors for PD-D

The identification of rare causal mutations for PD and PD-D has been extremely successful over the last 10 years, yet the search for genetic variants that alter risk for disease has been more difficult. The primary work in this area has been done in PD cohorts that include patients both with and without dementia; this is primarily because such cohorts are easier to collect and more readily available. In the instances where PD-D has been separated out as a distinct entity, the sample size tends to be quite small. As geneticists now clearly appreciate, cohorts of several thousand cases are required to discover novel genetic loci that exert a small effect in complex diseases, and thus success for PD-D in this area will require a concerted effort to collect larger sample sizes.

APOE

The *APOE* ε4 allele is probably the best-known genetic risk factor in adult-onset human disease. This variant confers substantial risk for AD: heterozygous carriers are approximately three times more likely and homozygous carriers eight times more likely to develop AD. Apolipoprotein E (ApoE) is a glycoprotein involved in the transport of lipoproteins, fat-soluble vitamins, and cholesterol into the lymph system and then into the blood. ApoE is synthesized and secreted by many tissues, primarily liver, brain, skin, and tissue macrophages, throughout the body, sites where it plays critically important roles [76]. The gene coding for ApoE resides on the long arm of chromosome 19 in a cluster with apolipoprotein C1 (*APOC1*) and apolipoprotein C2 (*APOC2*). It is a polymorphic gene with three major alleles, which translate into three isoforms of the protein, ApoE-ε3, ApoE-ε2, and ApoE-ε4. These isoforms differ from each other by amino acid substitutions at positions 112 and 158 [77].

Although genetic variability at *APOE* is neither necessary nor sufficient for the development of AD, its risk has been shown to be dose dependent and correlated with the age at onset of the disease [78]. Given the robust association between ApoE and AD it has been hypothesized that a similar relationship exists with PD-D and DLB. Several studies have evaluated the role of ApoE in PD-D, with contradictory results [79–82]. As previously noted, however, these studies are individually of quite limited sample size. A meta-analysis of the studies published between 1966 and 2004 concluded that the *APOE* ε4 allele appears to be associated with a higher prevalence of dementia in PD (with an increased odds ratio of 1.6) [83]. *APOE* ε4 has been clearly associated with DLB, lending further support for the idea that PD-D, DLB, and AD are, at least in part, members of an aetiological spectrum of disorders.

GBA

Mutations in both copies of the glucocerebrosidase gene (*GBA*), encoding a lysosomal enzyme known to cleave the glycolipid glucocerebroside into glucose and ceramide, cause autosomal recessive Gaucher's disease. Interestingly, heterozygous variants in *GBA* have been shown to increase the risk for the development of PD. Clinical observation of patients and relatives of patients with Gaucher's disease indicates that they seem to present with PD more often than expected, leading to the identification of variants in *GBA* as a risk for PD. This association was first identified in the Ashkenazi Jewish population [84] and later confirmed by a large worldwide meta-analysis [85] showing that carriers of a single *GBA* mutant allele were at around a five-fold greater risk for PD.

PD associated with *GBA* risk alleles was found to be clinically similar to idiopathic PD and possibly associated with greater rates of bradykinesia, resting tremor, rigidity, and cognitive changes. Additionally, mutations in *GBA* have also been found in DLB patients [86–89], confirming an association between genetic variability at this locus, parkinsonism, and dementia. Further evidence implicating *GBA* in the development of dementia in PD came from a study performing a genetic screen of the whole *GBA* gene in a cohort of UK PD patients. Cognitive decline or dementia was observed in 48% of PD patients carrying *GBA* alterations, thus suggesting that mutations in *GBA* might increase the risk of developing cognitive impairment in individuals suffering from PD [90]. Similar findings were revealed in a Spanish population: after sequencing *GBA* in 225 PD patients, variants in this gene were associated with a significant risk of dementia during the clinical course of PD [91]. More recently *GBA* mutations have been shown to influence the natural history of PD in a community-based incident cohort from the UK. *GBA* mutations were found to be present at a frequency of 3.5% (higher than the prevalence of other genetic mutations know to be associated with PD). Although no significant differences were found in the clinical features present in PD cases with and without *GBA* variants at baseline, the hazard ratio for progression to dementia was significantly greater in carriers of *GBA* variants after a median of 6 years' follow-up. In PD patients with *GBA* mutations, the risk of progression to dementia was found to be more than five times that of patients without such mutations [92].

Other genetic risk factors for PD-D

The primary catalyst for the investigation of genetic risk factors associated with PD-D comes from previous association with AD, PD, or DLB. Given the previously mentioned sample size requirements and the numerous confounders in candidate gene association studies, robust genetic associations in these diseases have been relatively few and far between. For a long time the most consistent genetic risk associations in PD have probably been those with common variants in *SNCA* and *MAPT*, although these have not been without controversy [93–95]. These associations were confirmed by genome-wide association studies (GWAS) in PD, which have also identified 22 additional loci conferring a low risk for the development of PD (*LRRK2, RAB7L1, BST1, HLA-DRB5, GAK, ACMSD, STK39, MCCC1, SYT11, CCDC62, FGF20, STX1B, GPNMB, SIPA1L2, INPP5F, MIR4697HG, GCH1, VPS13C, SCARB2, RIT2, DDRGK1, SREBF*) [96, 97].

Most of the studies evaluating the role of genetic variants in the risk of developing PD-D have focused on *MAPT* and *SNCA* and have mostly failed to find significant associations [93, 98, 99]. Divergent results suggesting that the tau inversion influences the development of cognitive impairment and dementia in patients with idiopathic PD were reported by Goris et al. [100] who studied 659 PD patients, 109 of whom were followed up for 3.5 years from diagnosis, and 2176 control subjects. Although only 11 of the incident cohort of 109 PD patients developed new-onset dementia during the 3.5 years of follow-up, H1 haplotype homozygotes presented a greater rate of cognitive decline than H2 haplotype carriers, assessed by the changes observed in MMSE per year [100]. Similarly, a case–control study investigating the role of genetic variability in *SNCA* showed no associations with PD-D. Six polymorphic loci (including the Rep1 microsatellite) in the promoter of the *SNCA* gene were examined in 114 PD-D patients and 114 patients with sporadic PD but no dementia [101]. In this case the absence of evidence does not imply evidence of absence; without exception these studies comprise relatively small case numbers, particularly when considering the number of patients with cognitive decline or dementia. It is therefore difficult to rule out variability at *SNCA* or *MAPT* as a risk factor for PD-D until well-powered comprehensive studies have been performed. Given the association between the *MAPT* haplotype and other dementias, parsimony would suggest an association with PD-D; however, time and well-structured analyses will tell.

Case–control analyses of variants in *COMT* [102], *CYPD6* [103], *MAOB* [104], *GSK3B* [100], *BCHE* [105], and *ESR1* [106] suggest that these loci present no significant risk for the development of PD-D. In contrast, the interaction between a *DCP1* insertion polymorphism and *APOE* ε4 was reported to increase the risk of PD with coexisting AD pathology [105]. A possible role for gene–toxin interactions in PD-D was also revealed when a high predicted probability for developing PD-D was established in PD patients carrying a particular *CYP2D6* allele who were exposed to pesticides [104].

Given the similarities between AD and PD it has been hypothesized that the same aetiological factors could be present in both diseases. A few studies have tested this hypothesis, with different conclusions: in a Korean population no significant associations were found between the AD susceptibility loci *ABCA7*, *APOE*, *CLU*, *CR1*, and *PICALM* and the susceptibility to PD [107]; similarly, the study of one polymorphism in *PICALM* in a small cohort of Greek PD patients also showed no significant association [108]; and a couple of studies have also hinted at a possible association between the p.R47H variant in *TREM2* and PD [109, 110]. An exploratory analysis revealed no association between *CR1* and *PICALM* and PD, but suggested an association with *CLU*. Interestingly this association was found to be stronger for PD-D than for PD without dementia [111]. This preliminary result supports the hypothesis that, similar to *APOE*, other genetic variants identified to be risk factors for the development of AD would also have a role in the development of PD-D. Genome-wide association with PD-D has only been reported once, and with relatively small cohorts of samples: Chung et al. [113] used *genome-wide association study* data from 443 PD cases from their previous report [112] and telephone interviews for follow-up assessments of motor and cognitive outcomes a median of 9 years after the initial assessment. From the 443 PD patients initially enrolled, follow-up data were available for 417, 44 of whom were considered to have cognitive impairment. No variant remained significant after Bonferroni correction, with single nucleotide polymorphisms (SNPs) in *CLRN3* and *C4orf26* showing the stronger associations [113]. Although this study was clearly underpowered it remains the only genome-wide study with a follow-up of cognitive outcomes. Additionally, a recent report [114] showed that loci that increase the risk of both PD and AD are not widespread, suggesting that the pathological overlap observed between these two diseases could happen 'downstream' of the primary susceptibility genes that increase the risk of each disease. A similarly well-designed study is needed to reveal real genetic risk factors for the development of PD-D at a genome-wide level.

Next steps in gene identification for dementia in PD

At the beginning of this chapter we said that identification of genetic factors for disease appears to be most successful when a relatively unbiased genome-wide approach can be taken rather than a focused candidate gene analysis. Technological limitations have previously made it unfeasible to take this kind of approach in association mapping (as opposed to linkage mapping), leaving candidate gene association work as the main practical alternative. However, the development of high-throughput genotyping platforms has made genome-wide association a realistic possibility. Such platforms are capable of accurately genotyping millions of SNPs in parallel and this method has now been successfully applied to identify risk loci in PD and several other complex disorders [96, 115, 116]. Successful identification by genome-wide association studies of genetic variability that confers risk for disease depends on many factors, including sample size, population homogeneity, and effect size (described comprehensively by Hardy and Singleton [117]). For this type of study the primary limitations for PD-D are sample size and agreement on the diagnostic criteria for this disorder. Even when common genetic risk loci for PD-D are identified, many challenges will exist; the most immediate will be fine mapping of these loci (i.e. a better understanding of the actual alleles that confer risk within the risk region) and mapping out the immediate effects of risk variants—which transcripts do they affect, do they alter expression, if so in which way, or do they alter splicing? There is also room for further genomic exploration of complex diseases like PD-D [117], including whole-exome/whole-genome sequencing in the rare cases where PD-D segregates in families, deep resequencing to identify rare risk variants, analysis of genomic copy number variation as a risk factor for disease, epigenetic assays to detect a role for this type of variation in disease, and deep sequence analysis to define whether somatic mutations may play a role in the development and progression of PD-D. All of these approaches offer unique insights and challenges, and the rapidly increasing availability of techniques to address these issues means that workers in this field should be preparing for the tasks ahead. The most obvious preparation would be the collection of large cohorts of well-characterized patients.

Conclusion

Dementia is more frequently observed in autosomal dominant forms of PD (particularly in cases caused by *SNCA* mutation) than in the recessive forms. The genetic basis of dementia occurring in apparently sporadic PD is less well understood, with variability in *APOE* and *GBA* being the most consistent genetic risk factors. The primary goal of disease genetics is to shed light onto the molecular aetiology of disease with an eye toward defining potential points for therapeutic intervention. Clearly there has been substantial progress in the genetics of PD (and implicitly PD-D); however, there is still a long way to go. The tools are now at hand to achieve a more complete understanding of the genetic basis of common complex diseases, including PD-D. Not only will a more complete genetic understanding of these diseases inform us about aetiology, but it is also likely to add more clarity to the idea that this disease is aetiologically similar to DLB and AD. There will certainly be challenges to a successful dissection of the genetic basis of PD-D, perhaps the most immediate of which is that of achieving sufficient sample size to detect and confirm a genuine genetic association; however, for the first time the route to success is relatively clear.

References

1. **Kitada T, Asakawa S, Hattori N, et al.** Mutations in the parkin gene cause autosomal recessive juvenile parkinsonism. Nature 1998; **392**: 605–8.
2. **Valente EM, Abou-Sleiman PM, Caputo V, et al.** Hereditary early-onset Parkinson's disease caused by mutations in PINK1. Science 2004; **304**: 1158–60.
3. **Bonifati V, Rizzu P, van Baren MJ, et al.** Mutations in the DJ-1 gene associated with autosomal recessive early-onset parkinsonism. Science 2003; **299**: 256–9.
4. **Zimprich A, Benet-Pagès A, Struhal W, et al.** A mutation in VPS35, encoding a subunit of the retromer complex, causes late-onset Parkinson disease. Am J Hum Genet 2011; **89**: 168–75.

5. **Vilariño-Guell C, Wider C, Ross OA, et al.**, VPS35 mutations in Parkinson disease. Am J Hum Genet 2011; **89**: 162–7.

6. **Deng H, Gao K, Jankovic J.** The VPS35 gene and Parkinson's disease. Mov Disord 2013; **28**: 569–75.

7. **Sharma M, Ioannidis JP, Aasly JO, et al.** A multi-centre clinico-genetic analysis of the VPS35 gene in Parkinson disease indicates reduced penetrance for disease-associated variants. J Med Genet 2012; **49**: 721–6.

8. **Polymeropoulos MH, Higgins JJ, Golbe LI, et al.** Mapping of a gene for Parkinson's disease to chromosome 4q21-q23. Science 1996; **274**: 1197–9.

9. **Polymeropoulos MH, Lavedan C, Leroy E, et al.**, Mutation in the alpha-synuclein gene identified in families with Parkinson's disease. Science 1997; **276**: 2045–7.

10. **Spillantini MG, Schmidt ML, Lee VM, et al.** Alpha-synuclein in Lewy bodies. Nature 1997; **388**: 839–40.

11. **Kruger R, Kuhn W, Müller T, et al.** Ala30Pro mutation in the gene encoding alpha-synuclein in Parkinson's disease. Nat Genet 1998; **18**: 106–8.

12. **Zarranz JJ, Alegre J, Gómez-Esteban JC, et al.** The new mutation, E46K, of alpha-synuclein causes Parkinson and Lewy body dementia. Ann Neurol 2004; **55**: 164–73.

13. **Proukakis C, Dudzik CG, Brier T, et al.** A novel alpha-synuclein missense mutation in Parkinson disease. Neurology 2013; **80**: 1062–4.

14. **Kiely AP, Asi YT, Kara E, et al.** Alpha-synucleinopathy associated with G51D SNCA mutation: a link between Parkinson's disease and multiple system atrophy? Acta Neuropathol 2013; **125**: 753–69.

15. **Singleton AB, Farrer M, Johnson J, et al.** Alpha-synuclein locus triplication causes Parkinson's disease. Science 2003; **302**: 841.

16. **Chartier-Harlin MC, Kachergus J, Roumier C, et al.** Alpha-synuclein locus duplication as a cause of familial Parkinson's disease. Lancet 2004; **364**: 1167–9.

17. **Farrer M, Kachergus J, Forno L, et al.** Comparison of kindreds with parkinsonism and alpha-synuclein genomic multiplications. Ann Neurol 2004; **55**: 174–9.

18. **Gwinn-Hardy K, Mehta ND, Farrer M, et al.** Distinctive neuropathology revealed by alpha-synuclein antibodies in hereditary parkinsonism and dementia linked to chromosome 4p. Acta Neuropathol 2000; **99**: 663–72.

19. **Kruger R, Kuhn W, Leenders KL, et al.** Familial parkinsonism with synuclein pathology: clinical and PET studies of A30P mutation carriers. Neurology 2001; **56**: 1355–62.

20. **Appel-Cresswell S, Vilarino-Guell C, Encarnacion M, et al.** Alpha-synuclein p.H50Q, a novel pathogenic mutation for Parkinson's disease. Mov Disord 2013; **28**: 811–13.

21. **Tokutake T, Ishikawa A, Yoshimura N, et al.** Clinical and neuroimaging features of patient with early-onset Parkinson's disease with dementia carrying SNCA p.G51D mutation. Parkinsonism Relat Disord 2014; **20**: 262–4.

22. **Lesage S, Anheim M, Letournel F, et al.** G51D alpha-synuclein mutation causes a novel parkinsonian-pyramidal syndrome. Ann Neurol 2013; **73**: 459–71.

23. **Markopoulou K, Wszolek ZK, Pfeiffer RF.** A Greek-American kindred with autosomal dominant, levodopa-responsive parkinsonism and anticipation. Ann Neurol 1995; **38**: 373–8.

24. **Markopoulou K, Wszolek ZK, Pfeiffer RF, et al.** Reduced expression of the G209A alpha-synuclein allele in familial Parkinsonism. Ann Neurol 1999; **46**: 374–81.

25. **Spira PJ, Sharpe DM, Halliday G, et al.** Clinical and pathological features of a Parkinsonian syndrome in a family with an Ala53Thr alpha-synuclein mutation. Ann Neurol 2001; **49**: 313–19.

26. **Bostantjopoulou S, Katsarou Z, Papadimitriou A, et al.** Clinical features of parkinsonian patients with the alpha-synuclein (G209A) mutation. Mov Disord 2001; **16**: 1007–13.

27. **Papapetropoulos S, Paschalis C, Athanassiadou A, et al.** Clinical phenotype in patients with alpha-synuclein Parkinson's disease living in Greece in comparison with patients with sporadic Parkinson's disease. J Neurol Neurosurg Psychiatry 2001; **70**: 662–5.

28. **Ahn TB, Kim SY, Kim JY, et al.**, Alpha-synuclein gene duplication is present in sporadic Parkinson disease. Neurology 2008; **70**: 43–9.

29. **Ibanez P, Bonnet AM, Débarges B, et al.** Causal relation between alpha-synuclein gene duplication and familial Parkinson's disease. Lancet 2004; **364**: 1169–71.

30. **Nishioka K, Hayashi S, Farrer MJ, et al.** Clinical heterogeneity of alpha-synuclein gene duplication in Parkinson's disease. Ann Neurol 2006; **59**: 298–309.

31. **Fuchs J, Nilsson C, Kachergus J, et al.** Phenotypic variation in a large Swedish pedigree due to SNCA duplication and triplication. Neurology 2007; **68**: 916–22.

32. **Ikeuchi T, Kakita A, Shiga A, et al.** Patients homozygous and heterozygous for SNCA duplication in a family with parkinsonism and dementia. Arch Neurol 2008; **65**: 514–19.

33. **Obi T, Nishioka K, Ross OA, et al.** Clinicopathologic study of a SNCA gene duplication patient with Parkinson disease and dementia. Neurology 2008; **70**: 238–41.

34. **Ross OA, Braithwaite AT, Skipper LM, et al.** Genomic investigation of alpha-synuclein multiplication and parkinsonism. Ann Neurol 2008; **63**: 743–50.

35. **Uchiyama T, Ikeuchi T, Ouchi Y, et al.** Prominent psychiatric symptoms and glucose hypometabolism in a family with a SNCA duplication. Neurology 2008; **71**: 1289–91.

36. **Nishioka K, Ross OA, Ishii K, et al.** Expanding the clinical phenotype of SNCA duplication carriers. Mov Disord 2009; **24**: 1811–19.

37. **Sironi F, Trotta L, Antonini A, et al.** Alpha-synuclein multiplication analysis in Italian familial Parkinson disease. Parkinsonism Relat Disord 2010; **16**: 228–31.

38. **Shin CW, Kim HJ, Park SS, et al.** Two Parkinson's disease patients with alpha-synuclein gene duplication and rapid cognitive decline. Mov Disord 2010; **25**: 957–9.

39. **Itokawa K, Sekine T, Funayama M, et al.**, A case of alpha-synuclein gene duplication presenting with head-shaking movements. Mov Disord 2013; **28**: 384–7.

40. **Muenter MD, Forno LS, Hornykiewicz O, et al.**, Hereditary form of parkinsonism–dementia. Ann Neurol 1998; **43**: 768–81.

41. **Sekine T, Kagaya H, Funayama M, et al.** Clinical course of the first Asian family with Parkinsonism related to SNCA triplication. Mov Disord 2010; **25**: 2871–5.

42. **Gwinn K, Devine MJ, Jin LW, et al.** Clinical features, with video documentation, of the original familial Lewy body parkinsonism caused by alpha-synuclein triplication (Iowa kindred). Mov Disord 2011; **26**: 2134–6.

43. **Kojovic M, Sheerin UM, Rubio-Agusti I, et al.** Young-onset parkinsonism due to homozygous duplication of alpha-synuclein in a consanguineous family. Mov Disord 2012; **27**: 1827–9.

44. **Kasten M, Klein C.** The many faces of alpha-synuclein mutations. Mov Disord 2013; **28**: 697–701.

45. **Cookson MR, Dauer W, Dawson T, et al.** The roles of kinases in familial Parkinson's disease. J Neurosci 2007; **27**: 11865–8.

46. **Paisan-Ruiz C, Jain S, Evans EW, et al.** Cloning of the gene containing mutations that cause PARK8-linked Parkinson's disease. Neuron 2004; **44**: 595–600.

47. **Zimprich A, Biskup S, Leitner P, et al.** Mutations in LRRK2 cause autosomal-dominant parkinsonism with pleomorphic pathology. Neuron 2004; **44**: 601–7.

48. **Farrer M, Stone J, Mata IF, et al.** LRRK2 mutations in Parkinson disease. Neurology 2005; **65**: 738–40.

49. **Bras JM, Guerreiro RJ, Ribeiro MH, et al.** G2019S dardarin substitution is a common cause of Parkinson's disease in a Portuguese cohort. Mov Disord 2005; **20**: 1653–5.

50. **Mata IF, Taylor JP, Kachergus J, et al.** LRRK2 R1441G in Spanish patients with Parkinson's disease. Neurosci Lett 2005; **382**: 309–11.

51. **Wszolek ZK, Vieregge P, Uitti RJ, et al.** German-Canadian family (family A) with parkinsonism, amyotrophy, and dementia—Longitudinal observations. Parkinsonism Relat Disord 1997; **3**: 125–39.

52. **Covy JP, Yuan W, Waxman EA, et al.** Clinical and pathological characteristics of patients with leucine-rich repeat kinase-2 mutations. Mov Disord 2009; **24**: 32–9.

53. Meeus B, Verstraeten A, Crosiers D, et al. DLB and PDD: a role for mutations in dementia and Parkinson disease genes? Neurobiol Aging 2012; **33**: 629.e5–629.e18.

54. Healy DG, Falchi M, O'Sullivan SS, et al. Phenotype, genotype, and worldwide genetic penetrance of LRRK2-associated Parkinson's disease: a case-control study. Lancet Neurol 2008; **7**: 583–90.

55. Di Fonzo A, Rohé CF, Ferreira J, et al., A frequent LRRK2 gene mutation associated with autosomal dominant Parkinson's disease. Lancet 2005; **365**: 412–15.

56. Aasly JO, Toft M, Fernandez-Mata I, et al. Clinical features of LRRK2-associated Parkinson's disease in central Norway. Ann Neurol 2005; **57**: 762–5.

57. Lesage S, Ibanez P, Lohmann E, et al. G2019S LRRK2 mutation in French and North African families with Parkinson's disease. Ann Neurol 2005; **58**: 784–7.

58. Goldwurm S, Zini M, Di Fonzo A, et al. LRRK2 G2019S mutation and Parkinson's disease: a clinical, neuropsychological and neuropsychiatric study in a large Italian sample. Parkinsonism Relat Disord 2006; **12**: 410–19.

59. Belarbi S, Hecham N, Lesage S, et al. LRRK2 G2019S mutation in Parkinson's disease: a neuropsychological and neuropsychiatric study in a large Algerian cohort. Parkinsonism Relat Disord 2010; **16**: 676–9.

60. Ben Sassi S, Nabli F, Hentati E, et al. Cognitive dysfunction in Tunisian LRRK2 associated Parkinson's disease. Parkinsonism Relat Disord 2012; **18**: 243–6.

61. Scott WK, Grubber JM, Conneally PM, et al. Fine mapping of the chromosome 12 late-onset Alzheimer disease locus: potential genetic and phenotypic heterogeneity. Am J Hum Genet 2000; **66**: 922–32.

62. Takao M, Ghetti B, Hayakawa I, et al. A novel mutation (G217D) in the Presenilin 1 gene (PSEN1) in a Japanese family: presenile dementia and parkinsonism are associated with cotton wool plaques in the cortex and striatum. Acta Neuropathol 2002; **104**: 155–70.

63. Piscopo P, Marcon G, Piras MR, et al. A novel PSEN2 mutation associated with a peculiar phenotype. Neurology 2008; **70**: 1549–54.

64. Ozawa T, Takano H, Onodera O, et al. No mutation in the entire coding region of the alpha-synuclein gene in pathologically confirmed cases of multiple system atrophy. Neurosci Lett 1999; **270**: 110–12.

65. Lincoln SJ, Ross OA, Milkovic NM, et al. Quantitative PCR-based screening of alpha-synuclein multiplication in multiple system atrophy. Parkinsonism Relat Disord 2007; **13**: 340–2.

66. Scholz SW, Houlden H, Schulte C, et al. SNCA variants are associated with increased risk for multiple system atrophy. Ann Neurol 2009; **65**: 610–14.

67. Al-Chalabi A, Dürr A, Wood NW, et al. Genetic variants of the alpha-synuclein gene SNCA are associated with multiple system atrophy. PLoS ONE 2009; **4**: e7114.

68. Yun JY, Lee WW, Lee JY, et al. SNCA variants and multiple system atrophy. Ann Neurol 2010; **67**: 554–5.

69. Robert M, Mathuranath, PS. Tau and tauopathies. Neurol India 2007; **55**: 11–16.

70. Hirokawa N. Microtubule organization and dynamics dependent on microtubule-associated proteins. Curr Opin Cell Biol 1994; **6**: 74–81.

71. Goedert M, Spillantini MG, Potier MC, et al. Cloning and sequencing of the cDNA encoding an isoform of microtubule-associated protein tau containing four tandem repeats: differential expression of tau protein mRNAs in human brain. EMBO J 1989; **8**: 393–9.

72. Gustke N, Trinczek B, Biernat J, et al. Domains of tau protein and interactions with microtubules. Biochemistry 1994; **33**: 9511–22.

73. Rademakers R, Hutton M. The genetics of frontotemporal lobar degeneration. Curr Neurol Neurosci Rep 2007; **7**: 434–42.

74. Mirra SS, Murrell JR, Gearing M, et al. Tau pathology in a family with dementia and a P301L mutation in tau. J Neuropathol Exp Neurol 1999; **58**: 335–45.

75. **Nasreddine ZS, Loginov M, Clark LN, et al.** From genotype to phenotype: a clinical pathological, and biochemical investigation of frontotemporal dementia and parkinsonism (FTDP-17) caused by the P301L tau mutation. Ann Neurol 1999; **45**: 704–15.

76. **Mahley RW, Rall SC Jr.** Apolipoprotein E: far more than a lipid transport protein. Annu Rev Genomics Hum Genet 2000; **1**: 507–37.

77. **Saunders AM, Strittmatter WJ, Schmechel D, et al.**, Association of apolipoprotein E allele epsilon 4 with late-onset familial and sporadic Alzheimer's disease. Neurology 1993; **43**: 1467–72.

78. **van Duijn CM, de Knijff P, Cruts M, et al.** Apolipoprotein E4 allele in a population-based study of early-onset Alzheimer's disease. Nat Genet 1994; **7**: 74–8.

79. **Parsian A, Racette B, Goldsmith LJ, et al.** Parkinson's disease and apolipoprotein E: possible association with dementia but not age at onset. Genomics 2002; **79**: 458–61.

80. **Marder K, Maestre G, Cote L, et al.** The apolipoprotein epsilon 4 allele in Parkinson's disease with and without dementia. Neurology 1994; **44**: 1330–1.

81. **Inzelberg R, Chapman J, Treves TA, et al.** Apolipoprotein E4 in Parkinson disease and dementia: new data and meta-analysis of published studies. Alzheimer Dis Assoc Disord 1998; **12**: 45–8.

82. **Pankratz N, Byder L, Halter C, et al.** Presence of an APOE4 allele results in significantly earlier onset of Parkinson's disease and a higher risk with dementia. Mov Disord 2006; **21**: 45–9.

83. **Huang X, Chen P, Kaufer DI, et al.** Apolipoprotein E and dementia in Parkinson disease: a meta-analysis. Arch Neurol 2006; **63**: 189–93.

84. **Aharon-Peretz J, Rosenbaum H, Gershoni-Baruch R.** Mutations in the glucocerebrosidase gene and Parkinson's disease in Ashkenazi Jews. N Engl J Med 2004; **351**: 1972–7.

85. **Sidransky E, Nalls MA, Aasly JO, et al.** Multicenter analysis of glucocerebrosidase mutations in Parkinson's disease. N Engl J Med 2009; **361**: 1651–61.

86. **Nalls MA, Duran R, Lopez G, et al.** A multicenter study of glucocerebrosidase mutations in dementia with Lewy bodies. J Am Med Assoc Neurol 2013; **70**: 727–35.

87. **Goker-Alpan O, Giasson BI, Eblan MJ, et al.** Glucocerebrosidase mutations are an important risk factor for Lewy body disorders. Neurology 2006; **67**: 908–10.

88. **Clark LN, Kartsaklis LA, Wolf Gilbert R, et al.** Association of glucocerebrosidase mutations with dementia with Lewy bodies. Arch Neurol 2009; **66**: 578–83.

89. **Nishioka K, Ross OA, Vilariño-Güell C, et al.** Glucocerebrosidase mutations in diffuse Lewy body disease. Parkinsonism Relat Disord 2011; **17**: 55–7.

90. **Neumann J, Bras J, Deas E, et al.** Glucocerebrosidase mutations in clinical and pathologically proven Parkinson's disease. Brain 2009; **132**: 1783–94.

91. **Seto-Salvia N, Pagonabarraga J, Houlden H, et al.** Glucocerebrosidase mutations confer a greater risk of dementia during Parkinson's disease course. Mov Disord 2012; **27**: 393–9.

92. **Winder-Rhodes SE, Evans JR, Ban M, et al.** Glucocerebrosidase mutations influence the natural history of Parkinson's disease in a community-based incident cohort. Brain 2013; **136**: 392–9.

93. **Zhang J, Song Y, Chen H, et al.** The tau gene haplotype h1 confers a susceptibility to Parkinson's disease. Eur Neurol 2005; **53**: 15–21.

94. **Farrer M, Maraganore DM, Lockhart P, et al.** Alpha-synuclein gene haplotypes are associated with Parkinson's disease. Hum Mol Genet 2001; **10**: 1847–51.

95. **Spadafora P, Annesi G, Pasqua AA, et al.** NACP-REP1 polymorphism is not involved in Parkinson's disease: a case-control study in a population sample from southern Italy. Neurosci Lett 2003; **351**: 75–8.

96. International Parkinson's Disease Genomics Consortium (IPDGC); Wellcome Trust Case Control Consortium 2 (WTCCC2). A two-stage meta-analysis identifies several new loci for Parkinson's disease. PLoS Genet 2011; **7**: e1002142.

97. Nalls MA, Plagnol V, Hernandez DG, et al. Imputation of sequence variants for identification of genetic risks for Parkinson's disease: a meta-analysis of genome-wide association studies. Lancet 2011; **377**: 641–9.

98. Zappia M, Annesi G, Nicoletti G, et al. Association of tau gene polymorphism with Parkinson's disease. Neurol Sci 2003; **24**: 223–4.

99. Ezquerra M, Campdelacreu J, Gaig C, et al. Lack of association of APOE and tau polymorphisms with dementia in Parkinson's disease. Neurosci Lett 2008; **448**: 20–3.

100. Goris A, Williams-Gray CH, Clark GR et al. Tau and alpha-synuclein in susceptibility to, and dementia in, Parkinson's disease. Ann Neurol 2007; **62**: 145–53.

101. De Marco EV, Tarantino P, Provenzano G, et al. Alpha-synuclein promoter haplotypes and dementia in Parkinson's disease. Am J Med Genet B Neuropsychiatr Genet 2008; **147**: 403–7.

102. Camicioli R, Rajput A, Rajput M, et al. Apolipoprotein E epsilon4 and catechol-O-methyltransferase alleles in autopsy-proven Parkinson's disease: relationship to dementia and hallucinations. Mov Disord 2005; **20**: 989–94.

103. Golab-Janowska M, Honczarenko K, Gawrońska-Szklarz B, et al. CYP2D6 gene polymorphism as a probable risk factor for Alzheimer's disease and Parkinson's disease with dementia. Neurol Neurochir Pol 2007; **41**: 113–21.

104. Hubble JP, Kurth JH, Glatt SL, et al. Gene-toxin interaction as a putative risk factor for Parkinson's disease with dementia. Neuroepidemiology 1998; **17**: 96–104.

105. Mattila KM, Rinne JO, Röyttä M, et al. Dipeptidyl carboxypeptidase 1 (DCP1) and butyrylcholinesterase (BCHE) gene interactions with the apolipoprotein E epsilon4 allele as risk factors in Alzheimer's disease and in Parkinson's disease with coexisting Alzheimer pathology. J Med Genet 2000; **37**: 766–70.

106. Isoe-Wada K, Maeda M, Yong J, et al. Positive association between an estrogen receptor gene polymorphism and Parkinson's disease with dementia. Eur J Neurol 1999; **6**: 431–5.

107. Chung SJ, Jung Y, Hong M, et al. Alzheimer's disease and Parkinson's disease genome-wide association study top hits and risk of Parkinson's disease in Korean population. Neurobiol Aging 2013; **34**: 2695.e1–2695.e7.

108. Kalinderi K, Bostantjopoulou S, Katsarou Z, et al., Lack of association of the PICALM rs3851179 polymorphism with Parkinson's disease in the Greek population. Int J Neurosci 2012; **122**: 502–605.

109. Benitez BA, Cruchaga C. TREM2 and neurodegenerative disease. N Engl J Med 2013; **369**: 1567–8.

110. Rayaprolu S, Mullen B, Baker M, et al. TREM2 in neurodegeneration: evidence for association of the p.R47H variant with frontotemporal dementia and Parkinson's disease. Mol Neurodegener 2013; **8**: 19.

111. Gao J, Huang X, Park Y, et al., An exploratory study on CLU, CR1 and PICALM and Parkinson disease. PLoS ONE 2011; **6**: e24211.

112. Maraganore DM, de Andrade M, Lesnick TG, et al. High-resolution whole-genome association study of Parkinson disease. Am J Hum Genet 2005; **77**: 685–93.

113. Chung SJ, Armasu SM, Biernacka JM, et al. Genomic determinants of motor and cognitive outcomes in Parkinson's disease. Parkinsonism Relat Disord 2012; **18**: 881–6.

114. Moskvina V, Harold D, Russo G, et al. Analysis of genome-wide association studies of Alzheimer disease and of Parkinson disease to determine if these 2 diseases share a common genetic risk. J Am Med Assoc Neurol 2013; **70**: 1268–76.

115. Hindorff LA, Sethupathy P, Junkins HA, et al. Potential etiologic and functional implications of genome-wide association loci for human diseases and traits. Proc Natl Acad Sci USA 2009; **106**: 9362–7.

116. Welter D, MacArthur J, Morales J, et al. The NHGRI GWAS Catalog, a curated resource of SNP-trait associations. Nucleic Acids Res 2014; **42**: D1001–D1006.

117. Hardy J, Singleton A. Genomewide association studies and human disease. N Engl J Med 2009; **360**: 1759–68.

Chapter 14

Neurochemical pathology of Parkinson's disease dementia and dementia with Lewy bodies

David Whitfield, Margaret Ann Piggott, Elaine K. Perry, and Paul T. Francis

Introduction

Whether neurotransmitter deficits and related changes in Parkinson's disease dementia (PD-D) differ in kind or degree compared with those in Parkinson's disease (PD) is an important question when considering the clinical manifestations they underlie. A detailed understanding of the functions of neurotransmitters and the consequences of their deficits can lead to rational drug design and treatment strategies appropriate for PD-D patients. In a wider context it is of interest to consider to what extent drugs that have some efficacy in people with Alzheimer's disease (AD) might work better or worse in those with PD-D. This chapter will review neurochemical pathology in transmitter systems in PD-D and potential associations with clinical symptoms.

Information on neurotransmitter make-up and receptors is gleaned most excitingly and usefully, in terms of guiding therapy, from in vivo imaging, but it is obtained in greater detail and with information on several parameters together from post-mortem investigation.

The original finding of Hornykiewicz and Ehringer [1] of reduced dopamine concentration in post-mortem striatal tissue from PD cases (first reported in the early 1960s and republished in English in 1998 [2]), and its replacement therapy [3, 4] were revolutionary developments. Neurochemists have sought with hope to discover similar apparently simple relationships between other disorders or symptoms and single transmitter systems, but often find that combinations of neurotransmitter changes are responsible. PD-D by definition evolves from levodopa-responsive PD, but even PD is more than a disorder of movement and a deficiency of dopamine [5].

Changes in neurotransmitter systems in PD-D

Dopamine: pre-synaptic dopaminergic measures

As the disease progresses, concentrations of dopamine and homovanillic acid continue to decline and are consequently further reduced in PD-D than in PD. The loss of dopamine follows a pattern which reflects neuron loss in the substantia nigra [6], progressively affecting areas of low calbindin immunostaining first. The ratio of homovanillic acid to dopamine (each measured as pmol/mg protein) is an index of dopamine turnover, which is elevated in PD to an average of 45 times normal in the putamen but is not increased significantly over controls in dementia with Lewy bodies (DLB) [7]. Although this study from 1999 was not prospective, within the PD cases analysed those who had cognitive problems recorded in their case notes ($n = 6$) had lower homovanillic acid/dopamine ratios than those without ($n = 9$) (8 ± 6 versus 50 ± 44; two-tailed t-test, $p = 0.04$). Increased turnover is one of the compensatory changes that occurs in PD and begins to fail in PD-D.

Reduced dopamine concentration is mirrored by dopamine transporter (DAT) density. This has been measured both in vitro and in vivo in PD-D, and is reliably shown to be reduced below PD levels (and is also lower than in DLB). 2β-Carbomethoxy-3β-(4-iodophenyl)-N-(3-fluoropropyl)-N-nortropane (FP-CIT) single-photon emission computed tomography (SPECT) shows DAT density in PD-D to be reduced by more than 50% compared with DLB or PD [8].

Loss of substantia nigra and DAT may not initially be symmetrical between hemispheres, and this is reflected by unilateral expression of symptoms, especially rigidity [9, 10], although there is still significant bilateral loss. Evolution to PD-D shows a reduction of dopamine markers to a similar extent bilaterally [8].

Given the huge reduction in dopamine transmission in PD-D affecting extrastriatal areas (the thalamus, nucleus accumbens, and probably cortical areas which are more difficult to investigate) there are consequent effects on more than motor function. The thalamus receives dopamine via nigrostriatal collaterals, which have been shown to have depleted dopamine transporter immuno-reactivity in the 1-methyl-4-phenyl-1,2,3,6-tetrahydropyridine (MPTP)-treated monkey model of PD [11]. Nigrothalamic dopamine is likely to be reduced in PD-D. Using ^{125}I-N-(3-iodoprop-(2E)-enyl)-2β-carbomethoxy-3β-(4′-methylphenyl)nortropane (PE2I) autoradiography, tracts from the substantia nigra bifurcating to course through both the globus pallidus and along the margin of the reticular nucleus of the thalamus can be visualized, and these tracts are at least 50% less dense in PD-D, DLB, and PD compared with controls. At these most posterior striatal levels, DAT were more extensively reduced in the caudate in PD-D than in PD and DLB, especially in the ventromedial section. At these caudal levels clinical correlations were, not surprisingly, with extrapyramidal symptoms, with greater reductions in the putamen and the tract along the reticular nucleus being associated with more severe Hoehn and Yahr stages and Unified Parkin-son's Disease Rating Scale scores. Comparing PD-D to DLB with a similar severity of movement disability (Hoehn and Yahr stage 3 only) there was greater loss of DAT in the ventromedial puta-men and medial caudate in PD-D, perhaps showing some residual efficacy of compensatory mechanisms in PD (which are not invoked in DLB). A report using fluorodopa PET imaging also suggests that dopaminergic depletion in the caudate contributes to cognitive impairment in PD patients [12], and a study of progression of decline in DAT in PD-D, PD, and DLB showed cor-relation with cognitive decline [13].

Post-synaptic dopaminergic measures

In post-mortem analysis in PD without dementia, dopamine D2 receptor density is upregulated by more than 70% in the striatum [7], a compensatory change tending to 'damp down' over-activity of striato-pallidal neurons. Although this study did not include prospective assessment, PD cases with cognitive problems recorded in their case notes had lower striatal D2 binding (particularly dorsally) than PD cases with unimpaired cognition. In the thalamus, D2 receptors were upregulated two-fold in all regions examined in PD compared with controls [14], but in PD-D D2 receptors showed upregulation compared with controls only in the motor thalamic ventrointermedius nucleus, which, while significant, was relatively modest [14]. Although there is some difficulty imaging D2 receptors in vivo due to the presence of intrinsic dopamine, positron emission tomography (PET) and SPECT have shown upregulation of striatal D2 receptors to be a very early event in PD [15, 16], with the levels falling over the years as disease progresses and with dopaminergic therapy [17], until D2 density falls back to control levels.

After the striatum and thalamus, the highest brain D2 densities are in the cortex, particularly the temporal cortex. Piggott et al. [14] found that D2 receptors in the temporal cortex in PD-D and DLB were significantly reduced by more than 40% (though not in AD). Reduced temporal cortical D2 density correlated with cognitive decline as measured by the Mini-Mental State Examination (MMSE) score (Fig. 14.1), but not with hallucinations or delusions, giving theoretical grounds for the deleterious effect that neuroleptics have on cognition in PD-D [18].

Dopaminergic medications are usually reported to have limited benefit in DLB, with a low likelihood of motor improvement and a risk of exacerbating psychosis [19]. One study found that levodopa challenge did not have clinically significant adverse cognitive effects in PD-D [20] and was needed for control of motor symptoms; expert opinion, however, is to withdraw dopamine agonists in PD-D as they may worsen psychosis.

In DLB, D2 striatal density was lowest in patients having severe neuroleptic sensitivity and was slightly higher in those who were tolerant of neuroleptic treatment [21, 22]; it may be that patients with a lower D2 density are more at risk of sudden catastrophic blockade due to the D2 antagonist action of neuroleptics. By this token, in PD-D the risk of neuroleptic blockade of D2 receptors must increase as disease progresses, and severe reactions to neuroleptics were found to occur as often in PD-D as in DLB [23].

A post-mortem analysis showed D1 receptors in the caudate to be reduced with cognitive impairment in PD, unrelated to the degree of Alzheimer pathology [24]. However, this is in contrast to a more recent study showing no relationship between cognitive impairment and the activity of DAT in the striatum [25].

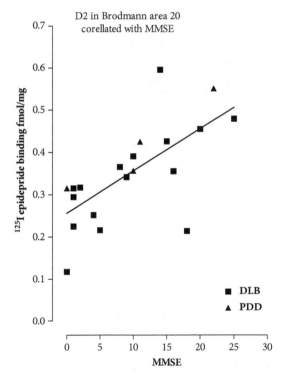

Fig. 14.1 Reduced temporal cortical D2 density is correlated with cognitive decline as measured by the MMSE score.

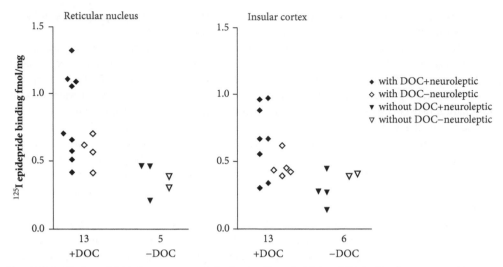

Fig. 14.2 In PD-D and DLB there was statistically significantly higher D2 binding (as measured by ^{125}I-epipride binding) in the reticular nucleus and insula cortex in patients with disturbances of consciousness (DOC). Roughly equal numbers of PD-D and DLB cases were studied. There was no effect of concurrent neuroleptic medication.

Although somewhat complicated by neuroleptic use, in PD-D and DLB there was statistically significantly higher thalamic D2 binding in patients with disturbances of consciousness, particularly in nuclei with a role in the maintenance of consciousness, including the reticular nucleus [14], and also in the insular cortex; there were roughly equal numbers of PD-D and DLB cases [14] (Fig. 14.2).

It is likely that D2 receptors located on gamma-aminobutyric acid (GABA)-ergic neurons in the reticular nucleus will, being inhibitory, help maintain thalamic and cortical activity; this may underlie fluctuations in cognitive functions. In an environment of reduced transmitter concentration, relatively higher numbers of D2 receptors may amplify small transmitter changes leading to variations in consciousness and attention. Similarly, there were more nicotinic receptors in some thalamic nuclei in patients with variations in consciousness [26] (see the section 'Nicotinic receptor changes'), possibly suggesting cholinergic and dopaminergic substrates for fluctuations, and combined cholinergic and dopaminergic therapy is required to treat disturbed consciousness in PD-D and DLB.

Acetylcholine

The major transmitter system associated with the symptoms of PD-D is the cholinergic system. Arising from the basal forebrain (including septal, diagonal band, and Meynert nuclei which constitute the cholinergic projections to the neocortex) the cholinergic system innervates all areas of the cerebral cortex including the hippocampus, and also the reticular nucleus of the thalamus. Cholinergic brainstem neurons (from the pedunculopontine and laterodorsal tegmental nuclei) innervate the thalamus and cerebellum. The highly cholinergic putamen and caudate nucleus do not receive inputs but have their own intrinsic cholinergic neurons (large striatal interneurons).

The importance of acetylcholine (ACh) and cholinergic deficits in cognitive impairment and dementia in general was recognized in the late 1970s [27], and a few years later in PD too

[28, 29]. In PD, initial reports indicated that there were no deficits in cholinergic parameters [30] and anticholinergic drugs were recommended to treat motor symptoms [31], although there were some near contemporaneous reports warning against the use of anticholinergics in PD [32]. Gradually the loss of other transmitters besides dopamine was recognized in patients with PD-D [33], with several early reports highlighting the significant reduction in both cholinergic basal forebrain neurons [34] and cortical choline acetyltransferase (ChAT) (the enzyme that synthesizes acetylcholine) and acetylcholinesterase (AChE) activities [29, 35]. Perry et al. [36] reported that PD-D, which had up until then generally been attributed to the presence of Alzheimer-type cortical pathology, actually usually occurs in the absence of substantial Alzheimer-type changes and is rather related to abnormalities in the cortical cholinergic system. This is supported by observations of the relative frequencies of Alzheimer-type and Lewy body pathology in a substantial cohort of post-mortem tissue, in which PD-D cases had considerably smaller amounts of AD pathology than DLB and AD cases. However, mixed pathology is still an important determinant of the progression of dementia and cognitive decline [37, 38].

Perry et al. [36] found extensive reductions of ChAT and less extensive reductions of AChE in all four cortical lobes in PD-D. ChAT reductions in the temporal cortex in PD-D correlated with the degree of mental impairment but not with the extent of plaque or tangle formation. In PD, but not AD, the decrease in neocortical (particularly temporal) ChAT correlated with the number of neurons in the nucleus of Meynert, suggesting that primary degeneration of these cholinergic neurons may be related to declining cognitive function in PD [36]. A further study by Mattila et al. [24] confirmed these findings, showing that cognitive impairment in PD correlated with ChAT activity in the temporal and prefrontal cortex and hippocampus, unrelated to Alzheimer pathology and additionally showing a correlation with the numbers of cortical Lewy bodies. In vivo PET measurement of AChE showed remarkable reductions in the entire cortex in PD-D [39]. In 2012 a study confirmed that thalamic cholinergic neurons are spared in AD compared with DLB and PD-D [40]. In another study in PD-D (but not in DLB) there were significant reductions in ChAT in the thalamic reticular, mediodorsal, and centromedian nuclei, associated with a long duration of parkinsonism and dementia [41]. It is now recognized that cholinergic losses are generally greater in PD-D than in AD, in terms of pre-synaptic cortical activities but also in the striatum and in the projection from the pedunculopontine nucleus to the thalamus. As in AD, there is consistent involvement of the nucleus basalis of Meynert, but with Lewy body pathology and more extensive cell loss [42]. In DLB too, the cortical ChAT and AChE losses (determined post mortem) exceed those in AD (except in the hippocampus) and are apparent early in the disease course [43].

Studies of the neurochemical pathology of PD-D had been pursued by Perry et al. in Newcastle for several years prior to 1989 [44], but investigations of the originally named senile dementia of Lewy body type were based on cases identified in retrospective pathological studies as atypical Alzheimer's. Since they had come to autopsy through psychiatric services, they included mainly individuals with few apparent extrapyramidal features [44] and were designated as DLB at the 1995 International Workshop Consortium on DLB [45]. By the later 1990s prospectively assessed clinical cohorts included patients with DLB similar to those in the previous pathological studies, as well as dementia cases with concurrent, or subsequently developed, extrapyramidal symptoms, or diagnosed levodopa-responsive PD of several to many years standing, allowing comparison of DLB with and without extrapyramidal symptoms and PD-D. While DLB and PD-D may be very similar there are documented differences clinically and pathologically, and it should not be assumed that significant findings in one will be replicated in the other.

In PD-D, in vivo SPECT imaging of the vesicular ACh transporter has shown considerable losses throughout the cortex, while in PD there was some reduction only in the parietal and occipital cortex [46]. Similarly, a PET study of AChE activity showed greater reduction in PD-D than in AD [47], with cortical AChE activity down 21% in PD-D compared with 13% in PD, correlating with measures of working memory, attention, and executive function, but not with the severity of motor symptoms [48]. The strong correlation of declining cholinergic measures with cognitive function was not the only finding; there were also increased symptoms of depression with greater reduction in cortical AChE activity as measured by PET in PD and PD-D [49].

In PD-D and DLB, patients with the greatest reductions in cholinergic measures are those most likely to have visual hallucinations. ChAT deficits are greater in some visual cortical areas in DLB patients with visual hallucinations than in those without, for example in Brodmann area 36 of the temporal cortex [50], and it may be that propensity to visual hallucinations is increased when much reduced ACh is combined with a relatively active serotonergic system [51].

Nicotinic receptor changes

Loss of nicotinic acetylcholine receptors (nAChR) in DLB is likely to reflect reduced cholinergic innervation (cortex and thalamus), dopaminergic innervation (striatum), and also attenuation of glutamatergic, GABA-ergic, and serotonergic neurons in the cortex, thalamus, and basal ganglia. Neocortical binding to nAChRs containing α4 and β2 subunits is reduced in PD, PD-D, and DLB [52, 53], and there is an apparent correlation between this nAChR deficit and reduction of ChAT reduction in the cortex [54].

In the striatum, nAChRs are more reduced in DLB and PD than in AD, notably of the α6-, α4-, β2-, and β3-containing subtypes [53]. Reduced nAChR binding in this region, which is at least in part on dopaminergic terminals, is as severe in DLB as in PD [53, 55], perhaps indicating that loss of these receptors occurs at a relatively early stage of nigrostriatal degeneration [55].

In contrast, α4β2-containing nAChRs visualized in vitro with [^{125}I]-5-IA85380 were not reduced in the thalamus in DLB (although there were reductions in PD) [26], but significant deficits were observed in patients without disturbances in consciousness [56]. Also in the temporal cortex, nAChR binding was relatively preserved in DLB patients with disturbed consciousness [57]. Since patients with disturbances of consciousness are able to be more alert at some times than at others, the neurotransmitter systems must be capable of supporting the higher level of awareness. In an analogous way to the suggested mechanism involving D2 receptors in thalamic nuclei with a role in fluctuation of consciousness; when cholinergic innervation is very low a higher density of nicotinic receptors may enable small transmitter fluctuations to lead to variations in consciousness and attention.

O'Brien et al. [58] used in vivo SPECT with [^{123}I]-5-IA85380 to show α4β2 nicotinic receptors in DLB; there were reductions in the frontal, temporal, and cingulate cortex and striatal regions but elevations in the occipital cortex which were greater in patients with a recent history of visual hallucinations. The muscarinic receptors M1 and M2/4 are particularly highly expressed in the visual cortex, as shown by autoradiography [59], and ^{123}I-iodo-quinuclidinyl-benzilate (^{123}I-QNB) SPECT showed that M1/M4 were elevated bilaterally in vivo in the occipital cortex in PD-D [60], which may contribute to visual disturbances in PD-D.

It is equivocal whether cortical α7-containing receptors are reduced generally in DLB [53, 54], but it is perhaps most likely to occur in DLB with hallucinations [61]. Reduced α7 receptor binding has also been noted in the reticular nucleus of the thalamus in DLB (in common with AD), a region innervated by cholinergic neurons from the basal forebrain [62].

Muscarinic receptor changes

Multiple muscarinic, G-protein-linked acetylcholine receptors (mAChRs; M1–M5) are expressed in the human brain, the most prevalent being M1 (in cortical regions) and M2 (widely distributed). Post-synaptically, there is less neuronal damage in PD-D and DLB than in AD [42]. Muscarinic M1 receptor modulation differs between DLB and AD. In severe AD M1 receptors are unchanged or slightly reduced and have defective coupling in the cortex, but in DLB M1 receptors have been reported to be upregulated in the temporal and parietal cortex [52], especially in cases with delusional symptoms [63], and higher in the frontal cortex in PD-D and DLB than in AD [64]. Similarly, immunohistochemistry indicates higher proportions of M1 in 'diffuse Lewy body disease' [65]. Additionally, coupling to G-protein second messenger systems is found to be preserved in DLB compared with AD in the temporal cortex [66], and in the frontal cortex in both PD-D and DLB [64]. In contrast to the neocortex, in PD-D and DLB striatal M1 receptor binding is reduced, in parallel with D2 receptors (M1 and D2 are distributed together, mainly on the same population of projection neurons from the striatum to the external globus pallidus) (see Fig. 14.3) [67]. This is possibly why cholinesterase inhibitor therapy tends not to provoke worsening of parkinsonism in PD-D and DLB patients.

Warren et al. [68] found M2 receptors to be elevated in the insular cortex in PD-D and DLB compared with controls, and they were significantly higher in PD-D than in DLB; this was significantly related to the severity and duration of extrapyramidal symptoms (Piggott, unpublished observations). Binding of M2 and M4 was higher in the cingulate cortex in PD-D and DLB compared with controls, and these increases were associated with visual hallucinations [69]. Raised M4 receptor density in the cingulate cortex was found to be related to impaired consciousness [69], and in the insular cortex it was related to the symptom of delusions. In contrast, M4 receptors were reduced in the mediodorsal thalamic nucleus in PD-D and DLB [70].

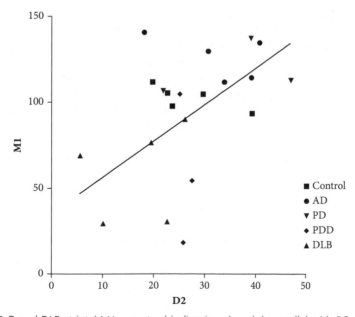

Fig. 14.3 In PD-D and DLB striatal M1 receptor binding is reduced, in parallel with D2 receptors.

Relationship between cholinergic medication and Alzheimer-type pathology

In PD long-term administration of drugs with an anticholinergic action is associated with increased Alzheimer-type pathology, with increased plaques and tangles [71]. Conversely, it has also been demonstrated that long-term exposure to nicotine (tobacco use) is associated with reduced AD pathology ($A\beta$ deposition) [72] and in the normal elderly to a greater preservation of neur on numbers in the substantia nigra. There is therefore a potential for the development of drugs which act selectively at muscarinic receptors, both neuroprotective (anti-Alzheimer pathology) M1 agonists [73] and therapeutically at other muscarinic receptor subtypes [74].

It was predicted in 1990 [75] 'that the cholinergic correlates of mental impairment in senile dementia of Lewy body type [and PD-D] together with the relative absence of cortical neurofibrillary tangles and evidence for postsynaptic cholinergic receptor compensation raise the question of whether this type of dementia may be more amenable to cholinotherapy than classical AD'. It was also recognized that the presence of visual hallucinations in the symptom profile would be diagnostic of greater cholinergic compromise [50, 51] and predicted a reliable response to cholinergic medication in these patients [76]. Activation of cholinergic receptors was recognized to be pro-cognitive, especially by improving attention [77, 78].

Glutamate

Excitatory amino acid transmission occurs between several components of the basal ganglia circuitry which are affected in PD-D, and excitotoxic mechanisms have been implicated in the progression of the disease. In PD there is increased output from the subthalamic nucleus, and glutamatergic drive from the subthalamic nucleus may be one of the compensatory mechanisms which begins to fail with disease progression to PD-D. Kashani et al. [79] found expression of the vesicular glutamate transporters VGLUT1 and VGLUT2 to be increased by 24 and 29%, respectively, in the putamen of patients with parkinsonism; by contrast, VGLUT1 was decreased in the prefrontal and temporal cortex of PD patients (by about 50%). The authors concluded that these findings demonstrate the existence of profound alterations of glutamatergic transmission in PD, which may contribute to the motor and cognitive impairments associated with the disease. A limitation of this study was that the extent of dementia was not assessed. There have been few investigations of glutamate markers in the Lewy body dementias. No change was shown in glutamate transporter protein in the cortex in two DLB cases [80], no change in *N*-methyl-D-aspartate (NMDA) receptor immunoreactivity in the entorhinal cortex and hippocampus [81], and no reduction in glutamate in cerebrospinal fluid (CSF) [82]. However, in other studies in DLB, GluR2/3 AMPA receptor immunoreactivity was decreased in the entorhinal cortex and hippocampus [81], and metabotropic mGluR1 and mGluR5 were reduced [83]. The mGluR5 receptor is increased in animal models of PD with dyskinesia [84] and seems to be reduced in the striatum and cortex in PD patients without dyskinesia compared with both PD with dyskinesia and controls. Further studies are needed to determine the extent of the changes in glutamate receptors in PD-D.

Zn^{2+} is released at glutamatergic terminals, where it acts as a neuromodulator of glutamatergic transmission and is important for the maintenance of cognition [85]. We have recently shown reductions in ZnT3 (see Fig. 14.4), the major ion pump responsible for controlling this release of Zn^{2+}, in the prefrontal cortex of PD-D patients [86].

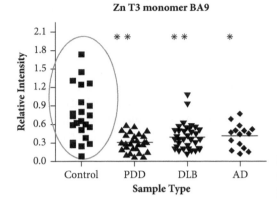

Fig. 14.4 ZnT3 levels are reduced in post-mortem tissue from PD-D, DLB, and AD patients relative to controls.

GABA

Anxiety, insomnia, and excessive daytime sleepiness are common complaints in PD-D and DLB, and may respond to treatment with benzodiazepines or modafinil which have GABA-ergic mechanisms. GABA-ergic components of the basal ganglia circuitry are likely to be affected in PD-D, but there are few published reports of GABA-ergic changes. Selective dendritic derangement of GABA-ergic medium spiny neurons in the striatum have been reported in late PD, and suggested to be linked to disrupted executive function [87, 88]. No difference in the GABA concentration in CSF was reported between DLB patients and a control group [82].

Serotonin (5-hydroxytryptamine, 5-HT)

Depression is a frequent symptom in PD-D and DLB, but a possible link between serotonin loss and depression remains to be clarified. The raphe nucleus is affected early in the course of PD [89], and Lewy body pathology and neuron loss have been reported in the raphe nucleus in DLB [90], although another study found no significant neuron loss [91]. Raphe neuron loss and reduced serotonin concentration in the striatum, pallidum, and cortex did not differ in PD with or without dementia [92], and similarly Perry et al. [93] did not find a correlation with dementia. Reduced serotonin has been reported in the striatum and cortex in DLB [90, 94, 95], but not in another study in the putamen [96]. Serotonin transporter binding is reduced by about 70% in the temporal and parietal cortex in DLB, with 5-HT$_{2A}$ receptors also reduced in the temporal cortex in DLB and PD-D [97]. There is little evidence that selective serotonin reuptake inhibitors are effective in depression in PD [98], and untreated PD patients with depression showed no differences in CSF serotonin metabolites compared with patients without depression [99]. DLB patients with a history of major depression actually had relatively higher serotonin transporter binding in the parietal cortex than those without [100], though serotonin transporters were at slightly lower density in PD-D/DLB than in controls.

PET imaging of 5-HT$_{1A}$ receptors (inhibitory autoreceptors) in the median raphe in PD showed a reduction (of 25%) in signal related to the presence of tremor but not to depression [101]. However, in vitro 5-HT$_{1A}$ receptors showed a significant increase (over 80%) in numbers in the temporal cortex (Brodmann area 36) in PD-D [102], and a significant elevation (68%) in cortical 5-HT$_{1A}$ receptors was found in PD-D/DLB patients with depression compared with non-depressed PD-D and DLB patients [102]. In a post-mortem autoradiographic study in PD (where cognitive function was not prospectively assessed) 5-HT$_{1A}$ receptors were increased in the frontal and temporal cortex compared with controls (although any relationship to depression was not assessed in this study) [103]. Hence, treatment of depression in DLB and PD-D may be more effective with incorporation of a 5-HT$_{1A}$ antagonist, to increase the efficacy of serotonin reuptake inhibitors.

Greater preservation of serotonergic function may be related to more behavioural and psychological symptoms such as aggression, anxiety, depressed mood, and agitation, while reduction of markers of serotonin activity may be related to cognitive impairment [104]; the balance between various transmitter systems is probably important [105]. Patients with visual hallucinations show a relative preservation of serotonin markers along with markedly reduced cholinergic parameters [51, 95, 97].

Noradrenaline

Degeneration of the locus coeruleus has been reported in PD, and suggested to be linked to symptoms of mood disorder and subtle cognitive changes [92, 106]. Using ^{11}C RTI-32 PET imaging to visualize dopamine and noradrenaline terminals, Remy et al. [107] found that reduced signal in the cingulate cortex, amygdala, thalamus, and locus coeruleus correlated with depression in PD compared with patients having equal motor disability but no depression. Noradrenergic loss is more extensive in PD-D than PD [33, 106, 108] and there are also reductions in DLB [109, 110]. Baloyannis et al. [111] found that noradrenergic losses were correlated with cognitive decline and morphological alteration of synapses in the locus coeruleus was more pronounced in PD-D than PD, while Szot et al. [110] found that neuron loss in the locus coeruleus correlated with cognitive decline. Szot et al. [110] also found evidence of compensation for the neuron loss in the remaining locus coeruleus neurons in AD and DLB, but in both disorders there was reduced α_{1D} and α_{2C} adrenergic receptor mRNA in the hippocampus. The density of α_2 adrenergic receptors was reported to be slightly increased in the frontal cortex in DLB [109]. Treatment with drugs active at α_1 or α_2 receptors has been suggested to improve spatial memory [112] or attention in PD [113] or PD-D [114].

Changes in the noradrenergic system in limbic areas may contribute to depression and to behavioural symptoms such as aggression and pacing, to cognitive decline in cortical areas, and to movement disorder in basal ganglia, but in the main these relationships have still to be investigated. In DLB, noradrenaline is much reduced in the putamen [90], which could mitigate motor symptoms.

Calcium

Several lines of evidence indicate the importance of calcium homeostasis in mechanisms of symptom generation and disease progression in PD and PD-D. In the cortex, neurons expressing calcium-binding proteins are more likely to be spared in DLB [115]. In the substantia nigra too the most vulnerable neurons are those with the lowest expression of calbindin [6]. In the substantia nigra, pacemaking activity is dependent on L-type calcium channels, while in the ventral tegmental area it depends on sodium channels [116]. It may be that calcium homeostasis is the key to selective vulnerability among neurons of the substantia nigra (and compared with neurons of the ventral tegmental area), since calcium concentration (via L-type calcium channels) together with cytosolic dopamine concentration and α-synuclein expression seem to be the three factors leading to neurotoxicity [117]. This is consistent with the observation that use of calcium channel antagonists to treat hypertension may confer a diminished risk of developing PD [118].

Fast oscillations in the gamma frequency in the cortex and thalamus have been implicated in attention, sensory processing, and memory, modulated by noradrenaline, dopamine, acetylcholine, and serotonin [119, 120]. In PD-D there is greater slowing of resting state brain oscillatory activity compared with PD, as detected by magneto-encephalography [119]. Calcium t-channels have a physiological function in thalamic oscillations [121, 122].

The status of calcium channels in the substantia nigra or cortex in PD-D is largely unknown; however, in a study carried out by Piggott et al. [123] in the 1980s, binding of nitredipine to L-type calcium channels in the temporal cortex was reported to be reduced in AD, but the greatest reduction (70%) was in cases which would today be more likely to be classified as DLB/PD-D.

Synaptic dysfunction in PD-D

Whilst the previous sections have addressed deficits of specific neurotransmitter systems, it is being increasingly recognized that synaptic changes on a more global level make a considerable contribution to the clinical and pathological features of PD-D and may underlie many of the neurochemical alterations. A number of the genes associated with PD have been linked to synaptic alterations. Garcia-Reitbock et al. [124] demonstrated that in transgenic mice expressing a truncated, more aggregation-prone form of α-synuclein there was a redistribution of SNARE (soluble N-ethylmaleimide-sensitive fusion protein attachment protein receptors) proteins at synapses in the striatum. This resulted in decreased vesicle release and dopamine signalling which was age-related. A more recent study from 2013 has shown that α-synuclein can affect dopamine homeostasis by influencing the localization of DAT to the membrane, and thus its functional activity [125]. Importantly this observation was again age-related, the authors finding that the ability of α-synuclein to direct DAT to the membrane was impaired in older mice.

Another link between α-synuclein and synaptic dysfunction was established when Burre et al. [126] demonstrated that α-synuclein is required for SNARE complex assembly through a chaperone-like activity involving binding to phospholipids and synaptobrevin-2. The authors emphasized the importance of this proof-reading faculty with increased age, when overburdened neurotransmitter systems would have increased susceptibility to a loss of this function, perhaps explaining some of the reported deficits in neurotransmitter release associated with α-synuclein. However, it is interesting to note that overexpression of α-synuclein (in a similar range to that found in gene duplication) caused a reduction in synaptic vesicle binding and release of neurotransmitters, including dopamine [127].

Another synaptic protein associated with PD-D through genetic risk, LRRK2, is likewise implicated in the synaptic vesicle machinery, where it is thought to contribute to the recycling of synaptic vesicles, and a loss of its kinase activity has been demonstrated to reduce synaptic transmission [128].

It has been suggested that dopaminergic neurons are particularly susceptible to synaptic vesicle deficits due to their distinctly large ratio of synaptic terminals to cell body [129]. This, coupled with observations that dopamine stabilizes α-synuclein protofibrils and is an oxidative stressor, raises the possibility that the selective vulnerability of dopaminergic neurons is due to these inherent properties.

Pre-synaptic α-synuclein pathology has been suggested to contribute to the synaptic dysfunction seen in LB-related dementias [130]. It was observed that this pathology, not visible using conventional techniques, was associated with the loss of dendritic spines in several cortical regions in DLB cases.

Conclusion

The best documented neurotransmitter changes in PD-D include loss of cholinergic markers and the progressive loss of dopamine. These deficits are associated with various changes in the related pre- and post-synaptic receptors. Alterations in serotonin, noradrenaline, and to lesser extent in other neurotransmitter systems have been reported; these are, however, less pronounced and need to be better elucidated. Neuropsychiatric and cognitive symptoms in PD-D are likely to be due to a combination of neurotransmitter deficits—particularly cholinergic and dopaminergic for cognitive dysfunction [131] (possibly with some noradrenergic influence); dopaminergic, noradrenergic, and serotonergic for depression [132]; and dopaminergic/serotonergic and cholinergic for visual hallucinations [51]. More generally there are emerging changes in synaptic machinery evident in PD-D that may also contribute to cognitive and behavioural symptoms. Clinical trials with treatment modalities such as mixed transmitter reuptake inhibitors for symptoms including depression and psychosis in PD-D are warranted [132, 133]. New possibilities for treatment targeting calcium channels [117] and perhaps synaptic dysfunction in general are also emerging.

References

1. **Ehringer H, Hornykiewicz O.** [Distribution of noradrenaline and dopamine (3-hydroxytyramine) in the human brain and their behavior in diseases of the extrapyramidal system.]. Klinische Wochenschrift 1960; **38**: 1236–9. (Original in German.)

2. **Ehringer H, Hornykiewicz O.** Distribution of noradrenaline and dopamine (3-hydroxytyramine) in the human brain and their behavior in diseases of the extrapyramidal system. Parkinsonism Relat Disord 1998; **4**: 53–7.

3. **McGeer PL, Zeldowicz LR.** Administration of dihydroxyphenylalanine to parkinsonian patients. Can Med Assoc J 1964; **90**: 463–6.

4. **Cotzias GC, Van Woert MH, Schiffer LM.** Aromatic amino acids and modification of parkinsonism. N Engl J Med 1967; **276**: 374–9.

5. **Archibald N, Burn D.** Parkinson's disease. Medicine 2008; **36**: 630–5.

6. **Damier P, Hirsch EC, Agid Y, et al.** The substantia nigra of the human brain—II. Patterns of loss of dopamine-containing neurons in Parkinson's disease. Brain 1999; **122**: 1437–48.

7. **Piggott MA, Marshall EF, Thomas N, et al.** Striatal dopaminergic markers in dementia with Lewy bodies, Alzheimer's and Parkinson's diseases: rostrocaudal distribution. Brain 1999; **122**: 1449–68.

8. **O'Brien JT, Colloby SM, Fenwick JP, et al.** Dopamine transporter loss visualized with FP-CIT SPECT in the differential diagnosis of dementia with Lewy bodies. Arch Neurol 2004; **61**: 919–25.

9. **Wenning GK, Donnemiller E, Granata R, et al.** ^{123}I-beta-CIT and ^{123}I-IBZM-SPECT scanning in levodopa-naive Parkinson's disease. Mov Disord 1998; **13**: 438–45.

10. **Tissingh G, Bergmans P, Booij J, et al.** Drug-naive patients with Parkinson's disease in Hoehn and Yahr stages I and II show a bilateral decrease in striatal dopamine transporters as revealed by [123I]beta-CIT SPECT. J Neurol 1998; **245**: 14–20.

11. **Freeman A, Ciliax B, Bakay R, et al.** Nigrostriatal collaterals to thalamus degenerate in parkinsonian animal models. Ann Neurol 2001; **50**: 321–9.

12. **Jokinen P, Brück A, Aalto S, et al.** Impaired cognitive performance in Parkinson's disease is related to caudate dopaminergic hypofunction and hippocampal atrophy. Parkinsonism Relat Disord 2009; **15**: 88–93.

13. **Colloby SJ, Williams ED, Burn DJ, et al.** Progression of dopaminergic degeneration in dementia with Lewy bodies and Parkinson's disease with and without dementia assessed using 123I-FP-CIT SPECT. Eur J Nucl Med Molec Imaging 2005; **32**: 1176–85.

14. **Piggott MA, Ballard CG, Dickinson HO, et al.** Thalamic D2 receptors in dementia with Lewy bodies, Parkinson's disease, and Parkinson's disease dementia. Int J Neuropsychopharmacol 2007; **10**: 231–44.

15. **Giobbe D, Castellano GC, Podio V.** Dopamine D2 receptor imaging with SPECT using IBZM in 16 patients with Parkinson disease. Ital J Neurol Sci 1993; **14**: 165–9.

16. **Antonini A, Schwarz J, Oertel WH, et al.** [^{11}C]raclopride and positron emission tomography in previously untreated patients with Parkinson's disease: influence of L-dopa and lisuride therapy on striatal dopamine D2-receptors. Neurology 1994; **44**: 1325–9.

17. **Antonini A, Schwarz J, Oertel WH, et al.** Long-term changes of striatal dopamine D2 receptors in patients with Parkinson's disease: a study with positron emission tomography and [11C]raclopride. Mov Disord 1997; **12**: 33–8.

18. **Piggott MA, Ballard CG, Rowan E, et al.** Selective loss of dopamine D2 receptors in temporal cortex in dementia with Lewy bodies, association with cognitive decline. Synapse 2007; **61**: 903–11.

19. **Goldman JG, Goetz CG, Brandabur M, et al.** Effects of dopaminergic medications on psychosis and motor function in dementia with Lewy bodies. Mov Disord 2008; **23**: 2248–50.

20. **Molloy SA, Rowan EN, O'Brien JT, et al.** Effect of levodopa on cognitive function in Parkinson's disease with and without dementia and dementia with Lewy bodies. J Neurol Neurosurg Psychiatry 2006; **77**: 1323–8.

21. **Piggott MA, Perry EK, Marshall EF, et al.** Nigrostriatal dopaminergic activities in dementia with Lewy bodies in relation to neuroleptic sensitivity: comparisons with Parkinson's disease. Biol Psych 1998; **44**: 765–74.

22. **Piggott MA, Perry EK, McKeith IG, et al.** Dopamine D2 receptors in demented patients with severe neuroleptic sensitivity [letter]. [Erratum in Lancet 1994; 343: 1170]. Lancet 1994; **343**: 1044–5.

23. **Aarsland D, Perry R, Larsen JP, et al.** Neuroleptic sensitivity in Parkinson's disease and parkinsonian dementias. J Clin Psychiatry 2005; **66**: 633–7.

24. **Mattila PM, Roytta M, Lonnberg P, et al.** Choline acetyltransferase activity and striatal dopamine receptors in Parkinson's disease in relation to cognitive impairment. Acta Neuropathol 2001; **102**: 160–6.

25. **Ziebell M, Andersen BB, Pinborg LH, et al.** Striatal dopamine transporter binding does not correlate with clinical severity in dementia with Lewy bodies. J Nucl Med 2013; **54**: 1072–6.

26. **Pimlott SL, Piggott M, Owens J, et al.** Nicotinic acetylcholine receptor distribution in Alzheimer's disease, dementia with Lewy bodies, Parkinson's disease, and vascular dementia: in vitro binding study using 5-[(^{125})I]-A-85380. Neuropsychopharmacology 2004; **29**: 108–16.

27. **Perry EK, Gibson PH, Blessed G, et al.** Neurotransmitter enzyme abnormalities in senile dementia. Choline acetyltransferase and glutamic acid decarboxylase activities in necropsy brain tissue. J Neurol Sci 1977; **34**: 247–65.

28. **Ruberg M, Ploska A, Javoy-Agid F, et al.** Muscarinic binding and choline acetyltransferase activity in Parkinsonian subjects with reference to dementia. Brain Res 1982; **232**: 129–39.

29. **Perry RH, Tomlinson BE, Candy JM, et al.** Cortical cholinergic deficit in mentally impaired Parkinsonian patients. Lancet 1983; **2**: 789–90.

30. **Aquilonius SM, Nystrom B, Schuberth J, et al.** Cerebrospinal fluid choline in extrapyramidal disorders. J Neurol Neurosurge Psychiatry 1972; **35**: 720–5.

31. **Sears ES.** Therapeutics of disordered movement. Am Fam Physician 1977; **16**: 145–54.

32. **de Smet Y, Ruberg M, Serdaru M, et al.** Confusion, dementia and anticholinergics in Parkinson's disease. J Neurol Neurosurg Psychiatry 1982; **45**: 1161–4.

33. **Mann DM, Yates PO.** Pathological basis for neurotransmitter changes in Parkinson's disease. Neuropathol Appl Neurobiol 1983; **9**: 3–19.

34. **Whitehouse PJ, Hedreen JC, White CL 3rd, et al.** Basal forebrain neurons in the dementia of Parkinson disease. Ann Neurol 1983; **13**: 243–8.

35. **Dubois B, Ruberg M, Javoy-Agid F, et al.** A subcortico-cortical cholinergic system is affected in Parkinson's disease. Brain Res 1983; **288**: 213–18.

36. **Perry EK, Curtis M, Dick DJ, et al.** Cholinergic correlates of cognitive impairment in Parkinson's disease: comparisons with Alzheimer's disease. J Neurol Neurosurg Psychiatry 1985; **48**: 413–21.

37. Attems J, Jellinger K. Neuropathological correlates of cerebral multimorbidity. Curr Alzheimer Res 2013; **10**: 569–77.

38. Dickson DW, Braak H, Duda JE, et al. Neuropathological assessment of Parkinson's disease: refining the diagnostic criteria. Lancet Neurol 2009; **8**: 1150–7.

39. Shinotoh H. [Imaging of brain acetylcholinesterase activity in dementias and extrapyramidal disorders]. Rinsho Shinkeigaku 2007; **47**: 822–5. (In Japanese.)

40. Kotagal V, Müller ML, Kaufer DI, et al. Thalamic cholinergic innervation is spared in Alzheimer disease compared to parkinsonian disorders. Neurosci Lett 2012; **514**: 169–72.

41. Ziabreva I, Ballard CG, Aarsland D, et al. Lewy body disease: thalamic cholinergic activity related to dementia and parkinsonism. Neurobiol Aging 2006; **27**: 433–8.

42. Tiraboschi P, Hansen LA, Alford M, et al. Cholinergic dysfunction in diseases with Lewy bodies. Neurology 2000; **54**: 407–11.

43. Tiraboschi P, Hansen LA, Alford M, et al. Early and widespread cholinergic losses differentiate dementia with Lewy bodies from Alzheimer disease. Arch Gen Psychiatry 2002; **59**: 946–51.

44. Perry RH, Irving D, Blessed G, et al. Senile dementia of Lewy body type. A clinically and neuropathologically distinct form of Lewy body dementia in the elderly. J Neurol Sci 1990; **95**: 119–39.

45. McKeith IG, Galasko D, Kosaka K, et al. Consensus guidelines for the clinical and pathologic diagnosis of dementia with Lewy bodies (DLB): report of the consortium on DLB international workshop. Neurology 1996; **47**: 1113–24.

46. Kuhl DE, Minoshima S, Fessler JA, et al. In vivo mapping of cholinergic terminals in normal aging, Alzheimer's disease, and Parkinson's disease. Ann Neurol 1996; **40**: 399–410.

47. Bohnen NI, Kaufer DI, Ivanco LS, et al. Cortical cholinergic function is more severely affected in parkinsonian dementia than in Alzheimer disease: an in vivo positron emission tomographic study. Arch Neurol 2003; **60**: 1745–8.

48. Bohnen NI, Kaufer DI, Hendrickson R, et al. Cognitive correlates of cortical cholinergic denervation in Parkinson's disease and parkinsonian dementia. J Neurol 2006; **253**: 242–7.

49. Bohnen NI, Kaufer DI, Hendrickson R, et al. Cortical cholinergic denervation is associated with depressive symptoms in Parkinson's disease and parkinsonian dementia. J Neurol Neurosurg Psychiatry 2007; **78**: 641–3.

50. Perry EK, Kerwin J, Perry RH, et al. Cerebral cholinergic activity is related to the incidence of visual hallucinations in senile dementia of Lewy body type. Dementia 1990; **1**: 2–4.

51. Perry EK, Marshall E, Kerwin J, et al. Evidence of a monoaminergic-cholinergic imbalance related to visual hallucinations in Lewy body dementia. J Neurochem 1990; **55**: 1454–6.

52. Perry EK, Smith CJ, Court JA, et al. Cholinergic nicotinic and muscarinic receptors in dementia of Alzheimer, Parkinson and Lewy body types. J Neural Transm 1990; **2**: 149–58.

53. Gotti C, Moretti M, Bohr I, et al. Selective nicotinic acetylcholine receptor subunit deficits identified in Alzheimer's disease, Parkinson's disease and dementia with Lewy bodies by immunoprecipitation. Neurobiol Dis 2006; **23**: 481–9.

54. Reid RT, Sabbagh MN, Corey-Bloom J, et al. Nicotinic receptor losses in dementia with Lewy bodies: comparisons with Alzheimer's disease. Neurobiol Aging 2000; **21**: 741–6.

55. Perry EK, Morris CM, Court JA, et al. Alteration in nicotine binding sites in Parkinson's disease, Lewy body dementia and Alzheimer's disease: possible index of early neuropathology. Neuroscience 1995; **64**: 385–95.

56. Pimlott SL, Piggott M, Ballard C, et al. Thalamic nicotinic receptors implicated in disturbed consciousness in dementia with Lewy bodies. Neurobiol Dis 2006; **21**: 50–6.

57. Ballard CG, Court JA, Piggott M, et al. Disturbances of consciousness in dementia with Lewy bodies associated with alteration in nicotinic receptor binding in the temporal cortex. Consciousness Cogn 2002; **11**: 461–74.

58. O'Brien JT, Colloby SJ, Pakrasi S, et al. Nicotinic alpha4beta2 receptor binding in dementia with Lewy bodies using [123]I-5IA-85380 SPECT demonstrates a link between occipital changes and visual hallucinations. NeuroImage 2008; **40**: 1056–63.

59. Piggott M, Owens J, O'Brien J, et al. Comparative distribution of binding of the muscarinic receptor ligands pirenzepine, AF-DX 384, (R,R)-I-QNB and (R,S)-I-QNB to human brain. J Chem Neuroanat 2002; **24**: 211–23.

60. Colloby SJ, Pakrasi S, Firbank MJ, et al. In vivo SPECT imaging of muscarinic acetylcholine receptors using (R,R) ^{123}I-QNB in dementia with Lewy bodies and Parkinson's disease dementia. NeuroImage 2006; **33**: 423–9.

61. Court JA, Ballard CG, Piggott MA, et al. Visual hallucinations are associated with lower alpha bungarotoxin binding in dementia with Lewy bodies. Pharmacol Biochem Behav 2001; **70**: 571–9.

62. Court J, Spurden D, Lloyd S, et al. Neuronal nicotinic receptors in dementia with Lewy bodies and schizophrenia: alpha-bungarotoxin and nicotine binding in the thalamus. J Neurochem 1999; **73**: 1590–7.

63. Ballard C, Piggott M, Johnson M, et al. Delusions associated with elevated muscarinic M1 receptor binding in dementia with Lewy bodies. Ann Neurol 2000; **48**: 868–76.

64. Warren NM, Piggott MA, Lees AJ, et al. Intact coupling of M1 receptors and preserved M2 and M4 receptors in the cortex in progressive supranuclear palsy: contrast with other dementias. J Chem Neuroanat 2008; **35**: 268–74.

65. Shiozaki K, Iseki E, Uchiyama H, et al. Alterations of muscarinic acetylcholine receptor subtypes in diffuse Lewy body disease: relation to Alzheimer's disease. J Neurol Neurosurg Psychiatry 1999; **67**: 209–13.

66. Perry E, Court J, Goodchild R, et al. Clinical neurochemistry: developments in dementia research based on brain bank material. J Neural Transm 1998; **105**: 915–33.

67. Piggott MA, Owens J, O'Brien J, et al. Muscarinic receptors in basal ganglia in dementia with Lewy bodies, Parkinson's disease and Alzheimer's disease. J Chem Neuroanat 2003; **25**: 161–73.

68. Warren NM, Piggott MA, Lees AJ, et al. The basal ganglia cholinergic neurochemistry of progressive supranuclear palsy and other neurodegenerative diseases. J Neurol Neurosurg Psychiatry 2007; **78**: 571–5.

69. Teaktong T, Piggott MA, McKeith IG, et al. Muscarinic M2 and M4 receptors in anterior cingulate cortex: relation to neuropsychiatric symptoms in dementia with Lewy bodies. Behav Brain Res 2005; **161**: 299–305.

70. Warren NM, Piggott MA, Lees AJ, et al. Muscarinic receptors in the thalamus in progressive supranuclear palsy and other neurodegenerative disorders. J Neuropathol Exp Neurol 2007; **66**: 399–404.

71. Perry EK, Kilford L, Lees AJ, et al. Increased Alzheimer pathology in Parkinson's disease related to antimuscarinic drugs.[see comment]. Ann Neurol 2003; **54**: 235–8.

72. Court JA, Johnson M, Religa D, et al. Attenuation of Abeta deposition in the entorhinal cortex of normal elderly individuals associated with tobacco smoking. Neuropathol Appl Neurobiol 2005; **31**: 522–35.

73. Fisher A. Cholinergic treatments with emphasis on m1 muscarinic agonists as potential disease-modifying agents for Alzheimer's disease. Neurotherapeutics 2008; **5**: 433–42.

74. Jakubik J, Michal P, Machova E, et al. Importance and prospects for design of selective muscarinic agonists. Physiol Res 2008; **57**(Suppl. 3): S39–S47.

75. Perry EK, Marshall E, Perry RH, et al. Cholinergic and dopaminergic activities in senile dementia of Lewy body type. Alzheimers Dis Assoc Disord 1990; **4**: 87–95.

76. Perry EK, Haroutunian V, Davis KL, et al. Neocortical cholinergic activities differentiate Lewy body dementia from classical Alzheimer's disease. NeuroReport 1994; **5**: 747–9.

77. Perry E, Walker M, Grace J, et al. Acetylcholine in mind: a neurotransmitter correlate of consciousness?[see comment]. Trends Neurosci 1999; **22**: 273–80.

78. **Voytko ML.** Cognitive functions of the basal forebrain cholinergic system in monkeys: memory or attention? Behav Brain Res 1996; **75**: 13–25.

79. **Kashani A, Betancur C, Giros B, et al.** Altered expression of vesicular glutamate transporters VGLUT1 and VGLUT2 in Parkinson disease. Neurobiol Aging 2007; **28**: 568–78.

80. **Scott HL, Pow DV, Tannenberg AE, et al.** Aberrant expression of the glutamate transporter excitatory amino acid transporter 1 (EAAT1) in Alzheimer's disease. J Neurosci 2002; **22**: RC206.

81. **Thorns V, Mallory M, Hansen L, et al.** Alterations in glutamate receptor 2/3 subunits and amyloid precursor protein expression during the course of Alzheimer's disease and Lewy body variant. Acta Neuropath 1997; **94**: 539–48.

82. **Molina JA, Gomez P, Vargas C, et al.** Neurotransmitter amino acid in cerebrospinal fluid of patients with dementia with Lewy bodies. J Neural Transm 2005; **112**: 557–63.

83. **Albasanz JL, Dalfo E, Ferrer I, et al.** Impaired metabotropic glutamate receptor/phospholipase C signaling pathway in the cerebral cortex in Alzheimer's disease and dementia with Lewy bodies correlates with stage of Alzheimer's-disease-related changes. Neurobiol Dis 2005; **20**: 685–93.

84. **Samadi P, Gregoire L, Morissette M, et al.** mGluR5 metabotropic glutamate receptors and dyskinesias in MPTP monkeys. Neurobiol Aging 2008; **29**: 1040–51.

85. **Adlard PA, Parncutt JM, Finkelstein DI, et al.** Cognitive loss in zinc transporter-3 knock-out mice: a phenocopy for the synaptic and memory deficits of Alzheimer's disease? J Neurosci 2010; **30**: 1631–6.

86. **Whitfield DR, Vallortigara J, Alghamdi A, et al.** Assessment of ZnT3 and PSD95 protein levels in Lewy body dementias and Alzheimer's disease: association with cognitive impairment. Neurobiol Aging 2014; doi: 10.1016/j.neurobiolaging.2014.06.015 [Epub ahead of print].

87. **Zaja-Milatovic S, Keene CD, Montine KS, et al.** Selective dendritic degeneration of medium spiny neurons in dementia with Lewy bodies. Neurology 2006; **66**: 1591–3.

88. **Zaja-Milatovic S, Milatovic D, Schantz AM, et al.** Dendritic degeneration in neostriatal medium spiny neurons in Parkinson disease. Neurology 2005; **64**: 545–7.

89. **Braak H, Ghebremedhin E, Rub U, et al.** Stages in the development of Parkinson's disease-related pathology. Cell Tissue Res 2004; **318**: 121–34.

90. **Langlais PJ, Thal L, Hansen L, et al.** Neurotransmitters in basal ganglia and cortex of Alzheimer's disease with and without Lewy bodies. Neurology 1993; **43**: 1927–34.

91. **Benarroch EE, Schmeichel AM, Low PA, et al.** Involvement of medullary regions controlling sympathetic output in Lewy body disease. Brain 2005; **128**: 338–44.

92. **Scatton B, Javoy-Agid F, Rouquier L, et al.** Reduction of cortical dopamine, noradrenaline, serotonin and their metabolites in Parkinson's disease. Brain Res 1983; **275**: 321–8.

93. **Perry EK, McKeith I, Thompson P, et al.** Topography, extent, and clinical relevance of neurochemical deficits in dementia of Lewy body type, Parkinson's disease, and Alzheimer's disease. Ann NY Acad Sci 1991; **640**: 197–202.

94. **Ohara K, Kondo N, Ohara K.** Changes of monoamines in post-mortem brains from patients with diffuse Lewy body disease. Prog Neuro-Psychopharmacol Biol Psychiatry 1998; **22**: 311–17.

95. **Perry EK, Marshall E, Thompson P, et al.** Monoaminergic activities in Lewy body dementia: relation to hallucinosis and extrapyramidal features. J Neural Transm 1993; **6**: 167–77.

96. **Piggott MA, Marshall EF.** Neurochemical correlates of pathological and iatrogenic extrapyramidal symptoms. In: Perry RH, McKeith IG, Perry EK (ed.) *Dementia with Lewy bodies: clinical, pathological, and treatment issues*. Cambridge: Cambridge University Press, 1996; pp. 449–67.

97. **Cheng AV, Ferrier IN, Morris CM, et al.** Cortical serotonin-S2 receptor binding in Lewy body dementia, Alzheimer's and Parkinson's diseases. J Neurol Sci 1991; **106**: 50–5.

98. **Ghazi-Noori S, Chung TH, Deane K, et al.** Therapies for depression in Parkinson's disease. Cochrane Database Syst Rev 2003(3): CD003465.

99. **Kuhn W, Muller T, Gerlach M, et al.** Depression in Parkinson's disease: biogenic amines in CSF of 'de novo' patients. J Neural Transm 1996; **103**: 1441–5.

100. **Ballard C, Johnson M, Piggott M, et al.** A positive association between 5HT re-uptake binding sites and depression in dementia with Lewy bodies. J Affect Disord 2002; **69**: 219–23.

101. **Doder M, Rabiner EA, Turjanski N, et al.** Tremor in Parkinson's disease and serotonergic dysfunction: an ^{11}C-WAY 100635 PET study. Neurology 2003; **60**: 601–5.

102. **Sharp SI, Ballard CG, Ziabreva I, et al.** Cortical serotonin 1A receptor levels are associated with depression in patients with dementia with Lewy bodies and Parkinson's disease dementia. Dement Geriatr Cogn Disord 2008; **26**: 330–8.

103. **Chen CP, Alder JT, Bray L, et al.** Post-synaptic 5-HT1A and 5-HT2A receptors are increased in Parkinson's disease neocortex. Ann NY Acad Sci 1998; **861**: 288–9.

104. **Halliday GM, McCann HL, Pamphlett R, et al.** Brain stem serotonin-synthesizing neurons in Alzheimer's disease: a clinicopathological correlation. Acta Neuropathol (Berl) 1992; **84**: 638–50.

105. **Lanari A, Amenta F, Silvestrelli G, et al.** Neurotransmitter deficits in behavioural and psychological symptoms of Alzheimer's disease. Mech Ageing Devel 2006; **127**: 158–65.

106. **Cash R, Dennis T, L'Heureux R, et al.** Parkinson's disease and dementia: norepinephrine and dopamine in locus ceruleus. Neurology 1987; **37**: 42–6.

107. **Remy P, Doder M, Lees A, et al.** Depression in Parkinson's disease: loss of dopamine and noradrenaline innervation in the limbic system. Brain 2005; **128**: 1314–22.

108. **Zweig RM, Cardillo JE, Cohen M, et al.** The locus ceruleus and dementia in Parkinson's disease. Neurology 1993; **43**: 986–91.

109. **Leverenz JB, Miller MA, Dobie DJ, et al.** Increased alpha 2-adrenergic receptor binding in locus coeruleus projection areas in dementia with Lewy bodies. Neurobiol Aging 2001; **22**: 555–61.

110. **Szot P, White SS, Greenup JL, et al.** Compensatory changes in the noradrenergic nervous system in the locus ceruleus and hippocampus of postmortem subjects with Alzheimer's disease and dementia with Lewy bodies. J Neurosci 2006; **26**: 467–78.

111. **Baloyannis SJ, Costa V, Baloyannis IS.** Morphological alterations of the synapses in the locus coeruleus in Parkinson's disease. J Neurol Sci 2006; **248**: 35–41.

112. **Riekkinen M, Jakala P, Kejonen K, et al.** The alpha2 agonist, clonidine, improves spatial working performance in Parkinson's disease. Neuroscience 1999; **92**: 983–9.

113. **Bedard MA, el Massioui F, Malapani C, et al.** Attentional deficits in Parkinson's disease: partial reversibility with naphtoxazine (SDZ NVI-085), a selective noradrenergic alpha 1 agonist. Clin Neuropharmacol 1998; **21**: 108–17.

114. **Coull JT.** Alpha$_2$-adrenoceptors in the treatment of dementia: an attentional mechanism? J Psychopharmacol 1996; **10**(Suppl. 3): 43–8.

115. **Gomez-Tortosa E, Sanders JL, Newell K, et al.** Cortical neurons expressing calcium binding proteins are spared in dementia with Lewy bodies. Acta Neuropathol 2001; **101**: 36–42.

116. **Chan CS, Guzman JN, Ilijic E, et al.** 'Rejuvenation' protects neurons in mouse models of Parkinson's disease. Nature 2007; **447**: 1081–6.

117. **Mosharov EV, Larsen KE, Kanter E, et al.** Interplay between cytosolic dopamine, calcium, and alpha-synuclein causes selective death of substantia nigra neurons.[see comment]. Neuron 2009; **62**: 218–29.

118. **Becker C, Jick SS, Meier CR.** Use of antihypertensives and the risk of Parkinson disease. Neurology 2008; **70**: 1438–44.

119. **Bosboom JL, Stoffers D, Stam CJ, et al.** Resting state oscillatory brain dynamics in Parkinson's disease: an MEG study. Clin Neurophysiol 2006; **117**: 2521–31.

120. **Bosboom JL, Stoffers D, Stam CJ, et al.** Cholinergic modulation of MEG resting-state oscillatory activity in Parkinson's disease related dementia. Clin Neurophysiol 2009; **120**: 910–15.

121. **Jones EG.** Synchrony in the interconnected circuitry of the thalamus and cerebral cortex. Ann NY Acad Sci 2009; **1157**: 10–23.

122. **Alexander GM, Carden WB, Mu J, et al.** The native T-type calcium current in relay neurons of the primate thalamus. Neuroscience 2006; **141**: 453–61.

123. **Piggott MA, Candy JM, Perry RH.** [³H]nitrendipine binding in temporal cortex in Alzheimer's and Huntington's diseases. Brain Res 1991; **565**: 42–7.

124. **Garcia-Reitbock P, Anichtchik O, Bellucci A, et al.** SNARE protein redistribution and synaptic failure in a transgenic mouse model of Parkinson's disease. Brain 2010; **133**: 2032–44.

125. **Kisos H, Ben-Gedalya T, Sharon R.** The clathrin-dependent localization of dopamine transporter to surface membranes is affected by α-synuclein. J Mol Neurosci 2014; **52**: 167–76.

126. **Burre J, Sharma M, Tsetsenis T, et al.** Alpha-synuclein promotes SNARE-complex assembly in vivo and in vitro. Science 2010; **329**: 1663–7.

127. **Nemani VM, Lu W, Berge V, et al.** Increased expression of alpha-synuclein reduces neurotransmitter release by inhibiting synaptic vesicle reclustering after endocytosis. Neuron 2010; **65**: 66–79.

128. **Piccoli G, Condliffe SB, Bauer M, et al.** LRRK2 controls synaptic vesicle storage and mobilization within the recycling pool. J Neurosci 2011; **31**: 2225–37.

129. **Esposito G, Ana Clara F, Verstreken P.** Synaptic vesicle trafficking and Parkinson's disease. Dev Neurobiol 2012; **72**: 134–44.

130. **Kramer ML, Schulz-Schaeffer WJ.** Presynaptic {alpha}-synuclein aggregates, not Lewy bodies, cause neurodegeneration in dementia with Lewy bodies. J Neurosci 2007; **27**: 1405–10.

131. **Calabresi P, Picconi B, Parnetti L, et al.** A convergent model for cognitive dysfunctions in Parkinson's disease: the critical dopamine-acetylcholine synaptic balance. Lancet Neurol 2006; **5**: 974–83.

132. **Poewe W.** Depression in Parkinson's disease. J Neurol 2007; **254**(Suppl. 5): 49–55.

133. **Ballard C, Day S, Sharp S, et al.** Neuropsychiatric symptoms in dementia: importance and treatment considerations. Int Rev Psychiatry 2008; **20**: 396–404.

Chapter 15

Pathological correlates of dementia in Parkinson's disease

Gonzalo J. Revuelta, Guttalu K. Kumaraswamy, and Carol F. Lippa

Introduction

The time-honoured original work by James Parkinson has been shown to be quite insightful in its ability to integrate a constellation of symptoms into a cohesive syndrome by observing a small group of patients. Parkinson understood that this disease affected more than just the motor system; however, he did not feel that pathological change extended to the encephalon, hence sparing the intellect [1]. With the advent of modern treatment, resulting in longer survival times, and detailed pathological examination of brains affected by Parkinson's disease (PD), it is now clear that pathological change does indeed extend to the encephalon, and subsequent cognitive dysfunction is not only common but of great consequence in this disease.

In early studies, definitions of cognitive dysfunction or dementia were not uniform, nor were the methods for their assessment. Adding to this complexity were patient populations which differed in terms of the pathology affecting them, co-morbidities, and age. Hence the reported prevalence of dementia in PD varied substantially, ranging from 3 to 78% [2]; newer studies reveal a prevalence rate of 30–40% [3–5].

Dementia associated with parkinsonism can be categorized clinically as PD dementia (PD-D) or dementia with Lewy bodies (DLB) depending on whether motor or cognitive symptoms, respectively, dominated the early stages of disease. It is becoming more apparent that there is a spectrum of clinical syndromes which, when correlated pathologically, have been found to range from pure forms linked exclusively to Lewy body-related pathology (LRP), as in diffuse Lewy body disease, to more heterogeneous forms with prominent Alzheimer's disease (AD)-related pathology (ARP), as in the Lewy body variant of AD (LBV).

The pathological changes responsible for cognitive dysfunction in PD are heterogeneous and complex. The principal pathological change is that of neuronal loss, or neurodegeneration. There are multiple underlying pathological features, including LRP, ARP, vascular pathology, or a combination of these. In this chapter we will review the current literature regarding these pathological changes and how they are thought to contribute to cognitive dysfunction in PD.

Lewy body pathology

Our knowledge of the underlying pathology in PD began with Frederic H. Lewy's discovery in 1912 of inclusion bodies in patients with PD [6]. These spherical filamentous inclusions, now known as Lewy bodies (LBs), have been at the centre of discussions about the pathology of this disease for over 100 years. In 1997, Polymeropoulos et al. [7] reported the discovery of a mutation

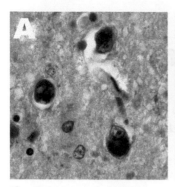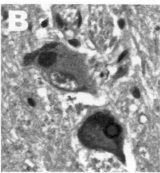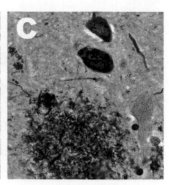

Fig. 15.1 Histopathological appearance of brain tissue from patients with Parkinson's disease dementia (PD-D). (A) Several cortical neurons at high power containing cortical Lewy bodies. Cortical Lewy bodies typically lack a halo, and they are the strongest pathological feature associated with PD-D. Their density also correlates with specific clinical features in some studies. (B) Nigral Lewy bodies in the cytoplasm of brainstem neurons. These are associated more closely with the motor features of PD. Nigral Lewy bodies usually contain a 'halo' that stains strongly for α-synuclein (images A and B are stained with antibodies directed against α-synuclein). (C) Modified silver stain to demonstrate Alzheimer's neurofibrillary tangles (top) and a senile plaque (bottom) in cortical brain tissue from the medial temporal lobe of a PD patient. Alzheimer's pathological features are not uncommon in PD-D patients, but do not correlate with dementia as closely as synuclein pathology (Lewy bodies and Lewy neurites).

in the gene coding for a pre-synaptic protein called α-synuclein in one Italian kindred and three unrelated Greek families with autosomal dominant PD. Following this finding, Spillantini et al. [8] found that LBs as well as dystrophic processes called Lewy neurites (LNs), with similar immunohistochemical properties to LBs, found in patients with idiopathic PD and DLB stained strongly for this protein, yielding clues about the composition of the inclusions. Shortly afterwards, Baba et al. [9] revealed that α-synuclein in LBs was aggregated into fibrils in both sporadic and genetic forms of PD. LBs have since been found to comprise more than 40 proteins, including ubiquitin, tau, heat shock proteins, neurofilaments, aggresomal proteins, and mitochondrial proteins, but α-synuclein is by far the most prominent [10].

Several neurodegenerative diseases have also been found to have inclusions which are immunoreactive for α-synuclein, including multiple system atrophy, pure autonomic failure, and neurodegeneration with brain iron accumulation type 1. These and others have joined the ranks of PD and DLB to form a new class of disease now referred to as the synucleinopathies [11].

In PD-D, LBs are abundant in cortical structures. Cortical LBs (CLBs) have been described as having a less distinct morphology, particularly when using haematoxylin and eosin staining, and they typically lack the distinctive halo which is classically found in LBs in the substantia nigra (SN) [10]. CLBs are the most specific pathological finding in PD-D and they have consistently been found to correlate with dementia [12–14] (see Fig. 15.1).

Alzheimer's disease-related pathology

Since 1907, when Alois Alzheimer identified neuritic plaques and neurofibrillary tangles (NFTs) as the principal pathological change in AD, much has been learned of these entities. Notable discoveries include the understanding of the ultrastructure of NFTs and neuritic plaques and their correlation with dementia in AD. Equally important has been the discovery of the hyperphos-phorylated tau protein as the major constituent of paired helical filaments and the discovery of the amyloid-beta (Aβ) peptide as the major component of amyloid plaques [15] (see Fig. 15.1). These findings have led to the classification of diseases in terms of their immunoreactivity for these proteins and have changed the way we think about these entities clinically. We now use the term amyloidopathy to refer to AD (both familial and sporadic forms), Down's syndrome, and a few others. Similarly, we use the term tauopathy to refer to frontotemporal dementia, progressive supranuclear palsy, corticobasal degeneration, and several other diseases. Other proteins have also been implicated in neurodegenerative diseases, including progranulin, transactive response DNA-binding protein 43, and others [16].

Plaques and tangles are clearly present relatively frequently in PD-D, but they are less often sig-nificant contributors to dementia. Many cases have been reported of a clinical and pathological picture of PD-D without any ARP. Furthermore, multiple studies have found them to be weak correlates for dementia in PD-D, as opposed to LRP [13]. However, subcortical accumulation of Aβ has been reported in PD-D and it is also linked to the faster progression to dementia [17, 18]. Although it correlates highly with LRP burden [19], the level of Aβ is unlikely to be a single neuro-pathological substrate in the progression to dementia. Cognitive impairment occurring at a later phase of PD and advanced age increase the likelihood of multiple pathologies being present. The brains of such patients are likely to demonstrate Aβ and tau pathologies as well as α-synuclein. Variants of two highly investigated genes, *APOE* and *MAPT*, linked to the risk of PD-D [19, 20], are also associated with Aβ aggregation [21] and increased tau expression [22], respectively, there-by suggesting a strong association of all three pathologies. A synergistic role has been proposed for Lewy body pathology as well as associated Aβ and tau pathology in the neurodegeneration causing PD-D [23]. The lower levels of ARP in comparison with AD and the predominance of Lewy body pathology in PD-D suggest that the observed ARP may be a factor contributing to Lewy body pathology, which is the central mechanism in the development of dementia.

Distribution of pathology and clinico-pathological correlation

Previous reports point to the SN as the primary site of neurodegeneration in PD, Tretiakoff [24] has been credited for this finding (in 1919). Since then, our understanding of the pathological changes in the SN has grown significantly. LRP is first found ventrally in the SN pars compacta (SNc), and then spreads to paranigral, medial, and dorsal areas. There is neuronal loss in conjunc-tion with LRP, specifically of melanized and dopaminergic neurons in area A9 of the SNc [25]. These pathological changes in A9, which result in decrease in dopamine, tyrosine hydroxylase, and dopamine transporter immunoreactivity in the striatum, correlate with the duration and severity of motor symptoms [26]. It is not clear, however, whether these neurochemical changes are directly related to LRP.

It has become evident that neurodegeneration in PD goes well beyond the SN, and in fact affects not only subcortical dopaminergic nuclei but also basal cholinergic structures, the dorsal motor nucleus of the vagus nerve, olfactory structures, raphe nuclei, the locus coeruleus, peduncolo-pontine nuclei, hypothalamic nuclei, spinal nuclei, and cortical structures. LRP, ARP, and vascular change are the principal pathologies thought to result in neuronal loss in these structures. Specif-ically, LRP has been documented in the striatum of patients with a variety of synucleinopathies [27]. It has been suggested that greater LRP burden in the SN is indicative of a predominant motor syndrome as in PD or PD-D, and conversely a greater LRP burden in the striatum is more indicative of an illness of predominantly dementing type such as DLB [28]. Furthermore, LRP often involves the peripheral nervous system, including autonomic nuclei, ganglia, and nerves subserving the vasculature, intestines, heart, and adrenal and salivary glands [25]. Of note, there have been reports of LBs in two patients with PD who had undergone transplantation of fetal mesencephalic dopaminergic neurons with long-term survival. Grafted cells in these two patients were not functionally impaired [29].

LRP has been described in both limbic (layer II) and neocortical structures (layers V and VI). Pathological change in specific structures within these areas has been studied meticulously in order to correlate clinical symptomatology with cortical LRP burden, and to differentiate between synucleinopathies. Of all the cortical areas studied, it appears that LRP burden in the parahippocampus is most indicative of dementia, although in DLB cases the pathology was more heterogeneous [30]. Similarly, in the entorhinal and anterior cingulate cortex (Brodmann area 24) LRP burden correlates well with cognitive deficits in patients with PD-D [14]. A high LRP burden in the parahippocampus and amygdala correlates well with early visual hallucinations. Furthermore, LRP in the inferior temporal cortical structures is associated with earlier onset of hallucinations, and therefore with a greater likelihood of developing DLB [31].

The diverse pathological findings previously described, which individually correlate with some clinical symptoms, have been consolidated in different ways in order to account for specific clinical syndromes. McKeith et al. [32] have devised and revised criteria for the pathological diagnosis of DLB, taking into account the extent of LRP in specific brain regions, as well as ARP, and rating pathological burden in a semi-quantitative fashion. In determining which clinical syndrome is most likely indicated by the pathological change being observed, the type of pathological change is as important as the distribution of such change. Therefore, the McKeith criteria assign a probability that the pathological change is consistent with the clinical syndrome of DLB, based not only on the LRP burden (which is directly related to the likelihood of the pathology representing clinical DLB) and the ARP (which is inversely related to the likelihood of the pathology representing clinical DLB [33]), but also on the areas involved. These criteria group cases into brainstem-predominant, limbic or transitional, and diffuse neocortical, and the likelihood that the pathological changes represent the clinical syndrome of DLB is greater with more rostral and lesser with more caudal changes [32, 33].

Disease progression

The question of whether the aforementioned pathological changes and their distribution actually follow a distinct course of progression is central to understanding the pathophysiology of LB-related dementia. Braak et al. [35] meticulously studied a series of brains from patients with clinical PD, incidental LBs and LNs, and controls. Working under the assumption that there was a coherent progression of disease in these cases, they organized the samples in a sequential manner, and subsequently developed a staging system for LRP in this patient population. The staging system that emerged proposed a caudo-rostral progression of pathological change, which began in the dorsal motor nucleus of the glossopharyngeal and vagus nerves, as well as the olfactory nucleus, and ascended to mesocortical and then neocortical structures. The first two stages are related to incidental Lewy body disease, the third and fourth stages to motor symptoms, and the later stages (five and six) to concurrent cognitive dysfunction. Later studies by the same authors were able to correlate cognitive dysfunction with this staging system of LRP in patients with PD [36].

Multiple counter-examples to this staging system have since been proposed, whereby sparing of caudal regions occurs with more rostral involvement, which implies that other pathological changes, apart from Lewy body pathology, may be contributing [25]. Further evidence of this notion is that the existence of LRP—to the extent that it meets the pathological criteria for diagnosis of DLB—may occur in the absence of a clinical dementing syndrome [37]. More recent revisions of this staging system propose that the early sites of LRP are the olfactory bulb and enteric plexus of the stomach, suggesting that a neurotrophic pathogen enters through the nasal or gastric mucosa and proceeds to the central nervous system via anterograde progression to temporal structures or through retrograde transport via peripheral ganglia, respectively [38].

A competing theory, which not only challenges Braak's proposed theory of disease progression but is also a unitary theory of pathophysiology for Lewy body diseases, identifies three distinct clinico-pathological subgroups. The first consists of a younger group of patients with a predominantly early motor phenotype, which is consistent with caudo-rostral progression of pathological change. The second subgroup consists of patients who suffered a more aggressive course of disease, with an early onset of dementia and concomitant early neocortical involvement. The third subgroup identified represents patients with later disease onset, and a subsequently shorter course, with a greater burden of pathological change that also tended to be more heterogeneous. This theory, and the data that support it, implies that a caudo-rostral progression of pathological change is only applicable to a subgroup of patients, and does not explain progression of disease in other subgroups, particularly those who follow a dementia-dominant clinical course [39].

In a critical evaluation Jellinger [40] questioned the predictive value of the current staging system, noting that there is little correlation between Braak LB stages and the neuronal cell loss as well as the clinical severity of dementia. Others have suggested a more informative semi-quantitative and quantitative assessment of Lewy body pathology over the existing topographical staging for a better correlation of the cognitive impairment and the underlying pathology [23]. A unified staging system was proposed during 2009 by the BrainNet Europe Consortium [41], which combined the brainstem, limbic, and neocortical stages as well as the Braak staging. As a result of a study involving 22 observers analysing 31 autopsy cases, this system incorporates a modified Braak staging [42] and a modified McKeith typing [43]. The staging process involves an assessment of 10 different areas of the brain—medulla, pons, midbrain, basal forebrain, striatum, hippocampus, cingulate gyri, temporal cortex, frontal cortex, and parietal cortex—for the presence or absence of α-synuclein immunoreactivity, LBs, and LNs. The pattern of distribution to assess the typical/atypical nature and presence or absence of amygdala-predominant type to assess the severity of LRP is also taken into consideration [41].

Aetiologies underlying neurodegeneration

From the information previously presented, we understand the pathology that is found in PD-D, where it occurs, how it may correlate with clinical symptoms, how it can be correlated with clinical syndromes, and how it progresses; nevertheless the mechanisms that underlie these pathological changes remain unclear. Several theories have been developed to explain why the pathological changes that take place in Lewy body diseases actually occur. At the root of this discussion is the assumption that the aggregation of α-synuclein in LBs is the central neuropathological feature of these diseases, and this is supported by the finding that mutations in the α-synuclein gene lead to parkinsonism, the finding of aggregated α-synuclein with abnormal nitration, phosphorylation, and ubiquitination, the development of neurodegeneration in α-synuclein transgenic animal models, and the aforementioned clinico-pathological correlation studies [28]. The finding that LBs are found in grafted neurons supports this assertion; however, the finding that LRP is present in patients without parkinsonism or cognitive dysfunction (incidental Lewy body disease) implies at least that LRP may not be the only mechanism underlying neurodegeneration in Lewy body diseases, which is certainly the case in more severe dementing syndromes such as DLB. Furthermore, some have theorized that there is a 'bystander' effect occurring when multiple pathologies such as LRP and ARP coexist and possibly augment one another in these disease entities. Recent studies suggest that a combination of Lewy body pathology and ARP rather than Lewy body pathology alone is the most robust pathological correlate of PD-D. Such a combination has been linked with faster progression of dementia, and the rate of progression also correlates with the Aβ burden [23, 44]. A combined assessment of α-synuclein, tau, and Aβ is a better predictor of the progression of dementia than α-synuclein alone [23]. Clinico-pathological studies using cerebrospinal fluid (CSF) analysis and in vivo positron emission tomography (PET) scanning with the ^{11}C-Pittsburgh-B compound shed some light on the role of ARP. CSF levels of tau and Aβ have been thoroughly investigated as biomarkers in AD [45, 46], and it is suggested that intra-parenchymal sequestration of Aβ results in its relatively reduced levels in CSF. Some studies specifically testing these biomarkers in PD-D revealed reduced CSF Aβ levels, and in vivo PET studies assessing amyloid burden showed less severe and less frequent amyloid accumulation in PD-D. It was noted that pre-dementia patients also showed reduced CSF levels of amyloid markers, whereas PD patents without dementia showed higher levels than patients with PD-D [47].

Others have suggested that the mere accumulation of abnormal proteins is not sufficient to account for the clinical symptoms, and instead an assessment of the neurochemical changes that occur as a result of the degeneration of neurons, particularly monoaminergic neurons, would more accurately represent the underlying pathophysiology. Other changes, including vascular and normal ageing changes, can contribute to the degeneration of these neurons to differing degrees [25].

If we accept the assumption that α-synuclein pathology is central to the pathophysiology of these diseases, it still remains unclear how exactly that occurs. The possibility of a direct toxic effect of α-synuclein has been proposed, but this remains unproven. Indeed, α-synuclein aggregates may be a by-product of compensatory biological processes that are neuroprotective. Other possible mechanisms underlying degeneration include overproduction of α-synuclein, dysfunction of chaperones and other components of the ubiquitin–proteosome system, inflammation, oxidative stress, excitotoxicity, mitochondrial dysfunction, growth factor deficiencies, prion-like mechanisms of cell injury, or a combination of these [48].

Conclusion

Dementia is common in PD, especially as the disease progresses and patients get older. In its pure form, dementia in PD occurs when LB pathology spreads to involve cortical and limbic structures. In addition, many PD-D patients have concurrent AD or vascular changes. Clinicians will observe slightly different cognitive features in the different pathological forms that occur across the PD-D spectrum. The regional distribution of pathology will correlate with symptoms. For example, patients with 'pure PD-D' solely associated with LB pathology are less likely to experience a primarily amnestic dementia. When amnesia is a prominent feature, concurrent AD pathology is likely, beginning in medial temporal lobe regions that are key for forming new memories. Overall, there is clinical and pathological heterogeneity amongst PD-D patients. With an eye toward aetiologically based treatments, it will become more important to identify the biological factors involved in the development of dementia in each PD patient.

References

1. **Parkinson J**. *An essay on the shaking palsy*. London: Whittingham & Rowland, 1817. [Annotated reprint in Med Classics 1938; **2**: 957–98.]

2. **Goldmann Gross R, Siderowf A, Hurtig HI**. Cognitive impairment in Parkinson's disease and dementia with Lewy bodies: a spectrum of disease. Neurosignals 2008; **16**: 24–34.

3. **Aarsland D, Andersen K, Larsen JP, et al**. Prevalence and characteristics of dementia in Parkinson disease: an 8-year prospective study. Arch Neurol 2003; **60**: 387–92.

4. **Cummings JL**. The dementias of Parkinson's disease: prevalence, characteristics, neurobiology, and comparison with dementia of the Alzheimer type. Eur Neurol 1988; **28**(Suppl. 1): 15–23.

5. **Emre M**. Dementia in Parkinson's disease: cause and treatment. Curr Opin Neurol 2004; **17**: 399–404.

6. **Lewy F**. Zür pathologischen Anatomie der Paralysis agitans. Dtsch Z Nervenheilk 1914; **1**: 50–5.

7. **Polymeropoulos MH, Lavedan C, Leroy E, et al**. Mutation in the alpha-synuclein gene identified in families with Parkinson's disease. Science 1997; **276**: 2045–7.

8. **Spillantini MG, Schmidt ML, Lee VM, et al**. Alpha-synuclein in Lewy bodies. Nature 1997; **388**: 839–40.

9. **Baba M, Nakajo S, Tu PH, et al**. Aggregation of alpha-synuclein in Lewy bodies of sporadic Parkinson's disease and dementia with Lewy bodies. Am J Pathol 1998; **152**: 879–84.

10. **Shults CW**. Lewy bodies. Proc Natl Acad Sci USA 2006; **103**: 1661–8.

11. **Galvin JE, Lee VM, Trojanowski JQ**. Synucleinopathies: clinical and pathological implications. Arch Neurol 2001; **58**: 186–90.

12. **Aarsland D, Perry R, Brown A, et al**. Neuropathology of dementia in Parkinson's disease: a prospective, community-based study. Ann Neurol 2005; **58**: 773–6.

13. **Hurtig HI, Trojanowski JQ, Galvin J, et al**. Alpha-synuclein cortical Lewy bodies correlate with dementia in Parkinson's disease. Neurology 2000; **54**: 1916–21.

14. **Kovari E, Gold G, Herrmann FR, et al**. Lewy body densities in the entorhinal and anterior cingulate cortex predict cognitive deficits in Parkinson's disease. Acta Neuropathol 2003; **106**: 83–8.

15. **Iqbal K, Grundke-Iqbal I**. Discoveries of tau, abnormally hyperphosphorylated tau and others of neurofibrillary degeneration: a personal historical perspective. J Alzheimers Dis 2006; **9**: 219–42.

16. **Boeve BF, Hutton M**. Refining frontotemporal dementia with parkinsonism linked to chromosome 17: introducing FTDP-17 (MAPT) and FTDP-17 (PGRN). Arch Neurol 2008; **65**: 460–4.

17. **Ballard C, Ziabreva I, Perry R, et al**. Differences in neuropathologic characteristics across the Lewy body dementia spectrum. Neurology 2006; **67**: 1931–4.

18. **Sabbagh MN, Adler CH, Lahti TJ, et al**. Parkinson disease with dementia: comparing patients with and without Alzheimer pathology. Alzheimer Dis Assoc Disord 2009; **23**: 295–7.

19. **Colom-Cadena M, Gelpi E, Charif S, et al**. Confluence of alpha-synuclein, tau, and beta-amyloid pathologies in dementia with Lewy bodies. J Neuropathol Exp Neurol 2013; **72**: 1203–12.

20. **Williams-Gray CH, Goris A, Saiki M, et al**. Apolipoprotein E genotype as a risk factor for susceptibility to and dementia in Parkinson's disease. J Neurol 2009; **256**: 493–8.

21. **Polvikoski T, Sulkava R, Haltia M, et al**. Apolipoprotein E, dementia, and cortical deposition of beta-amyloid protein. N Engl J Med 1995; **333**: 1242–7.

22. **Laws SM, Friedrich P, Diehl-Schmid J, et al**. Fine mapping of the MAPT locus using quantitative trait analysis identifies possible causal variants in Alzheimer's disease. Mol Psychiatry 2007; **12**: 510–17.

23. **Compta Y, Parkkinen L, O'Sullivan SS, et al**. Lewy- and Alzheimer-type pathologies in Parkinson's disease dementia: which is more important? Brain 2011; **134**: 1493–505.

24. **Tretiakoff C**. Contribution a l'etude de l'anatomie pathologique du locus niger de Soemmering avec quelques dedutions relatives a la pathogenie des troubles du tonus musculaire et de la maladie de Parkinson. Thesis. University of Paris, 1919.

25. **Jellinger KA**. A critical reappraisal of current staging of Lewy-related pathology in human brain. Acta Neuropathol 2008; **116**: 1–16.

26. **Ma SY, Roytta M, Rinne JO, et al.** Correlation between neuromorphometry in the substantia nigra and clinical features in Parkinson's disease using dissector counts. J Neurol Sci 1997; **151**: 83–7.

27. **Duda JE, Giasson BI, Mabon ME, et al.** Novel antibodies to synuclein show abundant striatal pathology in Lewy body diseases. Ann Neurol 2002; **52**: 205–10.

28. **Lippa CF, Duda JE, Grossman M, et al.** DLB and PDD boundary issues: diagnosis, treatment, molecular pathology, and biomarkers. Neurology 2007; **68**: 812–19.

29. **Li JY, Englund E, Holton JL, et al.** Lewy bodies in grafted neurons in subjects with Parkinson's disease suggest host-to-graft disease propagation. Nat Med 2008; **14**: 501–3.

30. **Harding AJ, Halliday GM.** Cortical Lewy body pathology in the diagnosis of dementia. Acta Neuropathol 2001; **102**: 355–63.

31. **Harding AJ, Broe GA, Halliday GM.** Visual hallucinations in Lewy body disease relate to Lewy bodies in the temporal lobe. Brain 2002; **125**: 391–403.

32. **McKeith IG, Dickson DW, Lowe J, et al.** Diagnosis and management of dementia with Lewy bodies: third report of the DLB Consortium. Neurology 2005; **65**: 1863–72.

33. **Merdes AR, Hansen LA, Jeste DV, et al.** Influence of Alzheimer pathology on clinical diagnostic accuracy in dementia with Lewy bodies. Neurology 2003; **60**: 1586–90.

34. **Fujishiro H, Ferman TJ, Boeve BF, et al.** Validation of the neuropathologic criteria of the third consortium for dementia with Lewy bodies for prospectively diagnosed cases. J Neuropathol Exp Neurol 2008; **67**: 649–56.

35. **Braak H, Del Tredici K, Rub U, et al.** Staging of brain pathology related to sporadic Parkinson's disease. Neurobiol Aging 2003; **24**: 197–211.

36. **Braak H, Rub U, Jansen Steur EN, et al.** Cognitive status correlates with neuropathologic stage in Parkinson disease. Neurology 2005; **64**: 1404–10.

37. **Colosimo C, Hughes AJ, Kilford L, et al.** Lewy body cortical involvement may not always predict dementia in Parkinson's disease. J Neurol Neurosurg Psychiatry 2003; **74**: 852–6.

38. **Hawkes CH, Del Tredici K, Braak H.** Parkinson's disease: a dual-hit hypothesis. Neuropathol Appl Neurobiol 2007; **33**: 599–614.

39. **Halliday G, Hely M, Reid W, et al.** The progression of pathology in longitudinally followed patients with Parkinson's disease. Acta Neuropathol 2008; **115**: 409–15.

40. **Jellinger KA.** A critical evaluation of current staging of alpha-synuclein pathology in Lewy body disorders. Biochim Biophys Acta 2009; **1792**: 730–40.

41. **Alafuzoff I, Ince PG, Arzberger T, et al.** Staging/typing of Lewy body related alpha-synuclein pathology: a study of the BrainNet Europe Consortium. Acta Neuropathol 2009; **117**: 635–52.

42. **Muller CM, de Vos RA, Maurage CA, et al.** Staging of sporadic Parkinson disease-related alpha-synuclein pathology: inter- and intra-rater reliability. J Neuropathol Exp Neurol 2005; **64**: 623–8.

43. **Leverenz JB, Hamilton R, Tsuang DW, et al.** Empiric refinement of the pathologic assessment of Lewy-related pathology in the dementia patient. Brain Pathol 2008; **18**: 220–4.

44. **Compta Y, Parkkinen L, Kempster P, et al.** The significance of alpha-synuclein, amyloid-beta and tau pathologies in Parkinson's disease progression and related dementia. Neurodegener Dis 2014; **13**: 154–6.

45. **Dubois B, Feldman HH, Jacova C, et al.** Research criteria for the diagnosis of Alzheimer's disease: revising the NINCDS-ADRDA criteria. Lancet Neurol 2007; **6**: 734–46.

46. **Dubois B, Feldman HH, Jacova C, et al.** Revising the definition of Alzheimer's disease: a new lexicon. Lancet Neurol 2010; **9**: 1118–27.

47. **Buongiorno M, Compta Y, Marti MJ.** Amyloid-beta and tau biomarkers in Parkinson's disease-dementia. J Neurol Sci 2011; **310**: 25–30.

48. **Brundin P, Li JY, Holton JL, et al.** Research in motion: the enigma of Parkinson's disease pathology spread. Nat Rev Neurosci 2008; **9**: 741–5.

Chapter 16

Epidemiology, diagnosis, and correlates of mild cognitive impairment in Parkinson's disease

Elise Caccappolo and Karen Marder

Introduction

Earlier work on mild cognitive impairment (MCI) in Parkinson's disease (PD) was constrained by a lack of standardized diagnostic criteria, and frequently applied established MCI criteria typically used in Alzheimer's populations [1, 2]. In the clinical context of memory impairment, the construct of MCI has been conceived as representing the prodromal stage of early Alzheimer's disease (AD) [3] given that a high proportion of people with amnestic MCI progress to AD. Petersen's [4] criteria for amnestic MCI require the presence of a memory complaint and objective memory impairment for age with all other cognitive domains being within normal limits, as well as preserved activities of daily living. As the criteria for MCI expanded to incorporate non-amnestic MCI as a separate clinical phenotype of MCI [2], the identification of multiple-domain MCI and single-domain non-memory MCI as constructs acknowledged the possibility of impaired performance in other cognitive domains, i.e. with no memory deficit and intact or minimally impaired functioning.

As the construct of MCI has been applied to PD, PD-MCI has been described as the earliest stage of cognitive decline [5] as well as a risk factor for dementia [6, 7], in much the same way as amnestic MCI may progress to AD. The application of the construct of MCI in PD differs from its use in predicting AD in that PD is, by definition, already diagnosed when cognitive deficits may be demonstrated by the patient [8]. In fact, subtle cognitive impairment may already be present at the time of diagnosis of PD [9–12]. Although PD patients are at a higher risk of developing cognitive impairment than controls, with a more rapid decline in those who do [5, 6, 13], the timing of cognitive decline to dementia is variable [14], as is the profile and pattern of impairment [15–17]. It is unclear whether all PD-MCI patients will eventually progress to dementia or whether other factors such as genetic mutations or concomitant disease may contribute to the development or more rapid progression of cognitive impairment. Longitudinal studies have identified a more significant rate of cognitive decline across domains in PD patients compared with age-matched healthy controls [18] and have found dementia in 78% of PD patients 8 years after diagnosis [19] and in as many as 83% after 20 years [20].

Frequency estimates of PD-MCI

The reported frequency of PD-MCI varies due to differences in the populations studied (e.g. sample size, demographics, and whether on or off medication at the time of testing), disease characteristics (e.g. the extent of motor impairment), the definition of MCI used, methods used to classify MCI (e.g. neuropsychological tests utilized, domains assessed, cut-off score used), types of studies performed (cross-sectional versus longitudinal), and other factors such as whether prevalence or incidence rates were examined. In 2011, the Movement Disorder Society (MDS) commissioned a Task Force to estimate the frequency and characteristics of PD-MCI and its rate of conversion to dementia [21], with the goal of developing formal diagnostic criteria for PD-MCI [22]. A review of the literature to 1 September 2010 was conducted through Medline using free search terms including 'Parkinson' and 'mild cognitive impairment'. Studies included in the review were those that examined at least 100 PD patients without dementia in cross-sectional studies or 50 patients in prospective studies, examined cognitive functioning by means of neuropsychological tests that assessed at least three of five cognitive domains, and used either normative values or a control group to compare the neuropsychological function of the PD group. Articles were excluded that did not clearly define impaired cognition or dementia or that included subjects with dementia, surgically treated PD, or other neurological diseases. The studies reviewed included six cross-sectional and two prospective studies with a total of 776 PD patients, resulting in a mean cross-sectional prevalence of 26.7% PD-MCI (range 18.9–38.2%), a finding similar to the 25.8% prevalence reported in a multicentre pooled analysis of eight PD cohorts totalling 1346 patients where MCI was defined as impairment (1.5 SD below controls or normative data) in at least one domain [23]. The MDS Task Force findings further indicated that the frequency of PD-MCI increases with age and disease duration, single-domain MCI occurs more frequently than multiple-domain MCI, and within single-domain MCI, non-amnestic MCI is diagnosed more frequently than amnestic MCI.

Another review of PD-MCI [24] excluded studies that used screening batteries as opposed to more thorough neuropsychological assessment as well as studies that did not provide specific MCI diagnostic criteria. Subsequently, three of the eight studies included in the MDS Task Force review were also included in this review and three were excluded, while eight additional studies were included, resulting in a review of 11 studies. In this review [24] prevalence rates of PD-MCI ranged from 15 to 62%, with common estimates of approximately 30%. Those studies with the highest prevalence rates defined MCI as impairment on one neuropsychological test, defined either as performance 1.5 SD below the mean or, in some cases, defined without a cut-off, while the lower rates were provided by studies that defined impairment as scores that were at least 2 SD below the mean. Consistent with the MDS Task Force analyses, single-domain impairment was more common than multiple-domain MCI, and non-amnestic MCI was more frequently diagnosed than amnestic MCI for both single- and multiple-domain MCI. More recent investigations of PD-MCI have reported similarly varied prevalence rates, with frequencies ranging from 9 to 47%, with mean prevalence rates around 30% [17, 25–27]. Table 16.1 gives a review of PD-MCI studies.

Diagnostic criteria for MCI

In light of the review of existing literature, the MDS Task Force developed operationalized diagnostic criteria for PD-MCI that were based on Petersen's MCI criteria, with modifications for the specific characteristics of PD [22]. The criteria proposed by the MDS Task Force for PD-MCI are in concert with criteria for PD dementia (PD-D), also developed by a MDS Task Force [28]. They provide inclusion and exclusion criteria, specifying guidelines for the comprehensiveness of neuropsychological testing, and recommend subtype classification for PD-MCI. Recognizing that

Table 16.1 Studies of the prevalence of MCI in PD

Study	Sample	Cognitive measures used	MCI definition	Findings/subtypes
Aarsland et al., 2009a,b [12]	Community sample of 196 drug-naïve PD patients. Mean age 67.6 (8.3) years. Mean duration 2.3 years	CVLT-II VOSP subtests Animal fluency Stroop colour word test	≥1.5 SD below Z-score in at least 1 of 3 domains	18.9% MCI 86.5% single domain 62.2% non-amnestic MCI—single domain 24.3% amnestic MCI—single domain 13.5% multiple domain 2.7% non-amnestic MCI—multiple domain 10.8% amnestic MCI—multiple domain
Aarsland et al., 2010b [23]	Multicentre sample of 1346 PD patients without dementia. Mean age 67.5 years. Mean duration 6.1 years	Tests differed by centre. Domains included attention/executive, visuospatial (assessed in 1141 subjects) and memory	≥1.5 SD below composite mean score of control or normative sample in at least 1 domain	26% MCI 11% non-amnestic single domain 9% amnestic single domain 1% non-amnestic multiple domain 5% amnestic multiple domain
Caviness et al., 2007b [7]	Clinical, brain bank sample of 71 PD patients without dementia. Mean age 74.6 years. Mean duration 9.2 years	Stroop color word test Trail Making Test Letter and category fluency tests Digit Span, forward and backward Auditory Verbal Learning Test Clock-drawing test Judgment of Line test	'Consistent pattern of impaired performance on neuropsychological measures that load on that cognitive domain'	21% MCI 42% MCI if 1.5 SD on single test criterion was used 9% non-amnestic single domain 5% amnestic single domain 5% non-amnestic single domain 5% non-amnestic multiple domain 2% amnestic multiple domain

Table 16.1 (continued) Studies of the prevalence of MCI in PD

Study	Sample	Cognitive measures used	MCI definition	Findings/subtypes
Dalrymple-Alford et al., 2011 [25]	Clinic-based sample of 143 PD patients. Mean age 69.8 years. Mean disease duration 8.7 years	Verbal fluency D-KEFS subtests Stroop test Trail Making Test Digits forward CVLT-IISF Rey Complex Figure Judgment of Line Orientation	2 sets of criteria: >1.5 SD below mean on two tests within one domain; >1.5 SD on one score in each of two domains	30% for first criterion 37% for second criteron
Foltynie et al., 2004[a] [74]	Clinic-based sample of 142 PD patients without dementia. Mean age 73.7 years. Mean duration 2.2 years	Category and letter fluency Modified Tower of London test CANTAB spatial resolution subtest CANTAB pattern recognition memory subtest	≥1 SD below normative data in ≥1 test	35.2% MCI 58.0% single domain 34.0% frontostriatal deficits— single domain 24% temporal lobe deficits—single domain 42% frontostriatal and temporal deficits—multiple domain
Goldman et al., 2012 [74]	Clinic-based sample of 128 PD-MCI patients. Mean age 72.9 years. Mean disease duration 7.3 years	Digit Span, forward and backward Oral version of Symbol Digit Modalities Test Category fluency (animals) Word list-learning test Boston Naming Test Similarities subtest Judgment of Line Orientation Intersecting pentagons from MMSE	Z-score ≤ –1.5 SD for 1 domain	47.7% non-amnestic single domain 24.2% amnestic multiple domain 18.8% amnestic single domain 9.5% non-amnestic multiple domain

Table 16.1 (continued) Studies of the prevalence of MCI in PD

Study	Sample	Cognitive measures used	MCI definition	Findings/subtypes
Hoops et al., 2009[a,b] [75]	Clinic based sample (2 sites) of 132 PD patients (17 with PD-D). Mean age 68.1 years. Mean duration 8.2 years	Hopkins Verbal Learning Test Tower of London Digit Span, backward Cube copying	≥1.5 SD below normative data on tests in at least 2 cognitive domains	20.0% MCI MCI subtypes not reported
Janvin et al., 2006[a,b] [5]	Community sample of 72 PD patients without dementia. Mean age 73.2 years. Mean duration 11.2 years	Benton Visual Retention Test Judgment of Line Test Stroop colour word test	≥1.5 SD below control group in ≥1 subtest	52.8% MCI 60.5% single domain 44.7% non-amnestic MCI—single domain 15.8% amnestic single domain 39.5% multiple domain
Monastero et al., 2012 [26]	Clinic based sample of 290 PD patients. Mean age 68.8 years. Mean duration not reported	Rey Auditory Learning Test Token test Naming subtest of Aachener Aphasia Battery Visual search Trail Making Test Phonemic fluency test Raven's Coloured Progressive Matrices Frontal Assessment Battery Copy drawing test Position discrimination subtest of the VOSP	Used 'modified Petersen's criteria': (1) single, non-memory = abnormal test score (under normality cut-off) in 1 non-memory test; (2) amnestic MCI = abnormal score on at least one standardized memory test; (3) amnestic multiple domain = 1 abnormal test in ≥2 domains, one being memory; (4) non-amnestic multiple domain = 1 abnormal test in ≥2 tests, excluding memory	53% MCI 55% amnestic MCI 45% non-amnestic MCI

Table 16.1 (continued) Studies of the prevalence of MCI in PD

Study	Sample	Cognitive measures used	MCI definition	Findings/subtypes
Mamikonyan et al., 2009[a,b] [76]	Clinic based sample of 106 PD patients. Mean age 64.6 years. Mean duration 6.5 years	Hopkins Verbal Learning Test Digit Span, forward and backward Tower of London test Stroop colour word test Category fluency	≥1.5 SD below normative mean on 2/3 memory or executive scores; below age cut-off on Digit Span backward or forward	29% MCI 18% single domain 11% multiple domain
Muslimovic et al., 2005[a] [9]	Clinic-based sample of 115 PD patients. Mean age 66.2 years. Mean duration 1.5 years	Trail Making Test Stroop colour word test Tower of London—Drexel test Wisconsin Card Sort Test—modified WAIS-R Digit Symbol subtest COWAT Category fluency WAIS III Similarities subtest Auditory Verbal Learning Test Rivermead Behavioral Learning Test WMS III Logical Memory subtest WAIS-R Digit Span subtest Boston Naming Test Judgment of Line Test Groningen spatial subtest Clock-drawing test	≥2 SD below normative data on ≥3 tests	23.5% MCI MCI subtypes not reported

Table 16.1 (continued) Studies of the prevalence of MCI in PD

Study	Sample	Cognitive measures used	MCI definition	Findings/subtypes
Naismith et al., 2010[b] [77]	Clinic-based sample of 61 PD patients. Mean age 64.5 years. Mean duration 6.2 years	Digit Span subtest Trail Making Test WMS III Logical Memory subtest Category and letter fluency	≥1.5 SD below NART score in at least 1 domain	62% MCI 37% single domain 25% multiple domain
Pai and Chan, 2001[a] [32]	Clinic-based sample of 102 non-demented PD pts Mean age = 68 Mean disease duration not reported	Cognitive Abilities Screening Instrument memory and executive subtests	≥1.5 SD below control group in ≥1 subtest	38.2% MCI MCI subtypes not reported
Pedersen et al., 2013 [27]	Population-based sample of 182 PD patients. Mean age 68 years. Mean disease duration 2.3 years	Stroop test Semantic verbal fluency test California Verbal Learning Test-II VOSP Silhouettes and Cube subtest	MDS PD-MCI Task Force criteria (2012)	20.3% MCI MCI subtypes not classified due to lack of language domain on testing
Poletti et al., 2012 [78]	Clinic-based sample of 121 PD patients. Mean age 66.6 years. Mean disease duration 1.2 years		MDS PD-MCI Task Force criteria (2012)	14.8% PD-MCI 38.9% single domain (5 non-amnestic, 2 amnestic) 61.1% were multidomain (6 non-amnestic, 5 amnestic)

Table 16.1 (continued) Studies of the prevalence of MCI in PD

Study	Sample	Cognitive measures used	MCI definition	Findings/subtypes
Sollinger et al., 2010[b] [79]	Clinic-based sample of 72 PD patients (34 cognitively intact, 38 MCI). Mean age of MCI patients 66 years. Mean disease duration 8.7 years	Judgment of Line test Pentagon drawing from MMSE Boston Naming Test Category and letter fluency Digit Span, forward Trailmaking Test Hopkins Verbal Learning Test Three-item recall from MMSE Spell 'world' backward from MMSE	Clinical judgement based on estimated pre-morbid abilities	53% MCI 19% non-amnestic single domain 13% amnestic single domain 8% non-amnestic multiple domain 13% amnestic multiple domain
Song et al., 2008[b] [80]	Clinic-based sample of 75 PD patients. Mean age 64.9 years. Mean disease duration 4.8 years	Digit Span test Letter cancellation Comprehension Repetition Boston Naming Test Reading Writing Body part identification Praxis testing Intersecting pentagons Rey Osterreith Figure Test	2 SD below control group mean in ≥1 test	15% MCI MCI subtypes not reported

Table 16.1 (continued) Studies of the prevalence of MCI in PD

Study	Sample	Cognitive measures used	MCI definition	Findings/subtypes
		Hopkins Verbal Learning Test		
		Stroop colour word test		
		Motor impersistence		
		Go–no go test		
		Fist edge palm		
		Category and letter fluency		
Williams-Gray et al., 2007a [81]		Animal fluency	≥1 SD below control group in ≥1 test	57.1% MCI frontostriatal single domain ('predominant')
		Letter fluency		
		Tower of London		
		CANTAB Pattern Recognition Memory subtest		
		MMSE pentagons		
		CANTAB Spatial Recognition Memory subtests		

CVLT, California Verbal Learning Test; VOSP, Visual Object and Space Perception Battery; D-KEFS, Delis–Kaplan Executive Function System; WAIS, Wechsler Adult Intelligence Scale; COWAT, Controlled Oral Word Association Test; WMS, Wechsler Memory Scale; MMSE, Mini-Mental State Examination; NART, National Adult Reading Test.

[a]Included in the Litvan et al. (2011) review [21].

[b]Included in the Troster (2011) review [24].

resources for a detailed neuropsychological assessment may not be available or practical, the MDS Task Force PD-MCI diagnostic guidelines provide two levels of diagnosis:

◆ Level I: diagnosis is based on a global cognitive scale or a limited number of cognitive tests and does not allow for subtyping of PD-MCI.

◆ Level II: requires use of more comprehensive neuropsychological testing that includes at least two tests for each of five cognitive domains, with impairment on at least two neuropsychological tests, i.e. either two impaired tests in one domain or one impaired test each in two domains. Impairment is defined as performance between 1 and 2 SD below norms that are age, education, gender, and culturally appropriate *or* significant decline on serial testing *or* significant decline from estimated pre-morbid levels of performance. Diagnosis of PD-MCI by level II criteria allows for subtyping. The single-domain subtype refers to impairment on two tests within a single domain while performance in other domains remains preserved. Specification of the affected domain(s) (e.g. executive, memory) is recommended whether classifying PD-MCI as single or multiple domain.

Table 16.2 summarizes the proposed MDS-Task Force PD-MCI criteria.

The absence of significant functional decline that results from cognitive change is a requirement for diagnosing MCI. While the MDS Task Force criteria do not specify how functional status should be assessed (e.g. via self- or informant report, observation, interview, or rating scales), any functional decline secondary to cognitive decline must be differentiated from that due to motor dysfunction, particularly given that the absence of significant functional decline due to cognitive change is the fundamental feature that differentiates MCI from dementia [29].

In addition to the diagnostic guidelines put forward by the MDS Task Force, an alternative set of preliminary criteria for research purposes was proposed by Troster [24]; attempts were made to make these consistent with drafted criteria for 'mild neurocognitive disorder' within the DSM-V and PD-D criteria developed by the MDS Task Force [28]. These preliminary criteria suggest two categories of PD-related cognitive impairment that do not fulfil the criteria for dementia. The first category refers to general PD-MCI, where impairment has been documented but is not specifically attributed to a particular aetiology, i.e. cognitive deficits may be due to PD or another condition, whether concomitant or not. Examples of such alternative conditions include depression, vascular impairment, or AD. The second category applies to MCI that can be attributed to PD with some certainty. For the latter condition use of the diagnostic label PCI (Parkinson cognitive impairment) is suggested so as to differentiate it from general MCI. For both categories, daily functioning, defined as instrumental activities of daily living, must remain intact. While similar to the PD-MCI criteria proposed by the MDS Task Force overall, Troster's research criteria differ in regard to the specification of the onset of cognitive decline, i.e. cognitive decline must occur either at the time of or after the development of motor symptoms for PD-MCI and at least 12 months following the development of motor symptoms for PCI. Furthermore, while the definition of cognitive impairment is similar in both sets of guidelines, Troster's research criteria provide a more specific designation of impairment as it relates to estimated pre-morbid intellectual function. Both sets of criteria define impairment as performance that falls between 1 and 2 SD below appropriate norms on two or more tests within a domain or one test in at least two domains; however, where the MDS criteria define impairment as 'significant decline from estimated premorbid levels or on serial testing', Troster's criteria for both PD-MCI, for which aetiology is not required, and PCI, which attributes impairment to a PD aetiology, specify a decline of at least 1 SD on a test or cognitive domain composite score relative to prior testing or a score >1.5 SD below quantitative pre-morbid estimates. Requirement for evidence of change over time via specific cut-off scores, defined as SDs below the mean, increases specificity.

Table 16.2 MDS Task Force diagnostic criteria for MCI in PD

I. Inclusion criteria

- ◆ Diagnosis of Parkinson's disease based on UK PD Brain Bank criteria

- ◆ Gradual cognitive decline (in the context of established PD) as reported by either the patient or informant *or* observed by the clinician

- ◆ Cognitive deficits identified on either formal neuropsychological testing *or* a scale of global cognitive abilities

- ◆ Cognitive deficits do not interfere significantly with functional independence; however, subtle difficulties on complex functional tasks may be present

II. Exclusion criteria

- ◆ Diagnosis of Parkinson's disease dementia based on UK PD Brain Bank criteria

- ◆ Other explanations for cognitive impairment such as delirium, stroke, major depression, metabolic abnormalities, adverse medication effects, or head trauma

- ◆ Other Parkinson's disease-associated co-morbid conditions such as motor impairment, severe anxiety, depression, excessive daytime sleepiness, or psychosis that significantly influence cognitive testing (as per the opinion of the clinician)

- ◆ Cognitive deficits do not interfere significantly with functional independence; however, subtle difficulties on complex functional tasks may be present

III. Specific guidelines for PD-MCI level I and level II categories

- ◆ Level I (abbreviated assessment)

  - Impairment on a scale of global cognitive abilities that has been validated for use in Parkinson's disease *or*

  - Impairment on two or more tests when a limited neuropsychological battery is used; that is, a battery that includes less than two tests within each of the following domains: attention and working memory, executive functioning, language, memory, and visuospatial functioning

  - Impairment on two or more tests when a limited neuropsychological battery is used; that is, the battery includes less than two tests within each of the five cognitive domains or fewer than five domains are assessed

- ◆ Level II (comprehensive assessment)

  - Neuropsychological assessment that includes two tests within each of the following domains: attention and working memory, executive functioning, language, memory, and visuospatial functioning

  - Impairment on two or more tests; that is, either two impaired test scores in one cognitive domain or one impaired test score in two different cognitive domains

  - Impairment on tests defined as:

    Performance 1–2 SD below appropriate norms *or*

    Significant decline over serial neuropsychological testing *or*

    Significant decline as compared to estimated premorbid levels

Table 16.2 (continued) MDS Task Force diagnostic criteria for MCI in PD

IV. Subtype classification for PD-MCI (optional although strongly suggested for research purposes; requires two tests for each of the five domains assessed)

◆ PD MCI single domain—abnormal scores on two tests within a single cognitive domain (domain should be specified), with other domains unimpaired *or*

• PD MCI multiple domain—abnormal scores on one or more tests within two or more cognitive domains (domains should be specified)

Litvan I, Goldman JG, Troster AI, et al. Diagnostic criteria for mild cognitive impairment in Parkinson's disease: Movement Disorder Society Task Force guidelines. Movement disorders : official journal of the Movement Disorder Society (2012); 27:3, 349–56.

Troster's criteria, like those proposed by the MDS Task Force, are supplemented by a list of suggested screening batteries and tests for assessing each cognitive domain. Unfortunately, neither set of criteria proposes specific normative data to be used in interpreting scores from recommended tests, such as norms collected on older adults (e.g. Mayo's Older American Normative Studies, MOANS) or for patients from varied cultural backgrounds, thus increasing the likelihood of variability.

The ability to diagnose PD-MCI and its subtypes via validated criteria will aid the identification of PD patients at high risk of conversion to dementia who may benefit from clinical trials of neuroprotective agents, it may guide decision-making in patients considering deep brain stimulation [30], and will help to characterize patient groups for research and assist caregivers with decision-making and planning [31]. At present, however, the predictive value of both sets of criteria has not yet been assessed with prospective studies in terms of determining future risk of converting to dementia and the risks poised posed by different MCI subtypes. Future research will need to focus on determining the prognostic utility of the construct of PD-MCI as well as the two sets of diagnostic criteria.

The pattern of cognitive impairment in PD-MCI

The cognitive profile associated with PD-MCI is characterized primarily by executive dysfunction, commonly identified as difficulties with planning, sequencing, cognitive flexibility, and problem-solving as well as deficits in working memory and attention [7, 9, 11, 32–34]. Memory impairment, of either the encoding or retrieval type, is common [17, 25, 31]. Procedural memory is also impaired [10]. Posterior cortical deficits may also occur early in the disease [6], with visuospatial deficits including poor visual organization and visual-construction [9, 35, 36], which has been found to predict cognitive decline and dementia 3 and 5 years, respectively, after baseline assessment [6, 37]. Language dysfunction is rarely reported in the PD population without dementia, with the exception of deficits in phonemic, semantic, and alternating fluency (e.g. shifting between types of categories or types of phonemic criteria), which have been found to decline over time [38] and with disease severity as measured by Hoehn and Yahr stage [39], as well as to predict a later diagnosis of dementia [6, 40].

Genetic and clinical correlates of PD-MCI

PD-MCI has been associated with various demographic and motor features, including advanced disease, longer disease duration, older age at onset, severe motor symptoms, depression, and male gender [12]. A developing literature exists on the relationship between genetic risk factors and cognition in PD. Studies examining correlations between mutations associated with PD and the development of dementia have yielded varying results, in part due to methodological constraints (e.g. cross-sectional study design, small sample size, screening tests used as opposed to traditional neuropsychological batteries). These are summarized in the following subsections.

LRRK2

Specific cognitive dysfunction associated with mutations in leucine-rich repeat kinase 2 (*LRRK2*), a common cause of genetic PD, have not been identified to date in cross-sectional studies [41–44]. Of note, *LRRK2* G2019S carriers are more likely to have the postural instability and gait disturbance (PIGD) phenotype, which is more likely to be associated with cognitive impairment. The PIGD phenotype, however, has not been associated with cognitive impairment in cross-sectional studies of *LRRK2* G2019S carriers [45].

Parkin

In cross-sectional studies, the cognitive function of carriers of a parkin (*PARK2*) mutation did not differ from that of non-carriers [46, 47]. However, parkin mutation carriers (heterozygous, compound heterozygous, homozygous) with a disease duration of more than 14 years demonstrated better cognitive performance in attention and executive function domains than non-carriers with similar disease durations [48], suggesting that, similar to motor impairment, cognitive impairment in this more purely dopaminergic (nigropathy) form of parkinsonism may be more slowly progressive.

GBA

Carriers of glucocerebrosidase (*GBA*) mutation demonstrate significantly worse cognitive function than non-carriers, particularly within the domains of memory and processing speed [49]. Likewise *GBA* mutation represents a risk factor for cognitive impairment and dementia [37], with impaired performance identified on tests of memory (verbal and non-verbal) and visuospatial function in *GBA* mutation carriers compared with non-carriers with PD [50]. PD patients who were *GBA* mutation carriers were more likely to be classified as having a Clinical Dementia Rating Scale score of 0.5 or 1 compared with non-carriers [50]. In autopsy studies [51, 52], *GBA* mutations were associated with cognitive impairment in PD cases that did not meet criteria for AD, suggesting an independent effect of *GBA* on cognition. This finding has been demonstrated in both patients with PD-D and dementia with Lewy bodies (DLB) [53, 54].

APOE, MAPT, COMT

While cross-sectional studies have yielded disparate results, two prospective cohort studies found no association between the *APOE* ε4 genotype and the development of dementia [55] or the rate of change on the Mini-Mental State Examination (MMSE) [56]. One study looked at the rate of change on the Mattis Dementia Rating Scale (MDRS) over time and showed that the ε4 allele was associated with a more rapid decline in MDRS scores (three points per year; hazard ratio 2.8) [57]. In the same study, the *MAPT* H1/H1 haplotype was associated with lower memory scores but was not associated with decline and *COMT* Met/Met was associated with higher attention scores and did not show decline over time [57].

Neuroimaging studies of MCI in PD

Structural imaging

Structural imaging has been used primarily to differentiate PD from PD-D, AD, and DLB. As reviewed by Duncan et al. [58], inclusion of PD-MCI patients compared with PD and controls has been limited (there have been only four studies with more than 20 PD-MCI subjects since 2010). These studies cannot be readily compared because of different definitions of PD-MCI. Nevertheless, no consistent findings based on atrophy measures have been reported. Newer techniques such as diffusion tensor imaging (DTI) and white matter hyperintensity burden have not revealed any differences between PD-MCI and PD in small studies.

Single-photon emission computed tomography

Traditionally, ^{99m}Tc-hexamethylpropylene amine oxime (HMPAO) has been used to differentiate DLB and AD, based on the decreased occipital perfusion in DLB and [^{123}I]-FP-CIT has been used to examine striatal dopamine transporter (DAT) loss. Only recently has DAT imaging with [^{123}I]-FP-CIT been used to examine early PD cases longitudinally. In the largest study to date, 491 cases with disease duration of 2.06 years and a MMSE score of 29.3 at baseline had a significantly increased odds ratio of 3.3 (95% CI 1.7–6.7) for cognitive impairment defined as a Montreal Cognitive Assessment score of <26 if they were in the lowest quartile for striatal binding compared with the highest quartile. When MMSE < 24 was the outcome, the odds ratio associated with cognitive impairment was 7.6 (95% CI 0.8–68.4) for individuals in the lowest quartile for striatal binding. Change from baseline in imaging after 22 months was independently associated with motor, cognitive, and behavioural outcomes [59].

Positron emission tomography (PET)

^{18}F-fluorodeoxyglucose (^{18}FDG) PET has been used to demonstrate a PD-related cognitive pattern (PDCP) characterized by reductions in frontal and parietal association areas and increase in cerebellar vermis that is distinct from the PD-related motor pattern, is reproducible, and is unaltered by PD treatment [60]. When compared with neuropsychological test scores, this pattern correlated with memory and executive performance and remained distinct from the PD-related motor pattern when 15 patients were followed over 48 months [61]. In a subsequent study [62], differences in regional metabolism were analysed for a group of 51 PD patients categorized by MCI subtype. MCI was diagnosed if performance on one or more cognitive domains (executive, language, visuospatial, memory) fell at least 1.5 SD below normative values; patients were classified as having no impairment or single- or multiple-domain MCI. When compared with PD patients who were cognitively normal and healthy controls, multiple-domain MCI patients exhibited metabolic reductions in the inferior parietal lobe and middle frontal gyrus, whereas patients with single-domain MCI did not differ from controls or cognitively normal PD patients. Hypermetabolism was found in the pons and cerebellum for all three MCI groups, which may indicate a compensatory response to dopaminergic deficiency in the striatum. In a new study [63], correlation between a single cluster in the caudate nucleus based on DAT binding and expression of the broadly distributed PDCP network points to the relevance of nigral dopaminergic input to the caudate. The study raised the possibility that both reduced dopaminergic input and the PDCP network play a role in cognitive impairment, possibly interacting with other neurotransmitter deficiencies, for example in the cholinergic system.

Acetylcholinesterase (AchE) PET imaging

Methyl-4-piperidyl acetate (MP4A) and related tracers have been used to study PD and PD-D, demonstrating cholinergic dysfunction comparable to or greater than that found in AD [64]. Poor performance on tests of attention and working memory, followed by executive function, correlated with loss of cortical cholinesterase activity in PD-D [65]. A study that measured both striatal fluorodopa (F-DOPA) uptake and MP4A found that PD patients without dementia had moderate cholinergic dysfunction, but those with PD-D had a severe cholinergic deficit affecting the entire cortex, presumably reflecting loss of ascending projections from the nucleus basalis of Meynert. Frontal and temporo-parietal F-DOPA and MP4A binding covaried in PD-D, suggesting a role for both cholinergic denervation and dopaminergic deficits in PD-D [66].

Amyloid imaging

Amyloid imaging has been used to distinguish AD and DLB from PD-D, with a higher amyloid burden being associated with AD and DLB [67]. In a longitudinal study of 46 PD cases without dementia followed for up to 5 years [68], amyloid burden, measured by retention of Pittsburgh compound B (PiB), did not differ between PD cases who were cognitively normal and those with PD-MCI at baseline. However, higher amyloid burden did predict cognitive decline and transition to MCI and dementia, independent of APOE ε4. Amyloid burden was correlated with executive impairment but did not correlate with motor decline. The authors suggested that amyloid burden may contribute to cognitive impairment both independently and by enhancing the toxicity of α-synuclein.

Cerebrospinal fluid (CSF) biomarkers

CSF biomarkers that are classically associated with AD including amyloid-beta peptide 1–42 ($A\beta_{1-42}$), total tau, and p-tau have been studied in DLB and PD-D compared with AD and controls. There are only a few longitudinal studies of CSF biomarkers in PD-MCI patients, and change in the level of these proteins over time and the combination of biomarkers as they relate to cognitive impairment has not been systematically examined in large samples. A comprehensive review of CSF biomarkers was published by Parnetti et al. in 2013 [69]. There have been no studies of biomarkers associated with cognitive impairment in pre-manifest PD in carriers of dominantly inherited mutations such as *LRRK2*, or in carriers of *GBA* mutations who are at high risk of DLB and PD-D [54]. The strongest evidence was found for a relationship between low CSF $A\beta_{1-42}$ and cognitive decline, suggesting an association between amyloid and cognitive decline in PD. Mean CSF $A\beta_{1-42}$ in PD has been reported to be lower than in healthy controls, but higher than in AD [70]. In a cross-sectional study, $A\beta_{1-42}$ levels decreased systematically from cognitively normal PD to PD-MCI to PD-D to AD [71]. A 19% reduction of CSF $A\beta_{1-42}$ was seen in newly diagnosed PD patients compared with controls in the Norwegian ParkWest study, and it correlated with memory performance [72]. A longitudinal study of 45 PD patients found that low CSF $A\beta_{1-42}$ was an independent predictor of cognitive decline, a level of <192 being associated with a 5.85 points/year decline on the MDRS; CSF total tau or p-tau were not associated with cognitive decline [73]. It is unclear to what extent changes in CSF DJ-1 or α-synuclein levels correlate with cognitive impairment, since these measures have not been assessed longitudinally in parallel with changes in cognitive function.

Conclusion

MCI occurs in patients with PD and can be detected using appropriate neuropsychological assessment. PD-MCI is often present in the early stages, with an estimated 25–30% prevalence at the time of diagnosis. Recently, operationalized diagnostic criteria for PD-MCI have been proposed. The cognitive profile of PD-MCI varies, but is generally characterized by impairment in executive function, memory, and visuospatial function, with language functions being less affected. The heterogeneous cognitive profile of patients with PD-MCI and the variable pattern of impairment over time require further study. Longitudinal studies utilizing proposed diagnostic criteria will help to validate them in terms of their predictive value regarding conversion to dementia as well as responsiveness to various therapeutic/preventive interventions.

References

1. Petersen RC, Smith GE, Waring SC, et al. Mild cognitive impairment: clinical characterization and outcome. Arch Neurol 1999; **56**: 303–8.
2. Winblad B, Palmer K, Kivipelto M, et al. Mild cognitive impairment—beyond controversies, towards a consensus: report of the International Working Group on Mild Cognitive Impairment. J Intern Med 2004; **256**: 240–6.
3. Petersen RC, Doody R, Kurz A, et al. Current concepts in mild cognitive impairment. Arch Neurol 2001; **58**: 1985–92.
4. Petersen RC. Mild cognitive impairment as a diagnostic entity. J Intern Med 2004; **256**: 183–94.
5. Janvin CC, Larsen JP, Aarsland D, et al. Subtypes of mild cognitive impairment in Parkinson's disease: progression to dementia. Mov Disord 2006; **21**: 1343–9.
6. Williams-Gray CH, Evans JR, Goris A, et al. The distinct cognitive syndromes of Parkinson's disease: 5 year follow-up of the CamPaIGN cohort. Brain 2009; **132**: 2958–69.
7. Caviness JN, Driver-Dunckley E, Connor DJ, et al. Defining mild cognitive impairment in Parkinson's disease. Mov Disord 2007; **22**: 1272–7.
8. Dubois B, Burn D, Goetz C, et al. Diagnostic procedures for Parkinson's disease dementia: recommendations from the movement disorder society task force. Mov Disord 2007; **22**: 2314–24.
9. Muslimovic D, Post B, Speelman JD, Schmand B. Cognitive profile of patients with newly diagnosed Parkinson disease. Neurology 2005; **65**: 1239–45.
10. Foltynie T, Goldberg TE, Lewis SGJ, et al. Planning ability in Parkinson's disease is influenced by the COMT Val(158)Met polymorphism. Mov Disord 2004; **19**: 885–91.
11. Janvin CC, Aarsland D, Larsen JP. Cognitive predictors of dementia in Parkinson's disease: a community-based, 4-year longitudinal study. J Geriatr Psychiatry Neurol 2005; **18**: 149–54.
12. Aarsland D, Bronnick K, Larsen JP, et al., Norwegian ParkWest Study Group. Cognitive impairment in incident, untreated Parkinson disease: the Norwegian ParkWest study. Neurology 2009; **72**: 1121–6.
13. Barone P, Aarsland D, Burn D, et al. Cognitive impairment in nondemented Parkinson's disease. Mov Disord 2011; **26**: 2483–95.
14. Aarsland D, Kvaloy JT, Andersen K, et al. The effect of age of onset of PD on risk of dementia. J Neurol 2007; **254**: 38–45.
15. Aarsland D, Muniz G, Matthews F. Nonlinear decline of mini-mental state examination in Parkinson's disease. Mov Disord 2011; **26**: 334–7.
16. Aarsland D, Andersen K, Larsen JP, et al. Risk of dementia in Parkinson's disease: a community-based, prospective study. Neurology 2001; **56**: 730–6.
17. Goldman JG, Litvan I. Mild cognitive impairment in Parkinson's disease. Minerva Med 2011; **102**: 441–59.
18. Broeders M, Velseboer DC, de Bie R, et al. Cognitive change in newly-diagnosed patients with Parkinson's disease: a 5-year follow-up study. J Int Neuropsychol Soc 2013; **19**: 695–708.
19. Aarsland D, Andersen K, Larsen JP, et al. Prevalence and characteristics of dementia in Parkinson disease: an 8-year prospective study. Arch Neurol 2003; **60**: 387–92.

20. **Hely MA, Reid WG, Adena MA, et al**. The Sydney multicenter study of Parkinson's disease: the inevitability of dementia at 20 years. Mov Disord 2008; **23**: 837–44.

21. **Litvan I, Aarsland D, Adler CH, et al**. MDS Task Force on mild cognitive impairment in Parkinson's disease: critical review of PD-MCI. Mov Disord 2011; **26**: 1814–24.

22. **Litvan I, Goldman JG, Troster AI, et al**. Diagnostic criteria for mild cognitive impairment in Parkinson's disease: Movement Disorder Society Task Force guidelines. Mov Disord 2012; **27**: 349–56.

23. **Aarsland D, Bronnick K, Williams-Gray C, et al**. Mild cognitive impairment in Parkinson disease: a multicenter pooled analysis. Neurology 2010; **75**: 1062–9.

24. **Troster AI**. A precis of recent advances in the neuropsychology of mild cognitive impairment(s) in Parkinson's disease and a proposal of preliminary research criteria. J Int Neuropsychol Soc 2011; **17**: 393–406.

25. **Dalrymple-Alford JC, Livingston L, MacAskill MR, et al**. Characterizing mild cognitive impairment in Parkinson's disease. Mov Disord 2011; **26**: 629–36.

26. **Monastero R, Di Fiore P, Ventimiglia GD, et al**. Prevalence and profile of mild cognitive impairment in Parkinson's disease. Neurodegener Dis 2012; **10**: 187–90.

27. **Pedersen KF, Larsen JP, Tysnes OB, et al**. Prognosis of mild cognitive impairment in early Parkinson disease: the Norwegian ParkWest study. J Am Med Assoc Neurol 2013; **70**: 580–6.

28. **Emre M, Aarsland D, Brown R, et al**. Clinical diagnostic criteria for dementia associated with Parkinson's disease. Mov Disord 2007; **22**: 1689–707; quiz 837.

29. **Han JW, Lee SB, Kim TH, et al**. Functional impairment in the diagnosis of mild cognitive impairment. Alzheimer Dis Assoc Disord 2011; **25**: 225–9.

30. **Massano J, Garrett C**. Deep brain stimulation and cognitive decline in Parkinson's disease: a clinical review. Front Neurol 2012; **3**: 66.

31. **Martinez-Horta S, Kulisevsky J**. Is all cognitive impairment in Parkinson's disease 'mild cognitive impairment'? J Neural Transm 2011; **118**: 1185–90.

32. **Pai MC, Chan SH**. Education and cognitive decline in Parkinson's disease: a study of 102 patients. Acta Neurol Scand 2001; **103**: 243–7.

33. **Siegert RJ, Weatherall M, Taylor KD, et al**. A meta-analysis of performance on simple span and more complex working memory tasks in Parkinson's disease. Neuropsychology 2008; **22**: 450–61.

34. **Kehagia AA, Barker RA, Robbins TW**. Neuropsychological and clinical heterogeneity of cognitive impairment and dementia in patients with Parkinson's disease. Lancet Neurol 2010; **9**: 1200–13.

35. **Seto-Salvia N, Sanchez-Quinto F, Carbonell E, et al**. Using the Neanderthal and Denisova genetic data to understand the common MAPT 17q21 inversion in modern humans. Hum Biol 2012; **84**: 633–40.

36. **Stella F, Gobbi LT, Gobbi S, et al**. Early impairment of cognitive functions in Parkinson's disease. Arq Neuropsiquiatr 2007; **65**: 406–10.

37. **Seto-Salvia N, Pagonabarraga J, Houlden H, et al**. Glucocerebrosidase mutations confer a greater risk of dementia during Parkinson's disease course. Mov Disord 2012; **27**: 393–9.

38. **Azuma T, Cruz RF, Bayles KA, et al**. A longitudinal study of neuropsychological change in individuals with Parkinson's disease. Int J Geriatr Psychiatry 2003; **18**: 1115–20.

39. **Riepe MW, Kassubek J, Tracik F, et al**. Screening for cognitive impairment in Parkinson's disease—which marker relates to disease severity? J Neural Transm 2006; **113**: 1463–8.

40. **Levy G, Jacobs DM, Tang MX, et al**. Memory and executive function impairment predict dementia in Parkinson's disease. Mov Disord 2002; **17**: 1221–6.

41. **Ben Sassi S, Nabli F, Hentati E, et al**. Cognitive dysfunction in Tunisian LRRK2 associated Parkinson's disease. Parkinsonism Relat Disord 2012; **18**: 243–6.

42. **Shanker V, Groves M, Heiman G, et al**. Mood and cognition in leucine-rich repeat kinase 2 G2019S Parkinson's disease. Mov Disord 2011; **26**: 1875–80.

43. **Belarbi S, Hecham N, Lesage S, et al**. LRRK2 G2019S mutation in Parkinson's disease: a neuropsychological and neuropsychiatric study in a large Algerian cohort. Parkinsonism Relat Disord 2010; **16**: 676–9.

44. Goldwurm S, Zini M, Di Fonzo A, et al. LRRK2 G2019S mutation and Parkinson's disease: a clinical, neuropsychological and neuropsychiatric study in a large Italian sample. Parkinsonism Relat Disord 2006; **12**: 410–19.

45. Alcalay RN, Mejia-Santana H, Tang MX, et al. Motor phenotype of LRRK2 G2019S carriers in early-onset Parkinson disease. Arch Neurol 2009; **66**: 1517–22.

46. Lohmann E, Thobois S, Lesage S, et al. A multidisciplinary study of patients with early-onset PD with and without parkin mutations. Neurology 2009; **72**: 110–16.

47. Caccappolo E, Alcalay RN, Mejia-Santana H, et al. Neuropsychological profile of parkin mutation carriers with and without Parkinson disease: the CORE-PD study. J Int Neuropsychol Soci 2011; **17**: 91–100.

48. Alcalay RN, Caccappolo E, Mejia-Santana H, et al. Cognitive and motor function in long-duration PARKIN-associated Parkinson disease. J Am Med Assoc Neurol 2014; **71**: 62–7.

49. Neumann J, Bras J, Deas E, et al. Glucocerebrosidase mutations in clinical and pathologically proven Parkinson's disease. Brain 2009; **132**: 1783–94.

50. Alcalay RN, Caccappolo E, Mejia-Santana H, et al. Cognitive performance of GBA mutation carriers with early-onset PD: the CORE-PD study. Neurology 2012; **78**: 1434–40.

51. Clark LN, Kartsaklis LA, Wolf Gilbert R, et al. Association of glucocerebrosidase mutations with dementia with Lewy bodies. Arch Neurol 2009; **66**: 578–83.

52. Tsuang D, Leverenz JB, Lopez OL, et al. GBA mutations increase risk for Lewy body disease with and without Alzheimer disease pathology. Neurology 2012; **79**: 1944–50.

53. Sidransky E, Nalls MA, Aasly JO, et al. Multicenter analysis of glucocerebrosidase mutations in Parkinson's disease. N Engl J Med 2009; **361**: 1651–61.

54. Nalls MA, Duran R, Lopez G, et al. A multicenter study of glucocerebrosidase mutations in dementia with Lewy bodies. J Am Med Assoc Neurol 2013; **70**: 727–35.

55. Kurz MW, Dekomien G, Nilsen OB, et al. APOE alleles in Parkinson disease and their relationship to cognitive decline: a population-based, longitudinal study. J Geriatr Psychiatry Neurol 2009; **22**: 166–70.

56. Williams-Gray CH, Goris A, Saiki M, et al. Apolipoprotein E genotype as a risk factor for susceptibility to and dementia in Parkinson's disease. J Neurol 2009; **256**: 493–8.

57. Morley JF, Xie SX, Hurtig HI, et al. Genetic influences on cognitive decline in Parkinson's disease. Mov Disord 2012; **27**: 512–18.

58. Duncan GW, Firbank MJ, O'Brien JT, et al. Magnetic resonance imaging: a biomarker for cognitive impairment in Parkinson's disease? Mov Disord 2013; **28**: 425–38.

59. Ravina B, Marek K, Eberly S, et al. Dopamine transporter imaging is associated with long-term outcomes in Parkinson's disease. Mov Disord 2012; **27**: 1392–7.

60. Huang C, Mattis P, Tang C, et al. Metabolic brain networks associated with cognitive function in Parkinson's disease. NeuroImage 2007; **34**: 714–23.

61. Huang C, Tang C, Feigin A, et al. Changes in network activity with the progression of Parkinson's disease. Brain 2007; **130**: 1834–46.

62. Huang C, Mattis P, Perrine K, et al. Metabolic abnormalities associated with mild cognitive impairment in Parkinson disease. Neurology 2008; **70**: 1470–7.

63. Niethammer M, Tang CC, Ma Y, et al. Parkinson's disease cognitive network correlates with caudate dopamine. NeuroImage 2013; **78**: 204–9.

64. Bohnen NI, Kaufer DI, Ivanco LS, et al. Cortical cholinergic function is more severely affected in parkinsonian dementia than in Alzheimer disease: an in vivo positron emission tomographic study. Arch Neurol 2003; **60**: 1745–8.

65. Bohnen NI, Kaufer DI, Hendrickson R, et al. Cognitive correlates of cortical cholinergic denervation in Parkinson's disease and parkinsonian dementia. J Neurol 2006; **253**: 242–7.

66. Hilker R, Thomas AV, Klein JC, et al. Dementia in Parkinson disease: functional imaging of cholinergic and dopaminergic pathways. Neurology 2005; **65**: 1716–22.

67. **Gomperts SN, Locascio JJ, Marquie M, et al.** Brain amyloid and cognition in Lewy body diseases. Mov Disord 2012; **27**: 965–73.

68. **Gomperts SN, Locascio JJ, Rentz D, et al.** Amyloid is linked to cognitive decline in patients with Parkinson disease without dementia. Neurology 2013; **80**: 85–91.

69. **Parnetti L, Castrioto A, Chiasserini D, et al.** Cerebrospinal fluid biomarkers in Parkinson disease. Nat Rev Neurol 2013; **9**: 131–40.

70. **Shi M, Bradner J, Hancock AM, et al.** Cerebrospinal fluid biomarkers for Parkinson disease diagnosis and progression. Ann Neurol 2011; **69**: 570–80.

71. **Montine TJ, Shi M, Quinn JF, et al.** CSF Aβ(42) and tau in Parkinson's disease with cognitive impairment. Mov Disord 2010; **25**: 2682–5.

72. **Alves G, Bronnick K, Aarsland D, et al.** CSF amyloid-beta and tau proteins, and cognitive performance, in early and untreated Parkinson's disease: the Norwegian ParkWest study. J Neurol Neurosurg Psychiatry 2010; **81**: 1080–6.

73. **Siderowf A, Xie SX, Hurtig H, et al.** CSF amyloid {beta} 1–42 predicts cognitive decline in Parkinson disease. Neurology 2010; **75**: 1055–61.

74. **Goldman JG, Weis H, Stebbins G, et al.** Clinical differences among mild cognitive impairment subtypes in Parkinson's disease. Mov Disord 2012; **27**: 1129–36.

75. **Hoops S, Nazem S, Siderowf AD, et al.** Validity of the MoCA and MMSE in the detection of MCI and dementia in Parkinson disease. Neurology 2009; **73**: 1738–45.

76. **Mamikonyan E, Moberg PJ, Siderowf A, et al.** Mild cognitive impairment is common in Parkinson's disease patients with normal Mini-Mental State Examination (MMSE) scores. Parkinsonism Relat Disord 2009; **15**: 226–31.

77. **Naismith SL, Pereira M, Shine JM, et al.** How well do caregivers detect mild cognitive change in Parkinson's disease? Mov Disord 2011; **26**: 161–4.

78. **Poletti M, Frosini D, Ceravolo R, et al.** Mild cognitive impairment in de novo Parkinson's disease according to movement disorder guidelines. Mov Disord 2012; **27**: 1706; author reply 1707.

79. **Sollinger AB, Goldstein FC, Lah JJ, et al.** Mild cognitive impairment in Parkinson's disease: subtypes and motor characteristics. Parkinsonism Relat Disord 2010; **16**: 177–80.

80. **Song IU, Kim JS, Jeong DS, et al.** Early neuropsychological detection and the characteristics of Parkinson's disease associated with mild dementia. Parkinsonism Relat Disord 2008; **14**: 558–62.

81. **Williams-Gray CH, Foltynie T, Brayne CEG, et al.** Evolution of cognitive dysfunction in an incident Parkinson's disease cohort. Brain 2007; **130**: 1787–1798.

Chapter 17

The pathophysiological and prognostic heterogeneity of mild cognitive impairment in Parkinson's disease

Sophie E. Winder-Rhodes, Roger A. Barker, and Caroline H. Williams-Gray

Introduction

It is now well established that cognitive deficits can occur in Parkinson's disease (PD) and that some of these develop into dementia. It is also apparent that these deficits vary, not only between patients but also in individual patients over time as their disease evolves and their medication requirements change. A better understanding of the neurobiological basis of the different types of cognitive deficits is important to enable us to better treat and advise patients about their significance. In particular, understanding which specific cognitive deficits are the earliest features of PD dementia (PD-D) would not only allow us to advise patients and their families that this much feared complication of PD is incipient, but would also offer a window of potential therapeutic opportunity for disease-modifying therapies, as and when they become available. This latter issue is of critical importance as the development of PD-D is associated with a significantly impaired quality of life and life expectancy.

The early cognitive deficits of PD have of late acquired the label 'PD-MCI' [1]. This term, borrowed from the field of Alzheimer's disease (AD), recognizes cognitive deficits in PD that do not meet the criteria for dementia but nevertheless are sufficient to affect activities of daily living. However, its use becomes problematic if it is considered as a unitary concept describing one condition which represents the prodromal stage of PD-D—a theory that has been disproved in AD. Indeed cognitive impairment in PD can arise for a range of different reasons including:

- disease processes leading to the development of PD-D;
- compensatory dynamic changes in diffuse transmitter networks which arise as cells are lost but which are not predictive of dementia;
- changes which can be exacerbated by drug therapies;
- disorders of mood which can blunt and affect cognitive performance;
- alterations in levels of vigilance linked to the common sleep problems of PD;
- abnormalities in the testing process itself and how cognitive impairment is defined, for example is it 1, 1.5, or 2 SD below the mean?
- disease processes that are not linked to PD but are typical of ageing, given that PD usually develops in old age.

In this chapter, we will consider the heterogeneity of mild cognitive impairment (MCI) in PD, and review evidence that different types of cognitive impairment vary in terms of their prognosis and relationship to the development of PD-D. We will then explore the pathophysiological mechanisms underlying these varying cognitive deficits. We will focus on two key methods which have been used to examine the basis of these deficits as they evolve in the early stages of PD: first, genetic association studies, which can examine the relationship between pre-determined variations in biological pathways of interest and the development of particular cognitive phenotypes; and secondly functional imaging studies investigating the anatomical and neurochemical basis of cognitive deficits in vivo, which have implicated multiple networks and neurotransmitter systems. By better defining the pathophysiological origins of various types of cognitive deficits in PD, we can refine what is meant by PD-MCI and by so doing preserve its utility for research and clinical practice.

Heterogeneity of MCI in PD

The most accurate estimates of the frequency of cognitive impairment in PD come from studies evaluating population-based cohorts of incident patients. Such studies have reported that, even at the time of diagnosis, between a fifth and a third of patients are cognitively impaired [2–4]. Executive deficits are particularly well described and are demonstrated on neuropsychological tasks sensitive to frontal lobe dysfunction including planning tests based on the 'Tower of London' task, tests of spatial working memory, and attentional set shifting [5–7]. There is some evidence that executive impairment may even occur prior to the onset of overt motor features. In a large epidemiological study, impaired performance on executive and judgement tasks was found to be associated with increased PD incidence over 8 years of follow-up [8]. Furthermore, among unaffected first-degree relatives of PD patients, those carrying the G2019S *LRRK2* mutation are cognitively impaired compared with non-carriers, specifically on executive tasks, presumably as a prodrome to later development of motor parkinsonism [9].

While executive impairments may be the earliest detectable deficits in PD, impairments across a range of cognitive domains including attention, explicit memory, and visuospatial function are demonstrable in PD patients without dementia [10]. It has been proposed that some of these deficits may be secondary to the executive dysfunction. For example, in contrast to AD, impaired recall in PD seems to improve with cueing, suggesting that memory impairment relates to a difficulty in retrieving information rather than storing it, which may reflect a deficiency in internally cued search strategies [11, 12]. Similarly, impaired performance on visuospatial tasks may reflect, at least in part, executive problems with sequential organization of behaviour [13]. However, a number of authors assessing large PD cohorts without dementia have demonstrated that patients can be stratified into subgroups according to their cognitive deficits, suggesting that deficits in different cognitive domains can occur independently of one another [2, 4, 14, 15].

Attempts have been made to standardize the characterization of early cognitive impairment in PD through the construct of 'PD-MCI'. The recently proposed Movement Disorder Society (MDS) criteria for PD-MCI allow subtyping according to the number of cognitive domains affected (attention and working memory, executive memory, language, and visuospatial) [1]. However, unbiased domain-specific subtyping requires detailed neuropsychological testing, with two tests in each of the five cognitive domains. Three studies have achieved this to date; they found that the majority of patients with PD-MCI meet criteria for 'multidomain' impairment (>90% in prevalent cohorts [16, 17]; 65% in a newly diagnosed cohort [18]). While 'multidomain' impairment can be further categorized according to the affected domains, large collaborative studies will be needed to provide enough power to perform such complex subtyping. For the time being, the true prevalence of domain-specific subtypes of PD-MCI remains to be firmly established. Nonetheless, it is clear that cognitive deficits in early PD are diverse, and this diversity suggests that multiple aetiopathologies may be involved.

Prognosis of early cognitive deficits in PD

It cannot be assumed that cognitive dysfunction in early PD is in all cases a prodrome of PD-D. While some early deficits may progress inexorably, and thus represent the early stages of the dementing process, other deficits may have an alternative aetiology and more favourable prognosis. Until recently, longitudinal studies measuring cognitive function in PD have reported rather disparate findings, with a range of neuropsychological deficits including executive deficits [19–21], impaired verbal fluency [21, 22], visuospatial problems [21], and memory and language dysfunction [20, 23] reported to predict the development of PD-D. The findings of these studies, however, have been limited by two main factors. First, the nature of the cohorts was suboptimal: they included patients at varying disease stages and were mostly hospital-based, and thus not necessarily representative of PD in the general population. Secondly, their findings were highly dependent on the particular selection of tests employed in each study. The lack of a standardized approach to neuropsychological testing inevitably introduces bias and makes any comparison between studies difficult.

The first of these problems has been addressed in recent years through the establishment of a number of prospective studies in population-based cohorts of newly diagnosed patients, enabling a better description of the pattern and temporal evolution of cognitive dysfunction in PD. To date, most of these studies remain in their early stages with limited longitudinal data [24–27]. However, the CamPaIGN study [2], the first and longest running of these incident population-based cohort studies, has recently reported its 10-year follow-up data [28]. This study has followed up a population-representative cohort of 142 patients with idiopathic PD in the county of Cambridgeshire, UK, with detailed clinical and neuropsychological assessments at approximately 2-yearly intervals. Analysis at multiple time points has shown that the two most significant early neuropsychological predictors of later dementia, independent of age and other potential confounding factors, are poor performance on tests of semantic fluency and pentagon copying [28–30]. A semantic fluency score of less than 20 words in 90 seconds at diagnosis was associated with a hazard ratio (HR) of 3.1 ($p = 0.005$) for dementia at 10 years (Cox survival analysis), while impaired pentagon copying at diagnosis was associated with a HR for dementia of 2.6 ($p = 0.001$). Phonemic fluency, however, was not associated with increased dementia risk, and this dissociation between semantic and phonemic fluency implicates the temporal lobe-based semantic system in early dementia, rather than the frontal lobe-based search and retrieval system which is common to fluency tasks in general. Pentagon copying is a mixture of visuospatial and constructional ability, widely accepted to depend on the integrity of the parietal lobe [31]. There was no association between 'frontostriatally based' executive tasks and later dementia, and in fact there was no significant deterioration in performance on executive tasks over time. On the basis of these findings, as well as the finding of dissociable relationships between certain genetic variants and different cognitive functions as discussed later, we have previously suggested that cognitive impairments in early PD can be segregated into two main types. Executive deficits, primarily due to dysfunction in dopaminergic frontostriatal networks, are likely to fluctuate with disease course and medication, and are not clearly associated with dementia. In contrast, more posterior cortically based deficits represent the early stages of a dementing process which is proposed to be non-dopaminergic and likely to be related to cortical Lewy body deposition, subcortical cholinergic cell loss, and possibly to Alzheimer's type changes [28].

Other authors have provided further support for the idea that there are dissociable cognitive syndromes in PD. Pagonabarraga et al. [32] used the PD-Cognitive Rating Scale, which characterizes 'subcortical' and 'cortical' cognitive deficits, in subgroups of PD patients with no cognitive impairment, MCI, and dementia. They found evidence for progressive frontal–subcortical impairment as the disease evolves, but the transition from MCI to dementia was marked by the addition of deficits with a cortical basis. Muslimovic et al. [33] conducted a large meta-analysis, including 901 PD patients without dementia, to evaluate changes in multiple cognitive domains over time. Over a mean follow-up of 29 months, there was a statistically significant decline in global cognitive ability, visuospatial function, and memory, but not in executive function, in keeping with the idea that posterior cortical deficits represent a progressive dementing process while executive impairments do not.

The second problem affecting the majority of longitudinal studies of cognition in PD is the lack of a standardized approach to neuropsychological testing and defining cognitive impairment. The MDS diagnostic criteria for PD-MCI were proposed to alleviate this problem [1]. However, their prognostic utility remains to be determined. In one of only two longitudinal studies so far using the PD-MCI criteria, Pedersen et al. [25] studied a population-based cohort of 182 patients with incident PD and reported that of the 20.3% meeting PD-MCI criteria at baseline, 27% had developed dementia by 3-year follow-up, compared with only 0.7% of patients without MCI. There were similar rates of conversion to dementia among those meeting PD-MCI criteria at 1 year from baseline. However, a significant proportion with PD-MCI reverted to normal cognition at 3-year follow-up (21.6% of those with PD-MCI at baseline and 19.4% of those with PD-MCI at 1-year follow-up). In a second study, Broeders et al. [18] studied a consecutive clinic-based sample of 123 patients with newly diagnosed PD, following up 73 of these to 5 years. With the caveat that there was significant attrition of more cognitively impaired patients, they found that of the 35% diagnosed with PD-MCI at baseline 26% had developed dementia at 5 years. While the majority of those developing dementia at 5 years had had a previous diagnosis of PD-MCI, 18% had been cognitively normal at the previous assessment. In keeping with the findings of Pedersen et al., some individuals with PD-MCI subsequently reverted to normal cognition, although the numbers were lower (9% between baseline and year 1, and 6% between baseline and year 5), possibly due to their more detailed neuropsychological assessment with higher specificity.

While the numbers in these studies have not been sufficient to formally calculate positive and negative predictive values, these data support the idea that PD-MCI as a single entity is not a useful construct for predicting later dementia. It is critical that future studies explore subtypes of cognitive impairment to establish which domains are the most informative in terms of predicting dementia. The PD-MCI criteria do allow for such subtyping (level II criteria), but only if a full neuropsychological battery is used with at least two tests in each of five cognitive domains [1]. Level II PD-MCI criteria were used by Broeders et al. [18], but the numbers were too small to explore associations between MCI subtypes and progression to dementia. The most common subtype of MCI at baseline was 'multidomain' (65.1%), which is not unexpected given that the proposed cognitive syndromes in PD are not mutually exclusive. However, this may limit future attempts to examine the prognostic value of PD-MCI subgroups, and deficits on individual cognitive tests may remain the most useful prognostic variables.

Genetic influences on cognition in PD

Genetic association studies can provide opportunities to assess the pathophysiological mechanisms underlying different aspects of cognitive impairment in PD. So far, genome-wide association studies have not included sufficiently detailed clinical data to investigate loci associated with particular cognitive phenotypes, but some useful insights have been gained from adopting a candidate gene approach. Four genes in particular have been implicated in cognition in PD: *COMT, MAPT, APOE*, and *GBA*.

COMT

The enzyme catechol-*O*-methyltransferase (COMT) is involved in the degradation of catecholamines and acts as the principal regulator of synaptic dopamine within the cortex, especially the prefrontal cortex. The common Val158Met polymorphism in the *COMT* gene results in a trimodal distribution of high (Val/Val), intermediate (Val/Met), and low (Met/Met) enzyme activity [34]. These differences in activity have demonstrable effects on executive function in health and disease and have been exploited in attempts to understand the role of dopaminergic dysfunction in cognitive impairment in PD and its development.

In individuals without PD, low-activity *COMT* genotypes—implying higher prefrontal dopamine levels—have been associated with enhanced performance in problem-solving tasks that are known to engage prefrontal networks [35]. Interestingly, the opposite trend has been observed in cross-sectional studies of patients with early PD. In a large cohort of 288 newly diagnosed patients, low-activity *COMT* genotypes (associated with putatively higher dopaminergic activity) were associated with inferior performance on the CANTAB one-touch Tower of London test of spatial planning [36]. This association was replicated in an early PD cohort, although with a small effect size [29]. However, subsequent studies of patients with more established disease have reported either no overall association between *COMT* genotype and executive function [37] or the same pattern as in controls, with low-activity genotypes predicting superior performance [38].

These seemingly disparate observations have been accommodated through an inverted U-shaped model, in which dopamine levels are related non-linearly to cognitive performance [39]. It is hypothesized that there is an optimal level of dopamine within the prefrontal cortex and both increases and decreases relative to that level become detrimental to neural efficiency. The effects of the COMT enzyme will therefore be contingent on its dopaminergic environment, which in turn is influenced by disease progression and exogenous dopaminergic therapy. It is speculated that the high-activity Val/Val variant is advantageous in early PD because of the existence of abnormally elevated dopamine in the prefrontal cortex [40]; the Val/Val variant helps to negate these high dopamine levels while, under these circumstances, the low-activity Met/Met variant is detrimental as it contributes to dopamine 'overload'. As disease progresses, it is expected that the relative disadvantage of the Met/Met genotype is lost as the hyperdopaminergic state subsides, offering a rationale for the observation that patients with the *COMT* Met/Met genotype improve on executive tasks over time while those with the Val/Val genotype do not (Fig. 17.1) [29].

The inverted U-shaped model predicts that increasing dopaminergic stimulation further with medication contributes to even greater executive impairments in PD patients with the low-activity Met/Met *COMT* genotype, presumably due to dopamine overload, but not in those with Val/Val genotypes [36, 37]. These hypothetical effects of medication have been demonstrated at a single subject level, emphasizing the concept that COMT works within a dynamic system. In line with the inverted U-shaped model, increasing dopamine through COMT inhibition in healthy

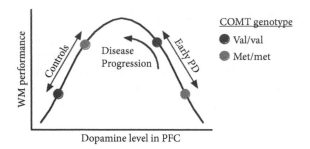

Fig. 17.1 Hypothesized inverted U-shaped relationship between working memory (WM) and dopaminergic activity in the prefrontal cortex (PFC). Predetermined factors influencing dopaminergic activity including disease state and *COMT* Val158Met genotype determine an individual's position on the curve, and hence predict their cognitive response to exogenous (drug-induced) changes in dopamine levels, as well as disease progression.

Williams-Gray CH, Evans JR, Goris A, et al, The distinct cognitive syndromes of Parkinson's disease: 5 year follow-up of the CamPaIGN cohort, Brain 2009, 132, 2958–69, by permission of Oxford University Press.

controls enhances executive function in individuals with the *COMT* Val/Val genotype but impairs performance in those with the Met/Met variant [41]; a similar direction of effect has been demonstrated using the Tower of London task in PD (authors' unpublished data). Hence it seems that increases as well as decreases in frontostriatal dopamine contribute to executive dysfunction in PD, and the cognitive response to medication is likely to vary as a function of individual differences in baseline dopaminergic state.

However, a consistent finding from longitudinal studies is that differences associated with variation in *COMT* are not linked to progressive global cognitive decline and dementia [28, 38]. This supports the hypothesis that although dopaminergic disturbances account for a proportion of the cognitive dysfunction in PD, other coexisting pathologies underlie progression to dementia.

MAPT

The *MAPT* gene encodes microtubule-associated protein tau which is widely expressed throughout the central nervous system and forms characteristic aggregates in several neurodegenerative diseases [42]. Mutations in *MAPT* lead to frontotemporal dementia with parkinsonism linked to chromosome 17 (FTDP-17) [43], while common variation in the *MAPT* gene is associated with the development of atypical parkinsonian syndromes, including progressive supranuclear palsy and corticobasal degeneration [44, 45]. There are two common extended haplotypes that incorporate the *MAPT* gene, H1 and H2, which are differentiated by a 900-kb genomic inversion. Association studies have now shown that the more common *MAPT* H1 haplotype is not only overrepresented in patients with PD but influences PD cognitive phenotype [28, 46]. In the CamPaIGN cohort, *MAPT* H1/H1 haplotype was associated with a strikingly increased rate of age-dependent cognitive decline over the first 3.5 years from diagnosis, as measured by rate of change in MMSE score; during this period, all subjects who developed dementia were H1 homozygotes [46]. After 10 years' follow-up of the same cohort, *MAPT* H1/H1 haplotype emerged as one of the key predictors of dementia after adjustment for age (HR 3.08) (Fig. 17.2) [28].

The association between *MAPT* H1 haplotype and dementia in PD has been replicated in a cross-sectional study of 102 patients [47]. Another study based on a prospective cohort of patients with established PD did not demonstrate any influence of H1 haplotype on global decline

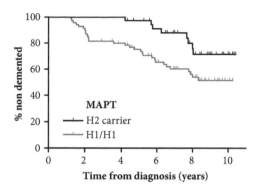

Fig. 17.2 Kaplan–Meier curve illustrating the cumulative probability of remaining free of dementia stratified by *MAPT* genotype in an incident PD cohort (CamPaIGN) followed for up to 10 years from diagnosis [28].

Reproduced from The CamPaIGN study of Parkinson's disease: 10-year outlook in an incident population-based cohort, Williams-Gray CH, Mason SL, Evans JR, et al, 84, 1258–64, ©2013 with permission from BMJ Publishing Group Ltd.

measured using the Mattis Dementia Rating Scale, but reported a detrimental effect of *MAPT* H1 haplotype specifically on tests of memory [38]. Our own cross-sectional functional MRI study of 37 PD patients without dementia (unpublished data discussed further in the subsection 'Non-dopaminergic networks') likewise found that H1 homozygotes had impaired visual recognition memory function compared with H2 haplotype carriers, implicating *MAPT* haplotype as a modulator of cognitive function that relies on the integrity of posterior cortical brain circuitry.

Evidence from post-mortem studies supports the concept that the *MAPT* H1 haplotype produces its cognitive effects by driving Lewy body pathology. In a study of 22 cases of dementia with Lewy bodies (DLB), matched for demographics and clinical variables, total Lewy body counts and α-synuclein deposits were significantly higher in the H1/H1 group (*n* = 12) than in the H2 carriers (*n* = 10) with no difference in Alzheimer's-type pathology [48]. In addition, in a post-mortem series of 762 cases with AD, Lewy body diseases, and vascular pathology, the *MAPT* H1 haplotype was associated with increased cortical Lewy body counts in frontal and parietal cortices but reduced Alzheimer's-type changes [49].

The mechanism by which *MAPT* impacts on protein aggregation in PD remains unclear, but the relative transcription of tau isoforms with three or four microtubule-binding domains (three- or four-repeat tau) has been shown to be altered in PD [50], and *MAPT* H1 or H1 subhaplotypes are associated with increased expression of total tau or of four-repeat tau [51–53]. Our own study [29] demonstrated that the H1 haplotype was associated with a 20% increase in four-repeat tau transcription in PD brains. Tau itself can interact and synergistically promote fibrilization of α-synuclein, the core component of Lewy bodies [54], and these proteins have been found to co-localize in brains with Lewy body pathology [55]. Interestingly, while variation in the α-synuclein gene (*SNCA*) has not been consistently linked to dementia outcome, an early follow-up of the CamPaIGN cohort revealed that the *MAPT* and *SNCA* risk alleles interacted to further increase the rate of early cognitive decline, supporting the concept of a synergistic pathological link between these proteins in vivo [46].

APOE

The association between variation in the apolipoprotein E gene (*APOE*) and Alzheimer's disease (AD) is well established [56]. Of the three alleles (ε2, ε3, and ε4), the *APOE* ε4 allele is associated with increased risk of AD and a younger age at disease onset, whereas *APOE* ε2 appears be protective. Given the phenotypic and pathological overlap between the two diseases, *APOE* has also been investigated as a candidate gene for susceptibility to PD-D; however, there has been a lack of consensus among studies to date.

Our own meta-analysis of 17 studies [57] suggested a modest association between increased *APOE* ε4 frequency and PD-D (*n* = 501) compared with PD without dementia (*n* = 1145; odds ratio 1.74; 95% CI 1.4–2.2). However, the reliability of this association is questionable for a number of reasons, including small study sizes, substantial variation in the criteria used to define dementia, significant heterogeneity of odds ratios between studies, and evidence of publication bias. In a large cohort of 2412 PD patients, *APOE* ε4 and *APOE* ε2 carrier status was not associated with either PD risk or MMSE score measured at an average of 7 years from disease onset [58].

Longitudinal studies of *APOE* have likewise produced inconsistent results. In a cohort of 212 patients with established PD and an average disease duration of 7 years, *APOE* ε4 carriers had a more rapid global cognitive decline than non-carriers as measured by their total score on the Mattis Dementia Rating Scale [38]. However, the CamPaIGN study found no effect of *APOE* genotype on either the overall rate of cognitive decline or the risk of dementia at any time point [28, 57]. Likewise, no significant associations between *APOE* ε4 and time to the onset of dementia were observed in a second study of 64 patients with prevalent PD followed longitudinally over a 12-year period [59]. It is possible that these inconsistencies relate to variations in pathological specificity, with concurrent Alzheimer's-type pathology accounting for some of the observed associations, particularly in older patients with longer disease durations. However, post-mortem studies have linked the *APOE* ε4 allele to cortical Lewy body disease in the absence of significant Alzheimer's type pathology, with a stronger association for DLB than PD-D [60], leading to the suggestion that in the presence of an α-synucleinopathy, *APOE* ε4 might accelerate the onset of dementia such that it precedes parkinsonism, via a mechanism independent of amyloid processing [60]. Hence exclusion of DLB cases may explain the lack of association between *APOE* ε4 and Lewy body disease in some studies, particularly in incident PD cohorts.

GBA

Mutations in the gene encoding the lysosomal enzyme glucocerebrosidase (*GBA*) cause Gaucher's disease, an autosomal recessive lysosomal storage disorder. The observation that patients with Gaucher's disease develop parkinsonism [61] in association with deposition of Lewy bodies in the brainstem and cortex [62] led to the hypothesis that *GBA* mutations may also contribute to the development of idiopathic PD. Over the past decade, this association has been firmly established: *GBA* mutations are significantly overrepresented even in seemingly sporadic PD, and are the most common single genetic cause of PD identified to date [63]. The mechanism underlying this association remains unclear; however, neuropathological studies have demonstrated that glucocerebrosidase co-localizes with Lewy bodies in mutation carriers, supporting the theory that mutant glucocerebrosidase may contribute to increased aggregation of α-synuclein [64]. On this basis, *GBA* mutations would also be expected to predispose to dementia in PD, and clinical comparisons have shown that this is indeed the case.

A recent cross-sectional study of 225 PD cases reported that dementia affected 50% of *GBA* mutation carriers (*n* = 22) versus 24% of non-carriers (*n* = 203), corresponding to an odds ratio for dementia of 5.8 (95% CI 1.98–17.2) after adjustment for age, disease duration, and gender [65]. This is in line with a prevalence of cognitive decline or dementia of 48% among *GBA* mutation carriers (*n* = 33) in a larger study of 790 pathologically confirmed PD cases. Neuropathological examination revealed more pronounced Lewy body pathology in the *GBA* mutation carriers than in the non-carriers, spreading into limbic and diffuse neocortical regions [66]. Another study which employed detailed cross-sectional neuropsychological assessment in early onset PD cases reported a higher frequency of memory and visuospatial impairments in those carrying a *GBA* mutation (*n* = 26) compared with non-carriers (*n* = 39) [67].

Our own work [68] has evaluated the influence of *GBA* mutations on cognitive phenotype in an unselected incident cohort (*n* = 121). Interestingly, at diagnosis *GBA* mutation carriers were clinically indistinguishable from non-carriers, with only a minor trend towards lower MMSE scores. However, over a 10-year follow-up period, *GBA* mutation carriers (*n* = 4) had an increased risk of developing dementia compared with non-carriers, after adjustment for *MAPT* genotype (HR 4.6; 95% CI 1.3–15.9). Furthermore, patients carrying more common *GBA* polymorphisms (*n* = 11), which have not consistently been associated with risk for PD, had a greater propensity than non-carriers to develop dementia (HR 3.3; 95% CI 1.1–10.0), suggesting that these variants may contribute to the heterogeneity of cognitive impairment in PD. Although *GBA* mutations are relatively rare and might only make a modest contribution to the overall burden of dementia in PD, they may provide important insights into the converging pathological mechanisms that contribute to this aspect of the disease.

Functional imaging

Functional imaging provides opportunities for visualizing networks that contribute to cognitive dysfunction in the living brain. Radiotracer imaging has the potential to demonstrate specific neurotransmitter disturbances that correlate with cognitive impairment, while functional magnetic resonance imaging (MRI) has a high spatial and temporal resolution to detect changes in brain function that map onto specific components of task performance.

Frontostriatal dysfunction

Given that the pathological hallmark of PD is degeneration of the ascending projections of midbrain dopaminergic neurons, the majority of functional imaging studies have concentrated on the role of frontostriatal circuitry in PD. Their findings have complemented decades of data from animal, pharmacological, and post-mortem studies emphasizing the contribution of dopaminergic disturbances to executive dysfunction in PD. Critically, the changes that underlie cognitive dysfunction have been shown to be distinct, such that executively impaired patients with early PD have differences in striatal and prefrontal activation compared with their cognitively unimpaired, but otherwise matched, counterparts [69]. An issue that remains unresolved is whether cognitive functions associated with the frontal lobe are impaired as an indirect consequence of impaired nigrostriatal dopaminergic function or a direct consequence of impaired mesocortical dopaminergic transmission.

The concept that frontally based deficits in PD are a consequence of abnormal outflow from the basal ganglia is supported by fluorodopa ([^{18}F]-DOPA) and [^{11}C]-raclopride positron emission tomography (PET) data, which have demonstrated correlations between caudate dopamine depletion and executive impairments (e.g. [70, 71]). Likewise, $H_2^{15}O$ PET and functional MRI studies have shown regional reductions in blood flow in the basal ganglia in the context of preserved cortical responses during working memory tasks in PD [72, 73]. Detailed PET correlation studies have even suggested that different task requirements are lateralized within the striatum, implying that the pattern of cognitive changes manifested by a patient with PD may reflect the side of dopamine loss [74].

Other studies, however, suggest that dopamine disturbances within the cortex have a more prominent role, but indicate that the relationship between cortical dopamine and cognitive function is complex. [^{18}F]-DOPA PET has showed increased dorsolateral prefrontal cortex dopamine in conjunction with reduced striatal dopamine in drug-naïve patients compared with controls, possibly as a compensatory mechanism [40, 75]. These cortical changes are related to performance: reaction time in tests of sustained attention correlated positively with [18F]-DOPA uptake in the dorsolateral prefrontal cortex while performance in a test of suppressed attention correlated negatively with [18F]-DOPA uptake in the medial frontal cortex and anterior cingulate [75]. Performance on the Tower of London planning task and a working memory task has been associated with abnormally high blood flow as measured with $H_2^{15}O$-PET in the right prefrontal and occipital cortices of patients off levodopa; levodopa normalized these disturbances to restore a pattern of blood flow similar to controls, and this correlated with change in performance [76]. It has been suggested that dopamine acting within the frontal cortex enables a focusing of activity of glutamatergic output neurons, which as a result respond more efficiently [77].

Imaging studies in PD patients genotyped for *COMT* Val158Met have provided further insights into the relationship between prefrontal dopamine and executive dysfunction. Using functional MRI in patients with PD, we demonstrated that impaired performance on both the Tower of London planning task and an attentional-control task in *COMT* Met homozygotes was associated with reduced blood oxygen level-dependent (BOLD) activation in frontoparietal networks (Fig. 17.3) without corresponding changes in striatal activation [78, 79]. These differences in activation were proposed to reflect differences in dopamine concentrations in the cortex, where COMT is the key mechanism of dopamine clearance, and [18F]-DOPA PET imaging has now provided supporting evidence for this. A study of 20 patients with early PD demonstrated reduced dopamine turnover and higher pre-synaptic dopamine levels across several frontal cortical areas in Met homozygotes (lower COMT enzyme activity), relative to Val homozygotes, with no apparent differences in the striatum [80]. These data collectively endorse a regionally specific effect of COMT on cortical dopamine and add weight to the idea that dopamine disturbances within the frontal cortex are capable of modulating the executive phenotype of PD.

Functional imaging also supports the concept that the inverted U-shaped relationship between dopamine levels and cognitive performance operates, at least in part, at a cortical level. Differential effects of *COMT* genotype on brain activation have been described in controls and PD patients on the same test of attentional control. In healthy volunteers, Val homozygotes had impaired set-formation ability and lower dorsolateral prefrontal cortex activation than Met homozygotes, while in PD patients, the opposite relationship was observed. This fits with the idea that PD patients, due to their cortical hyperdopaminergic state, sit further to the right of the inverted U-shaped curve where homozygosity for Met becomes detrimental due to presumed dopamine overload (Fig. 17.1) [81].

Although cortical and striatal disturbances are not mutually exclusive, the differing results of these cognitive neuroimaging studies in PD may reflect the heterogeneity observed within the patient population. The patients who have been included in studies vary over multiple dimensions that are known to impact on cognitive performance as well as brain function, including age, gender, dopaminergic medication, and, as we are now aware, genetic variation. It is also apparent that the relative impacts of cortical and striatal dopamine on performance depend on the specific demands of the task. It is theorized that cognitive stability benefits from increases in tonic prefrontal cortex dopaminergic transmission and reductions in phasic striatal dopaminergic transmission. In contrast, cognitive flexibility benefits from potentiated phasic striatal dopaminergic transmission and reduced tonic dopaminergic transmission in the prefrontal cortex. In addition, dorsal and ventral frontostriatal circuits contribute to the control of distinct types of representations [82]. By considering these differences in future studies we may be able to resolve some of the apparent inconsistencies described in PD.

(a)

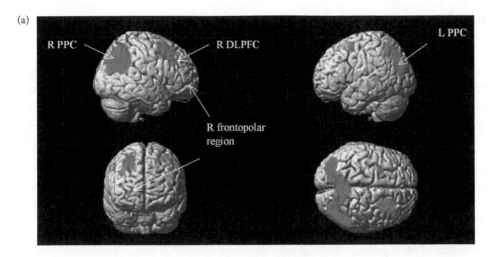

(b)

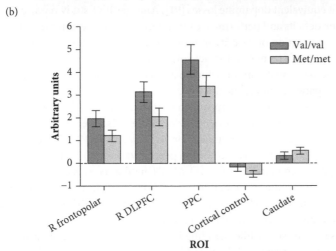

Fig. 17.3 Functional MRI was used to measure the effect of *COMT* Val158Met genotype on brain activation during performance of the Tower of London planning task in patients with early PD (*n* = 31). (A) BOLD activation during planning versus a control task (subtracting) in the whole cohort. Areas of signal change above a threshold of *p* = 0.05 after false discovery rate correction for whole brain volume are shown rendered onto a canonical brain image. PPC, posterior parietal cortex; DLPFC, dorsolateral pre*frontal cortex.* (B) Activity in Val (*n* = 16) versus Met (*n* = 15) homozygotes in regions of interest as indicated in (A). There was significant underactivation of the frontoparietal network activated by the planning task in Met versus Val homozygotes, as well as an impairment in behavioural performance (not shown).

Non-dopaminergic networks

Changes occurring outside of frontostriatal dopaminergic networks also impact on the cognitive phenotype of the disease. More widespread cortical hypometabolism has been described in PD patients with cognitive impairment than in those without, notably affecting parietal, occipital, and temporal lobes [83, 84]. Comparisons of patients with single- and multiple-domain MCI suggest that the degree and topography of hypometabolism reflects the extent of cognitive dysfunction [83, 84]. A serial imaging study in which 23 PD patients without dementia were followed longitudinally with fluorodeoxyglucose PET reported that progression to dementia was associated with more marked hypometabolism in the occipital lobe and posterior cingulate at baseline [85]. This provides further support for the hypothesis that more posterior cortical deficits are key manifestations of incident dementia in PD.

Post-mortem studies have provided evidence of cholinergic dysfunction in patients with PD [86, 87] and have identified greater acetylcholine reductions in the frontal cortex of PD-D patients than in their cognitively unimpaired counterparts [88]. Similarly PET imaging studies have demonstrated more prominent cholinergic disturbances in PD-D patients compared with those without dementia [89, 90], but equivalent dopamine losses [91]. Another PET study reported correlations between acetylcholine deficits and performance on attentional and executive tests in PD, but no relationship with disease duration or severity of motor features [91]. Thus, accumulating evidence suggest that cholinergic deficits play a distinct role in the cognitive profile of PD, and this is endorsed by the improvements in cognition which have been reported in clinical trials of cholinesterase inhibitors in PD patients with dementia [92].

Genetic imaging provides a novel bottom-up approach to understanding the substrates of cognitive impairment in PD, potentially even before behavioural deficits emerge. Based on our previous findings that *MAPT* H1/H2 haplotype impacts on progression to PD-D, we recently used functional MRI to explore the effects of this common genetic variant on brain function in patients without objective cognitive impairment. The H1 *MAPT* haplotype was associated with impaired memory recall ability and reduced medial temporal lobe activation during memory encoding. This effect was present in controls but accentuated in patients with PD with additional age-dependent effects. These data implicate *MAPT* as a more general modifier of brain function even prior to clinical onset of disease, while shedding light on the networks and tau-related mechanisms that contribute to the emergence of dementia in PD.

Conclusion

The use of cohorts of patients followed from disease onset has been invaluable in better understanding the natural history of treated PD, including the evolution of cognitive dysfunction in the disease. Using this approach we have described that there are two independent syndromes of cognitive impairment, one of which is a harbinger of a dementia and the other a consequence of disordered dopamine networks (Fig. 17.4). We and others have investigated genetic variations associated with these cognitive syndromes, and shown that PD patients, especially more elderly ones, who carry the H1/H1 *MAPT* genotype and/or a heterozygous mutation in *GBA* develop dementia earlier in their disease course—presumably because these genetic variants drive the disease process. Understanding how this occurs will be vital in better treating it, but these observations support the idea that PD can be better thought of not so much as a single disorder or a disorder that has many different subtypes, but as a disease process that can run at different speeds. In other words, it is likely that all patients with PD will eventually develop a dementia, with a final common pathophysiological pathway in everyone,

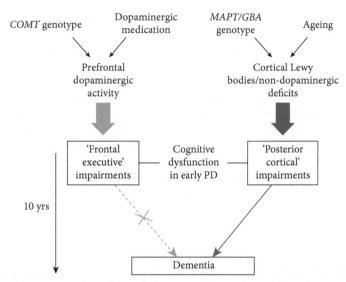

Fig. 17.4 Schematic representation of two distinct cognitive syndromes in early PD, and their hypothesized aetiological pathways. 'Frontal executive' impairments are caused by alterations in dopaminergic activity within frontostriatal networks, which are in turn influenced by dopaminergic medication and *COMT* genotype, and are not associated with global cognitive decline or dementia. In contrast, 'posterior cortical' type cognitive impairments do not have a dopaminergic basis, but reflect the early stages of an age-dependent dementing process influenced by genetic variations in *MAPT* and *GBA*, which is likely to involve cortical Lewy body deposition.

Williams-Gray CH, Evans JR, Goris A, et al, The distinct cognitive syndromes of Parkinson's disease: 5 year follow-up of the CamPaIGN cohort, Brain 2009, 132, 2958–69, by permission of Oxford University Press.

but in some it develops within 5 years of disease onset whereas in others it takes over 25 years. The key is in understanding the major determinants driving the rate of pathology and thus disease burden and expression.

However, as we have discussed, not all cognitive deficits in PD are linked to protein aggregation in cortical neurons and dementia, rather some are due to changes in neurotransmitter networks that arise as a compensatory response to the disease process. For example, as the nigrostriatal dopamine pathway fails other neighbouring dopaminergic pathways (mesolimbic, mesocortical) become upregulated as the whole dopaminergic network tries to maintain its level of activity. The consequence is that in the more intact dopaminergic projections there is a relative overdose of dopamine in cortical and ventral striatal areas which can be further exacerbated by the use of dopaminergic medication to treat the nigrostriatal loss. Understanding this, and how genetic variants (e.g. in *COMT*) affect the central handling of synaptic dopamine, may lead to a better use of pharmacological agents in patients, not only in terms of which patients to treat but also at what point in the disease process.

This complexity of pathophysiological processes underlying the different types of cognitive impairment in PD highlights the danger implicit in the recent adoption of the term PD-MCI. This concept has merit, but only if it is understood to be a short-hand way of saying that the patient does not have dementia but does have some cognitive problems. It is not defining a discrete entity either clinically or pathophysiologically; it does not provide any prognostic index to the patient's problems; and it does not have a single therapeutic solution. In time it may be refined, in particular to specify subtypes and their prognosis, and may ultimately be restricted to describe those patients who are developing incipient PD-D; if so then the term will have more merit, especially as we move towards an era of disease-modifying therapies.

In summary we have tried to highlight the complex changes that arise within the central nervous system of treated patients with PD as a result of evolving pathology and compensatory mechanisms. All of this plays out in a brain that may have developed in subtly different ways as a result of common genetic variations, which fundamentally alters the expression of the pathological processes of PD. Important targets for future research will be to understand whether genes associated with disease states affect the brain developmentally, and how they drive the disease process at a cellular and network level. Only by carefully defining the different types of cognitive impairment in PD can we hope to start to do this, and by so doing we may be able to fundamentally change how we treat this common complication in patients.

References

1. **Litvan I, Goldman JG, Troster AI, et al**. Diagnostic criteria for mild cognitive impairment in Parkinson's disease: Movement Disorder Society Task Force guidelines. Mov Disord 2012; **27**: 345–56.
2. **Foltynie T, Brayne CE, Robbins TW, et al**. The cognitive ability of an incident cohort of Parkinson's patients in the UK. The CamPaIGN study. Brain 2004; **127**: 550–60.
3. **Elgh E, Domellof M, Linder J, et al**. Cognitive function in early Parkinson's disease: a population-based study. Eur J Neurol 2009; **16**: 1278–84.
4. **Aarsland D, Bronnick K, Larsen JP, et al**. Cognitive impairment in incident, untreated Parkinson disease: the Norwegian ParkWest study. Neurology 2009; **72**: 1121–6.
5. **Owen AM, James M, Leigh PN, et al**. Fronto-striatal cognitive deficits at different stages of Parkinson's disease. Brain 1992; **115**: 1727–51.
6. **Robbins TW, James M, Owen AM, et al**. Cognitive deficits in progressive supranuclear palsy, Parkinson's disease, and multiple system atrophy in tests sensitive to frontal lobe dysfunction. J Neurol Neurosurg Psychiatry 1994; **57**: 79–88.
7. **Owen AM**. Cognitive dysfunction in Parkinson's disease: the role of frontostriatal circuitry. Neuroscientist 2004; **10**: 525–37.
8. **Ross GW, Abbott RD, Petrovitch H, et al**. Pre-motor features of Parkinson's disease: the Honolulu-Asia Aging Study experience. Parkinsonism Relat Disord 2012; **18**(Suppl. 1): S199–S202.
9. **Thaler A, Mirelman A, Gurevich T, et al**. Lower cognitive performance in healthy G2019S LRRK2 mutation carriers. Neurology 2012; **79**: 1027–32.
10. **Litvan I, Aarsland D, Adler CH, et al**. MDS task force on mild cognitive impairment in Parkinson's disease: Critical review of PD-MCI. Mov Disord 2011; **26**: 1814–24.
11. **Helkala EL, Laulumaa V, Soininen H, et al**. Recall and recognition memory in patients with Alzheimer's and Parkinson's disease. Ann Neurol 1988; **24**: 214–17.
12. **Pillon B, Deweer B, Agid Y, et al**. Explicit memory in Alzheimer's, Huntington's, and Parkinson's diseases. Arch Neurol 1993; **50**: 374–9.
13. **Stern Y, Mayeux R, Rosen J, et al**. Perceptual motor dysfunction in Parkinson's disease: a deficit in sequential and predictive voluntary movement. J Neurol Neurosurg Psychiatry 1983; **46**: 145–51.
14. **Janvin CC, Larsen JP, Aarsland D, et al**. Subtypes of mild cognitive impairment in Parkinson's disease: progression to dementia. Mov Disord 2006; **21**: 1343–9.
15. **Mamikonyan E, Moberg PJ, Siderowf A, et al**. Mild cognitive impairment is common in Parkinson's disease patients with normal Mini-Mental State Examination (MMSE) scores. Parkinsonism Relat Disord 2009; **15**: 226–31.

16. **Goldman JG, Holden S, Bernard B, et al**. Defining optimal cutoff scores for cognitive impairment using Movement Disorder Society Task Force criteria for mild cognitive impairment in Parkinson's disease. Mov Disord 2013; **28**: 1972–9.

17. **Marras C, Armstrong MJ, Meaney CA, et al**. Measuring mild cognitive impairment in patients with Parkinson's disease. Mov Disord 2013; **28**: 626–33.

18. **Broeders M, de Bie RM, Velseboer DC, et al**. Evolution of mild cognitive impairment in Parkinson disease. Neurology 2013; **81**: 346–52.

19. **Janvin CC, Aarsland D, Larsen JP**. Cognitive predictors of dementia in Parkinson's disease: a community-based, 4-year longitudinal study. J Geriatr Psychiatry Neurol 2005; **18**: 149–54.

20. **Levy G, Jacobs DM, Tang MX, et al**. Memory and executive function impairment predict dementia in Parkinson's disease. Mov Disord 2002; **17**: 1221–6.

21. **Mahieux F, Fenelon G, Flahault A, et al**. Neuropsychological prediction of dementia in Parkinson's disease. J Neurol Neurosurg Psychiatry 1998; **64**: 178–83.

22. **Jacobs DM, Marder K, Cote LJ, et al**. Neuropsychological characteristics of preclinical dementia in Parkinson's disease. Neurology 1995; **45**: 1691–6.

23. **Hobson P, Meara J**. Risk and incidence of dementia in a cohort of older subjects with Parkinson's disease in the United Kingdom. Mov Disord 2004; **19**: 1043–9.

24. **Domellof ME, Elgh E, Forsgren L**. The relation between cognition and motor dysfunction in drug-naive newly diagnosed patients with Parkinson's disease. Mov Disord 2011; **26**: 2183–9.

25. **Pedersen KF, Larsen JP, Tysnes OB, et al**. Prognosis of mild cognitive impairment in early Parkinson disease: the Norwegian ParkWest study. J Am Med Assoc Neurol 2013; **70**: 580–6.

26. **Yarnall AJ, Breen DP, Duncan GW, et al**. Characterising Mild Cognitive Impairment In Incident Parkinson's Disease: the ICICLE-PD Study [abstract]. Mov Disord 2013; **28**: 505.

27. **Caslake R, Taylor K, Scott N, et al**. Age-, gender-, and socioeconomic status-specific incidence of Parkinson's disease and parkinsonism in North East Scotland: the PINE study. Parkinsonism Relat Disord 2013; **19**: 515–21.

28. **Williams-Gray CH, Mason SL, Evans JR, et al**. The CamPaIGN study of Parkinson's disease: 10-year outlook in an incident population-based cohort. J Neurol Neurosurg Psychiatry 2013; **84**: 1258–64.

29. **Williams-Gray CH, Evans JR, Goris A, et al**. The distinct cognitive syndromes of Parkinson's disease: 5 year follow-up of the CamPaIGN cohort. Brain 2009; **132**: 2958–69.

30. **Williams-Gray CH, Foltynie T, Brayne CE, et al**. Evolution of cognitive dysfunction in an incident Parkinson's disease cohort. Brain 2007; **130**: 1787–98.

31. **Di Renzi E**. Visuospatial and constructional disorders. In: Feinberg TE, Farah MJ (ed.) *Behavioural neurology and neuropsychology*. New York: McGraw-Hill, 1997; pp. 297–307.

32. **Pagonabarraga J, Kulisevsky J, Llebaria G, et al**. Parkinson's disease-cognitive rating scale: a new cognitive scale specific for Parkinson's disease. Mov Disord 2008; **23**: 998–1005.

33. **Muslimovic D, Schmand B, Speelman JD, et al**. Course of cognitive decline in Parkinson's disease: a meta-analysis. J Int Neuropsychol Soc 2007; **13**: 920–32.

34. **Chen J, Lipska BK, Halim N, et al**. Functional analysis of genetic variation in catechol-O-methyltransferase (COMT): effects on mRNA, protein, and enzyme activity in postmortem human brain. Am J Hum Genet 2004; **75**: 807–21.

35. **Barnett JH, Jones PB, Robbins TW, et al**. Effects of the catechol-O-methyltransferase Val(158)Met polymorphism on executive function: a meta-analysis of the Wisconsin Card Sort Test in schizophrenia and healthy controls. Mol Psychiatry 2007; **12**: 502–9.

36. **Foltynie T, Goldberg TE, Lewis SG, et al**. Planning ability in Parkinson's disease is influenced by the COMT val158met polymorphism. Mov Disord 2004; **19**: 885–91.

37. **Hoogland J, de Bie RM, Williams-Gray CH, et al**. Catechol-O-methyltransferase val158met and cognitive function in Parkinson's disease. Mov Disord 2010; **25**: 2550–4.

38. **Morley JF, Xie SX, Hurtig HI, et al**. Genetic influences on cognitive decline in Parkinson's disease. Mov Disord 2012; **27**: 512–18.

39. **Cools R, D'Esposito M**. Inverted-U-shaped dopamine actions on human working memory and cognitive control. Biol Psychiatry 2011; **69**: e113–e125.

40. **Rakshi JS, Uema T, Ito K, et al**. Frontal, midbrain and striatal dopaminergic function in early and advanced Parkinson's disease. A 3D [(18)F]dopa-PET study. Brain 1999; **122**: 1637–50.

41. **Farrell SM, Tunbridge EM, Braeutigam S, et al**. COMT Val(158)Met genotype determines the direction of cognitive effects produced by catechol-O-methyltransferase inhibition. Biol Psychiatry 2012; **71**: 538–44.

42. **Goedert M, Spillantini MG**. Pathogenesis of the tauopathies. J Mol Neurosci 2011; **45**: 425–31.

43. **Spillantini MG, Murrell JR, Goedert M, et al**. Mutation in the tau gene in familial multiple system tauopathy with presenile dementia. Proc Natl Acad Sci USA 1998; **95**: 7737–41.

44. **Baker M, Litvan I, Houlden H, et al**. Association of an extended haplotype in the tau gene with progressive supranuclear palsy. Hum Mol Genet 1999; **8**: 711–15.

45. **Houlden H, Baker M, Morris HR, et al**. Corticobasal degeneration and progressive supranuclear palsy share a common tau haplotype. Neurology 2001; **56**: 1702–6.

46. **Goris A, Williams-Gray CH, Clark GR, et al**. Tau and alpha-synuclein in susceptibility to, and dementia in, Parkinson's disease. Ann Neurol 2007; **62**: 145–53.

47. **Seto-Salvia N, Clarimon J, Pagonabarraga J, et al**. Dementia risk in Parkinson disease: disentangling the role of MAPT haplotypes. Arch Neurol 2011; **68**: 359–64.

48. **Colom-Cadena M, Gelpi E, Marti MJ, et al**. MAPT H1 haplotype is associated with enhanced alpha-synuclein deposition in dementia with Lewy bodies. Neurobiol Aging 2013; **34**: 936–42.

49. **Wider C, Ross OA, Nishioka K, et al**. An evaluation of the impact of MAPT, SNCA and APOE on the burden of Alzheimer's and Lewy body pathology. J Neurol Neurosurg Psychiatry 2012; **83**: 424–9.

50. **Tobin JE, Latourelle JC, Lew MF, et al**. Haplotypes and gene expression implicate the MAPT region for Parkinson disease: the GenePD Study. Neurology 2008; **71**: 28–34.

51. **Kwok JB, Teber ET, Loy C, et al**. Tau haplotypes regulate transcription and are associated with Parkinson's disease. Ann Neurol 2004; **55**: 329–34.

52. **Rademakers R, Melquist S, Cruts M, et al**. High-density SNP haplotyping suggests altered regulation of tau gene expression in progressive supranuclear palsy. Hum Mol Genet 2005; **14**: 3281–92.

53. **Myers AJ, Pittman AM, Zhao AS, et al**. The MAPT H1c risk haplotype is associated with increased expression of tau and especially of 4 repeat containing transcripts. Neurobiol Dis 2007; **25**: 561–70.

54. **Giasson BI, Forman MS, Higuchi M, et al**. Initiation and synergistic fibrillization of tau and alpha-synuclein. Science 2003; **300**: 636–40.

55. **Ishizawa T, Mattila P, Davies P, et al**. Colocalization of tau and alpha-synuclein epitopes in Lewy bodies. J Neuropathol Exp Neurol 2003; **62**: 389–97.

56. **Farrer LA, Cupples LA, Haines JL, et al**. Effects of age, sex, and ethnicity on the association between apolipoprotein E genotype and Alzheimer disease. A meta-analysis. APOE and Alzheimer Disease Meta Analysis Consortium. J Am Med Assoc 1997; **278**: 1349–56.

57. **Williams-Gray CH, Goris A, Saiki M, et al**. Apolipoprotein E genotype as a risk factor for susceptibility to and dementia in Parkinson's disease. J Neurol 2009; **256**: 493–8.

58. **Federoff M, Jimenez-Rolando B, Nalls MA, et al**. A large study reveals no association between APOE and Parkinson's disease. Neurobiol Dis 2012; **46**: 389–92.

59. **Kurz MW, Dekomien G, Nilsen OB, et al**. APOE alleles in Parkinson disease and their relationship to cognitive decline: a population-based, longitudinal study. J Geriatr Psychiatry Neurol 2009; **22**: 166–70.

60. **Tsuang D, Leverenz JB, Lopez OL, et al**. APOE epsilon4 increases risk for dementia in pure synucleinopathies. J Am Med Assoc Neurol 2013; **70**: 223–8.

61. **Capablo JL, Saenz de Cabezon A, Fraile J, et al.** Neurological evaluation of patients with Gaucher disease diagnosed as type 1. J Neurol Neurosurg Psychiatry 2008; **79**: 219–22.

62. **Wong K, Sidransky E, Verma A, et al.** Neuropathology provides clues to the pathophysiology of Gaucher disease. Mol Genet Metab 2004; **82**: 192–207.

63. **Velayati A, Yu WH, Sidransky E.** The role of glucocerebrosidase mutations in Parkinson disease and Lewy body disorders. Curr Neurol Neurosci Rep 2010; **10**: 190–8.

64. **Goker-Alpan O, Stubblefield BK, Giasson BI, et al.** Glucocerebrosidase is present in alpha-synuclein inclusions in Lewy body disorders. Acta Neuropathol 2010; **120**: 641–9.

65. **Seto-Salvia N, Pagonabarraga J, Houlden H, et al.** Glucocerebrosidase mutations confer a greater risk of dementia during Parkinson's disease course. Mov Disord 2011; **27**: 393–9.

66. **Neumann J, Bras J, Deas E, et al.** Glucocerebrosidase mutations in clinical and pathologically proven Parkinson's disease. Brain 2009; **132**: 1783–94.

67. **Alcalay RN, Caccappolo E, Mejia-Santana H, et al.** Cognitive performance of GBA mutation carriers with early-onset PD: the CORE-PD study. Neurology 2012; **78**: 1434–40.

68. **Winder-Rhodes SE, Evans JR, Ban M, et al.** Glucocerebrosidase mutations influence the natural history of Parkinson's disease in a community-based incident cohort. Brain 2013; **136**: 392–9.

69. **Lewis SJ, Dove A, Robbins TW, et al.** Cognitive impairments in early Parkinson's disease are accompanied by reductions in activity in frontostriatal neural circuitry. J Neurosci 2003; **23**: 6351–6.

70. **Sawamoto N, Piccini P, Hotton G, et al.** Cognitive deficits and striato-frontal dopamine release in Parkinson's disease. Brain 2008; **131**: 1294–302.

71. **Rinne JO, Portin R, Ruottinen H, et al.** Cognitive impairment and the brain dopaminergic system in Parkinson disease. Arch Neurol 2000; **57**: 470–5.

72. **Dagher A, Owen AM, Boecker H, et al.** The role of the striatum and hippocampus in planning: a PET activation study in Parkinson's disease. Brain 2001; **124**: 1020–32.

73. **Owen AM, Doyon J, Dagher A, et al.** Abnormal basal ganglia outflow in Parkinson's disease identified with PET. Implications for higher cortical functions. Brain 1998; **121**: 949–65.

74. **Cheesman AL, Barker RA, Lewis SJ, et al.** Lateralisation of striatal function: evidence from 18F-dopa PET in Parkinson's disease. J Neurol Neurosurg Psychiatry 2005; **76**: 1204–10.

75. **Bruck A, Aalto S, Nurmi E, et al.** Cortical 6-[18F]fluoro-L-dopa uptake and frontal cognitive functions in early Parkinson's disease. Neurobiol Aging 2005; **26**: 891–8.

76. **Cools R, Stefanova E, Barker RA, et al.** Dopaminergic modulation of high-level cognition in Parkinson's disease: the role of the prefrontal cortex revealed by PET. Brain 2002; **125**: 584–94.

77. **Mattay VS, Berman KF, Ostrem JL, et al.** Dextroamphetamine enhances 'neural network-specific' physiological signals: a positron-emission tomography rCBF study. J Neurosci 1996; **16**: 4816–22.

78. **Williams-Gray CH, Hampshire A, Barker RA, et al.** Attentional control in Parkinson's disease is dependent on COMT val 158 met genotype. Brain 2008; **131**: 397–408.

79. **Williams-Gray CH, Hampshire A, Robbins TW, et al.** Catechol O-methyltransferase val158met genotype influences frontoparietal activity during planning in patients with Parkinson's disease. J Neurosci 2007; **27**: 4832–8.

80. **Wu K, O'Keeffe D, Politis M, et al.** The catechol-O-methyltransferase Val158Met polymorphism modulates fronto-cortical dopamine turnover in early Parkinson's disease: a PET study. Brain 2012; **135**: 2449–57.

81. **Fallon SJ, Williams-Gray CH, Barker RA, et al.** Prefrontal dopamine levels determine the balance between cognitive stability and flexibility. Cereb Cortex 2013; **23**: 361–9.

82. **Cools R.** Dopaminergic modulation of cognitive function-implications for L-DOPA treatment in Parkinson's disease. Neurosci Biobehav Rev 2006; **30**: 1–23.

83. **Huang C, Mattis P, Perrine K, et al.** Metabolic abnormalities associated with mild cognitive impairment in Parkinson disease. Neurology 2008; **70**: 1470–7.

84. **Hosokai Y, Nishio Y, Hirayama K, et al.** Distinct patterns of regional cerebral glucose metabolism in Parkinson's disease with and without mild cognitive impairment. Mov Disord 2009; **24**: 854–62.

85. **Bohnen NI, Koeppe RA, Minoshima S, et al.** Cerebral glucose metabolic features of Parkinson disease and incident dementia: longitudinal study. J Nucl Med 2011; **52**: 848–55.

86. **Arendt T, Bigl V, Arendt A, et al.** Loss of neurons in the nucleus basalis of Meynert in Alzheimer's disease, paralysis agitans and Korsakoff's disease. Acta Neuropathol 1983; **61**: 101–8.

87. **Aubert I, Araujo DM, Cecyre D, et al.** Comparative alterations of nicotinic and muscarinic binding sites in Alzheimer's and Parkinson's diseases. J Neurochem 1992; **58**: 529–41.

88. **Ruberg M, Rieger F, Villageois A, et al.** Acetylcholinesterase and butyrylcholinesterase in frontal cortex and cerebrospinal fluid of demented and non-demented patients with Parkinson's disease. Brain Res 1986; **362**: 83–91.

89. **Hilker R, Thomas AV, Klein JC, et al.** Dementia in Parkinson disease: functional imaging of cholinergic and dopaminergic pathways. Neurology 2005; **65**: 1716–22.

90. **Shimada H, Hirano S, Shinotoh H, et al.** Mapping of brain acetylcholinesterase alterations in Lewy body disease by PET. Neurology 2009; **73**: 273–8.

91. **Bohnen NI, Kaufer DI, Hendrickson R, et al.** Cognitive correlates of cortical cholinergic denervation in Parkinson's disease and parkinsonian dementia. J Neurol 2006; **253**: 242–7.

92. **Emre M, Aarsland D, Albanese A, et al.** Rivastigmine for dementia associated with Parkinson's disease. N Engl J Med 2004; **351**: 2509–18.

Chapter 18

Spectrum of Lewy body dementias: relationship of Parkinson's disease dementia to dementia with Lewy bodies

Clive Ballard, Sara Garcia-Ptacek, Inger van Steenoven, and Dag Aarsland

Introduction

Dementia with Lewy bodies (DLB) and Parkinson's disease (PD) with dementia (PD-D) are characterized by parkinsonism and a dementia syndrome typically dominated by attentional, visuospatial, and executive dysfunction and relatively well-preserved memory. Additional key symptoms are visual hallucinations (VH), cognitive fluctuations, severe neuroleptic sensitivity, and sleep disturbances such as excessive daytime sleepiness and rapid eye movement (REM) sleep behaviour disorder (RBD; a parasomnia manifested by vivid, often frightening dreams associated with simple or complex behaviour during REM sleep) [1].

The distinction between DLB and PD-D as operationally defined within the standardized clinical criteria for DLB depends entirely upon the duration of parkinsonism prior to dementia. An arbitrary cut-off of 1 year was chosen in the original consensus criteria for the clinical diagnosis of DLB [2]. Thus, PD-D would be diagnosed if dementia occurred more than 1 year after the onset of parkinsonism, whereas dementia prior to, or within, 1 year after the onset of parkinsonism would be classified as DLB. The third report of the DLB Consortium [1] revised the operationalized diagnostic criteria for DLB. That report highlighted the unresolved issues in the relationship between DLB and PD-D by emphasizing the overall clinical and pathological similarities of the conditions, but at the same time maintaining the arbitrary 1-year rule for distinguishing the two syndromes for research studies, where a distinction is necessary. For clinical practice it was recommended that PD-D should be diagnosed if dementia emerges in the context of clinically diagnosed PD, independent of the time interval. The importance of further research to resolve 'boundary issues' was also highlighted, but several key conceptual questions still remain unresolved. For example: are these conditions distinct or part of the same spectrum? If they are distinct, is the arbitrary 1-year rule a meaningful distinction between clinical entities with different clinical presentations? Addressing these issues is critical if we are to take forward our understanding of this spectrum of conditions in establishing biological markers, determining prognostic indicators, and, most importantly, in designing appropriate intervention studies and developing treatment paradigms across the dementias associated with Lewy bodies (LBs).

Studies directly comparing DLB and PD-D patients probably represent the best approach for resolving 'boundary issues', but methodological limitations have precluded clear conclusions in many of the comparative studies. For example, critical issues have included the selection of participants (i.e. whether community-based or hospital-based), whether participants were matched for severity of dementia, sample size, sensitivity, and other psychometric properties of the tests used to characterize them, and diagnostic criteria and methods of diagnosis (e.g. diagnosis based on autopsy, prospective clinical assessment, or retrospective chart review). In addition, many studies comparing neuropathology or neurochemistry in PD and DLB have not specified whether PD patients had dementia or not, and, if so, separately described the PD-D patients.

The aim of the current chapter is to summarize similarities and differences between DLB and PD-D from the best available information.

Comparative neuropathological, neurochemical, and biomarker studies

Neuropathology

DLB and PD-D cannot be differentiated by neuropathology alone, in particular since only patients with end-stage disease usually come to autopsy. Both syndromes are associated with less cortical atrophy than occurs in Alzheimer's disease (AD). Medial temporal lobe structures are abnormal in both DLB and PD-D, although the severity of hippocampal atrophy is less marked than that seen in AD. Both DLB and PD-D have similar, significant atrophy and pathology in the amygdala [3].

Limbic and cortical LBs are the main substrate of the dementia syndrome in DLB and PD-D [4–6]. Several studies have suggested that in many cortical regions the amount of LB pathology does not differentiate DLB from PD-D or PD [5, 6]. By contrast, data from the Newcastle Brain Bank (Table 18.1) indicate more pronounced cortical LB pathology in DLB compared with PD-D in a range of cortical areas, although the prolonged duration of PD prior to dementia in this cohort may explain the magnitude of disparity in cortical LB pathology [7]. Other work has suggested a more specific regional pattern of differences in LB density, with higher densities in para-hippocampal and inferior temporal cortices in DLB compared with PD-D [8]. In both DLB and PD-D, cortical LB pathology has an impact upon phenotype. For example, the density of temporal lobe LBs in DLB correlates with the early occurrence of the characteristic, well-formed VH, and cortical and limbic LBs have been linked to visual misidentifications [8–10]. In PD-D increasing LB densities in limbic and frontal cortices correlate with the severity of dementia [8, 10, 11].

Although LBs are the core pathological characteristics of DLB and PD-D, patients also show extracellular amyloid-beta (Aβ) plaques and intracellular neurofibrillary tangles. The density of amyloid plaques has generally been reported to be higher in DLB than in PD-D [5, 12], with the density of Aβ-positive plaques in many DLB patients being equivalent to that found in AD. Amyloid deposits, detected by Pittsburgh compound B (PIB) imaging with positron emission tomography (PET), are linked to cognitive impairment in DLB [13]. Other studies have linked cognitive impairment to LB pathology [4]. While the amount of Aβ deposition and number of cortical LBs are correlated with the severity of dementia in DLB, there is ongoing debate about whether this is the case in PD-D [5, 14], with one study suggesting that a combination of LB pathology and AD pathology is a robust pathological correlate of dementia in PD rather than any single pathology alone [14]. Amyloid burden seems higher in DLB than PD-D [13], and higher in PD-D than in PD. Neurofibrillary tangles are typically substantially less pronounced than in AD, but may nevertheless influence the clinical phenotype, particularly in DLB [15, 16].

Table 18.1 Comparison of Lewy body pathology between dementia with Lewy bodies (DLB) and Parkinson's disease with dementia (PD-D)

	DLB (*n* = 29)	PD-D (*n* = 11)	Evaluations
Age (years)	79.9 ± 4.8	74.2 ± 4.3	$t = 3.3, p = 0.002$*
Female	17	5	$X^2 = 0.6, p = 0.46$
MMSE score closest to death	9.6 ± 9.1	12.2 ± 9.4	$t = 0.7, p = 0.47$
Duration of dementia (years)	2.6 ± 1.8	2.1 ± 1.3	$t = 0.9, p = 0.35$
Duration of parkinsonism (years)	1.2 ± 1.4	9.9 ± 6.9	$t = 6.5, p < 0.0001$**
Frontal Lewy body density	1.2 ± 1.5	0.4 ± 0.3	$t = 2.5, p = 0.02$*
Transentorhinal Lewy body density	3.8 ± 2.9	1.8 ± 1.0	$t = 3.1, p = 0.004$*
Anterior cingulate Lewy body density	2.5 ± 2.4	1.4 ± 1.1	$t = 2.0, p = 0.049$*

*: $p < 0.05$, **: $p < 0.001$

Ballard C, Ziabreva I, Perry R, et al, Neurology, Differences in neuropathologic characteristics across the Lewy body dementia spectrum, 67, 11, 1931–1934 ©2006, with kind permission from Wolters Kluwer.

LB scoring is based on a semi-quantitative scale form 0–4.

One study has reported a marked LB-type pathology in the striatum in DLB, but not in PD. PD-D patients had striatal degeneration intermediate between PD and DLB [17]. By contrast, a preliminary report focusing on striatal pathology in 28 brains, including 7 PD, 7 PD-D, and 14 DLB, has indicated that striatal α-synuclein pathology is similar in PD-D and DLB. Amyloid plaques were also of similar severity in the striatum in the two conditions [18].

Since clinically the main difference between DLB and PD-D is the different timing of dementia and parkinsonism, each with different biological underpinnings, it is likely that any pathological differences between the two syndromes are most pronounced early in the disease course and reflect different regional onset and progression with a similar end stage. Methodological difficulties make this hypothesis difficult to test. According to one influential hypothesis, the progression of α-synuclein pathology in PD is characterized by being systematic, beginning in the brainstem and moving rostrally in predefined stages, with neocortical involvement in stages 5 and 6 [19]. Whereas this pattern of progression is found in many PD patients, the pattern in DLB suggests that the neocortex is involved from the onset of disease, and that some cases do not involve brainstem pathology. Emerging data are, however, not consistent with a unitary concept of the pathogenesis of LB pathology. Cases with subcortical pathology but no brainstem involvement [20], and cases with very high diffuse LB load that either occur at onset of clinical disease or rapidly infiltrate the brain, with accompanying rapidly progressive clinical symptoms and short survival [21, 22], have been reported. Exploration of the cellular causes of these different clinical and pathological subtypes, broadly corresponding to younger patients with a slowly progressing motor parkinsonism and elderly subjects with more rapidly progressive disease, is a high priority.

Overall, studies consistently indicate higher amyloid pathology in DLB than in PD-D, but the literature is highly variable, with markedly discrepant findings related to cortical LB pathology and striatal pathology. One study from our group, examining the relationship between LB pathology and the number of years of PD prior to dementia as a spectrum, demonstrated that there was substantially less cortical LB pathology in patients with long-standing PD prior to dementia than in DLB patients, but that the differences were less pronounced in patients with 1–5 years of PD before dementia developed [7]. This study would support the concept of a continuum of LB disease rather than two distinct entities, and the different duration of PD-D in different studies may explain some of the discrepancies in results.

Of note, one interesting study identified differential expression of α-synuclein, parkin, and synphilin isoforms in different LB diseases, suggesting the possibility that different molecular mechanisms lead to similar neuropathological changes and that there are subtle disease-specific differences between DLB and PD [23].

Involvement of α-synuclein in the peripheral autonomic nervous system is also found [24]. In a recent brain bank study with 28 donors, α-synuclein aggregates were found in all DLB and PD cases in the stellate and sympathetic ganglia, vagus nerve, gastrointestinal tract, adrenal glands, heart, and genitourinary tract, with a craniocaudal gradient of α-synuclein burden in the paravertebral sympathetic chain and gastrointestinal tract. Interestingly, although brain LB pathology differed between PD and DLB cases, peripheral α-synuclein aggregates did not [24]. This also reinforces the potential utility of cardiac [^{123}I]-metaiodobenzylguanidine (MIBG) scintigraphy, which quantifies post-ganglionic sympathetic activity [25].

Cerebrospinal fluid (CSF)

Studies of CSF have consistently shown characteristic changes of Aβ and tau peptides in AD, but the initial studies focusing on DLB and PD-D showed conflicting results. In PD patients with and without dementia, baseline Aβ peptide 1–42 (Aβ$_{1-42}$) might predict cognitive decline [26] and might be lower in a subset of PD patients with cognitive decline without dementia or PD-D [27]. An oxidated variant of Aβ$_{1-40}$ relative to the sum of Aβ peptides may be predominant in DLB compared with PD [28], although others have found a reduction in mean Aβ$_{1-42}$ in DLB [29]. Another study reported significantly reduced Aβ$_{1-42}$ in DLB compared with PD-D, whereas total and phosphorylated tau did not differ significantly [30]. A recent CSF biomarker study in DLB and PD-D supported the lower levels of Aβ$_{42}$ in DLB compared with PD-D. However, this study reported higher levels of total tau in DLB and the combination of both biomarkers showed a better discrimination than either biomarker alone. Moreover, in DLB but not PD-D the CSF profile was significantly correlated with cognitive performance on the Mini-Mental State Examination (MMSE) [31].

α-Synuclein aggregates are the pathological hallmark of DLB and PD-D, and appear to be the pathological substrate most closely related to progressive cognitive decline in these individuals. α-Synuclein is therefore a potentially attractive biomarker. In one study, patients with PD, multiple system atrophy, and DLB had lower CSF α-synuclein than patients with AD or other neurological disorders, although discrimination was best for PD-D [29]. However, others found similar or higher levels of total α-synuclein in the CSF of AD and DLB patients, thus questioning the relevance of this measure as a specific biomarker of LB disease, suggesting that it could rather be a marker of neurodegeneration [32]. The key may lie in the type of α-synuclein and its ratio in proportion to other proteins: other species, such as oligomeric or phosphorylated α-synuclein, may be more specific markers of DLB and PD. For example, one autopsy study demonstrated similar levels of total α-synuclein in DLB and AD, but higher levels of soluble oligomers of α-synuclein in DLB compared with AD [33], while another study showed that taking into account the oligomer/total α-synuclein ratio enhanced the discrimination between PD and AD [34]. Along this line, another study identified a 24-kDa protein that was recognized by α-synuclein in patients with LB disease but not in controls, and which appeared to correlate with cognition [35].

Other CSF biomarkers could add to the picture. Patients with PD and DLB have lower CSF uric acid than controls, while patients with PD without dementia have higher uric acid than those with DLB [36]. CSF levels of transthyretin, a clearance protein, are upregulated in AD and have been associated with clearance of Aβ and α-synuclein. In a recent study in patients with PD, PD-D, and DLB, CSF transthyretin levels were higher than in controls and negatively correlated with $Aβ_{1-42}$, total tau, and phosphorylated tau [36].

Although recent progress has been made in the measurement of α-synuclein and other biomarkers in the CSF, prospective studies with sufficient numbers of patients comparing PD-D and DLB are lacking. Longitudinal studies in this field will play an important role in furthering our understanding of the similarities and differences in the evolution of pathology in DLB and PD-D.

Neurochemistry

The majority of studies of the neurochemistry of DLB and PD-D have explored the dopamine and acetylcholine systems in neuropathological studies and some functional neuroimaging studies. The findings overall suggest a similar profile of changes in the two dementias, but with some specific differences that may relate to phenotype. Although changes in nigrostriatal dopamine are found in both syndromes, the severity and distribution of changes differ, with more marked nigral cell loss in PD-D than DLB—although this may be related to differences in disease duration. Importantly, there appears to be post-synaptic dopaminergic upregulation in PD but not in DLB, which may translate to the increased risk for neuroleptic sensitivity reactions found in a DLB patient group [37]. However, the interpretation of this study is difficult as there was no distinction between PD patients with and without dementia, and neuroleptic sensitivity is also prevalent in patients with PD and PD-D [38]. In addition to the well-known reductions in dopamine, marked cholinergic deficits have been reported in both DLB and PD-D in autopsy and PET studies. Cortical cholinergic deficits, secondary to cell loss of forebrain nuclei, are pronounced in DLB and PD-D to a greater extent than in AD [39, 40], and are associated with decreased performance on tests of attentional and executive functioning, but not with memory tests [41]. In addition, cholinergic deficits have also been reported in selected thalamic nuclei in PD-D [42]. In the insular cortex the cholinergic deficits were more marked in PD-D than DLB [43]. In DLB, but probably not in PD-D, there is a correlation between VH and cholinergic deficits in the temporal cortex [44, 46]. In addition, there is evidence linking cholinergic changes, in particular nicotinic modulation of thalamocortical circuitry, with disturbed consciousness in patients with DLB [45]. Neuroimaging studies using single-photon emission computed tomography (SPECT) ligands have also reported cholinergic receptor changes in DLB and PD-D, with increased muscarinic [47] and reduced nicotinergic binding in both dementias. One multitracer PET study compared patients with DLB, PD-D, and PD [48]. All patient groups showed reduced fluorodopa (FDOPA; a tracer for pre-synaptic dopaminergic functioning) uptake in the striatum and in the limbic and associative prefrontal areas. A severe reduction in binding of methyl-4-piperidyl acetate (MP4A; a ligand for neuronal acetylcholine esterase) and fluorodeoxyglucose (FDG; a ligand for energy metabolism) was found in patients with PD-D and with DLB [48]. Data from our group showed significantly higher frontal serotonin 5-HT1A receptor-binding density in DLB compared with PD-D, suggesting distinct neurochemical features of the two dementias [49].

Direct comparisons between DLB and PD-D patients have not yet been undertaken for a number of key neurochemical systems such as noradrenaline and glutamate. In addition, the association between neurochemical changes and clinical symptoms has rarely been explored. Studying the relationship between the time from onset of PD to dementia, we found that those with early dementia (i.e. less than 10 years after onset of PD) had similar morphological and neurochemical changes to those with DLB, whereas PD patients with late-onset dementia had less morphological cortical pathology (LBs, amyloid plaques, neurofibrillary tangles) but more severe cholinergic deficits in the temporal cortex [7].

Comparative studies of clinical features in PD-D and DLB

Cognitive deficits

The overall profile of cognitive deficits is similar in the two syndromes, with both PD-D and DLB patients exhibiting significantly more marked executive and attentional deficits, fluctuating attention, and less severe memory deficits than those with AD [50]. Some studies have reported more pronounced executive dysfunction in DLB than in PD-D, in particular in patients with mild dementia [51, 52]. In addition, more pronounced auditory attentional disturbances were identified in PD-D compared with DLB [53]. The finding of more pronounced differences between DLB and PD-D in early rather than later disease is consistent with the electroencephalogram (EEG) findings [54]. A study of pre-pulse inhibition, a paradigm which enables the study of basic attention processes independent of task understanding and deliberate participation, demonstrated more pronounced impairment in DLB than PD-D [55]. A recent study has shown that the more pronounced cognitive impairment in DLB compared with PD-D is already present in the mild cognitive impairment stage of the two diseases [56]. Although studies based on group means provide important information, comparison of group means may disguise heterogeneity within the groups. Indeed, evidence has demonstrated that subgroups with different cognitive profiles exist in PD and in PD-D: the majority of patients have an executive–visuospatial-dominant profile, whereas others have a memory-dominant profile [57, 58]. Similarly, some DLB patients, probably those with more abundant AD-type changes, may lack the characteristic pattern of neuropsychological deficits usually associated with LB diseases.

Neuropsychiatric symptoms

One of the core characteristics of DLB and PD-D is the high prevalence of neuropsychiatric symptoms (Table 18.2). The profile of neuropsychiatric symptoms is also similar in DLB and PD-D. Persistent VH are the most frequent neuropsychiatric symptom [16, 40, 59–62]. Although misidentification syndromes and delusions are also common and have a similar phenomenology in both DLB and PD-D patients [63], they may be more prevalent in DLB than in PD-D, possibly due to the morphological and/or neurochemical differences reported in the subsection on Neurochemistry. Depression is also common in both dementias [59–61]. Psychotic symptoms and depression are more frequent in DLB and PD-D than among people with AD, and the characteristic neuropsychiatric profile in DLB is less pronounced in those with more severe AD-type lesions [15, 16]. Apathy, with reduced initiative and motivation, and anxiety are also common neuropsychiatric symptoms. DLB patients more often reported symptoms of anxiety compared with AD patients [64].

Parkinsonism

A proportion of DLB patients do not suffer from parkinsonism (29%), sometimes even over a prolonged dementia of 5 years or more. However, parkinsonism is more frequently present in DLB than among patients with AD or vascular dementia (VaD) [65]. In the most detailed comparative study of parkinsonism to date, Burn et al. [66] found that DLB patients had less severe parkinsonism than people with PD-D, but a similar severity of motor deficits compared with PD patients without dementia. The severity of parkinsonism, however, appears to progress similarly in both conditions [65]. The majority of patients with DLB will develop characteristics of parkinsonism, including generalized slowing and postural and gait disturbances [67]. There are some subtle but important differences between DLB, PD-D, and PD in the key parkinsonian signs and symptoms. Postural instability and gait disturbance (PIGD), predominantly mediated by non-dopaminergic lesions, is more pronounced in DLB and PD-D than in PD patients without dementia, whereas the opposite is true for tremor [66]. In addition, parkinsonian features tend to be more symmetrical in PD-D [68]. In a prospective study, those who had PIGD-dominant PD at baseline, or who developed this after having tremor-dominant PD initially, had a higher risk of dementia compared than those who maintained a tremor-dominant phenotype [69]. Importantly, parkinsonism is a key factor explaining the functional impairment in DLB [70] as well as PD-D.

Cognitive and functional decline

Only one study has directly compared the course of cognitive decline in PD-D and DLB. This study reported that DLB and PD-D patients had a similar rate of decline on cognition over 2 years [71]. There are some indications that the course of disease is more severe in PD-D and DLB than in AD, although few longitudinal comparative studies have been done. The cognitive decline in PD-D [61] and DLB [72] seems to be similar to that in AD, but, consistent with the complex clinical symptoms in DLB, functional decline and mortality [72] progress more rapidly in DLB than in AD.

Structural and functional imaging

MIBG

Cardiac scintigraphy with $[^{123}I]$-MIBG enables the quantification of post-ganglionic cardiac sympathetic innervation, and several studies have demonstrated reduced cardiac uptake compared with mediastinal uptake in DLB and PD, as opposed to AD [73]. In one meta-analysis MIBG distinguished two diagnostic clusters: one including PD, individuals with RBD, and DLB, the second including AD, multiple system atrophy (MSA), progressive supranuclear palsy (PSP), VaD, and frontotemporal dementia [74]. Patients with PD-D or DLB have lower cardiac $[^{123}I]$-MIBG uptake than those with PD, in parallel with reduced cardiovascular autonomic function [75]. Direct comparative studies of DLB and PD-D are needed to complete the picture, with better

Table 18.2 Psychotic symptoms in dementia with Lewy bodies (DLB), Parkinson's disease with dementia (PD-D), and Alzheimer's disease (AD)

Symptom	DLB (*n* = 98)	PD-D (*n* = 48)	AD (*n* = 40)
Visual	71 (72%)	24 (50%)	10 (25%)
Auditory	37 (38%)	10 (21%)	4 (10%)
Delusions	56 (57%)	14 (29%)	12 (30%)

Data from Ballard et al. (1999) [62] and Aarsland et al. (2001) [59].

information needed to enable the interpretation of results in patients with concurrent cardiovascular disease.

Magnetic resonance imaging (MRI)

Using structural MRI, the typical finding in DLB is relative preservation of hippocampal and medial temporal lobe volumes in comparison with AD. Other cortical and subcortical changes have also been reported in DLB, including in the substantia innominata, hypothalamus, and dorsal midbrain [76]. Similar changes have been reported in PD-D. However, the two studies comparing grey matter in PD-D and DLB by MRI have conflicted, one reporting no differences [77] whereas the other found more pronounced cortical atrophy in DLB than in PD-D [78]. A further study focusing on voxel-based morphometry of grey and white matter densities between DLB and PD-D showed decreased grey matter density in PD-D in bilateral dorsolateral prefrontal, temporal, occipital, posterior cingular, and right parietal cortical areas compared with controls [79]. DLB showed similar changes but more pronounced atrophy, with significantly decreased grey matter density in left occipital, parietal, and striatal areas compared with PD-D. White matter analyses showed decreased density in PD-D and DLB compared with controls, with a greater decrease in DLB compared with PD-D. Additionally, the relative decrease of white matter relative to grey matter was more pronounced in DLB.

MRI diffusion tensor tractography shows significantly lower fractional anisotropy in the anterior cingulate fasciculi in PD-D and PD compared with controls, and this value correlated with the MMSE score [80]. A recent study showed that among patients with VH, DLB patients had more atrophy in pre-motor bilateral regions than PD-D patients, and the severity of hallucinations correlated with the intensity of grey matter volume reduction in the right inferior frontal gyrus and left precuneus only in DLB patients [81].

SPECT

SPECT studies of cerebral cortical blood flow have demonstrated characteristic patterns in DLB and PD-D. Cerebral perfusion deficits are confined mainly to either the parietal or occipital regions or both in DLB as compared with AD, whereas reductions in all cortical areas have been reported in PD-D [82]. Comparative studies have reported slightly different regional patterns of cerebral blood flow in DLB and PD-D. In one study, DLB patients had a more markedly reduced blood flow in the frontal lobe [83]. In another study, the pattern was similar, but DLB patients had a more pronounced overall reduction of cerebral blood flow than PD-D patients [84]. Longitudinal studies have reported a progressive reduction of frontal lobe blood flow in PD [85]. One study found no significant change in PD-D [86], while another found significantly reduced perfusion in the right posterior cingulate, right precuneus, and left posterior cingulate in PD-D patients relative to PD. Furthermore, in the longitudinal follow-up of this study patients who developed PD-D at the time of the second scan had significantly reduced right inferior parietal lobule perfusion [87]. Few studies have explored the associations between regional functional changes and specific clinical features. A longitudinal study reported correlations between increase in perfusion in the midline posterior cingulate and a decrease in the severity of hallucinations, and between fluctuations of consciousness and increased thalamic and decreased inferior occipital perfusion [88].

SPECT functional imaging studies of dopamine transporter loss, visualized with tracers such as $[^{123}I]$-N-3-fluoropropyl-2-β-carbomethoxy-3-β-(4-iodophenyl)-nortropane (FP-CIT) SPECT, have identified characteristic patterns in DLB and PD-D compared with PD patients without dementia, people with AD, and normal controls. Characteristic differences are evident in the nigrostriatal dopamine system, demonstrating striatal abnormalities in PD and DLB, compared with AD and healthy controls [89, 90]. A slightly different pattern in DLB and PD has been suggested, with PD and PD-D patients showing more left–right asymmetry and a more posterior striatal degeneration than DLB patients [89, 90]. A similar rate of decline of striatal binding in PD-D and DLB has been shown [91]. The differences in the pattern of asymmetry are consistent with what has been reported in clinical studies of parkinsonism with regard to its symmetry [68].

PIB imaging

The development of the ^{11}C-labelled amyloid ligand PIB as a biomarker of cortical Aβ deposition has enabled in vivo assessment of amyloid burden. Although there is some variation, the overall picture is that DLB patients have PIB binding that is similar to or less pronounced than AD patients, whereas PD-D patients have similar [92] or lower [93] PIB binding than DLB patients, consistent with pathological findings. The validity of PIB binding as a marker of amyloid pathology in DLB and PD-D was supported in a study finding reduced $Aβ_{1-42}$ in those patients with pathological binding. The overall conclusion to date is that PD-D has a lower amyloid burden than DLB, and DLB somewhat less than AD [13, 38, 93]. PIB binding correlates with cognition in DLB but not with motor symptoms [13].

Electrophysiology

Characteristic EEG changes have been reported in patients with DLB, such as slowing of background activity and frequency variability. Two studies included both PD-D and DLB patients. In one study of patients with early and mild dementia [54], patients with DLB and PD-D had more posterior slowing and frequency variation than AD and healthy control subjects. At baseline, the changes were more common and severe in DLB than in PD-D, although at the 2-year follow-up, the changes in PD-D had become more pronounced. Interestingly, two subgroups of PD-D with and without cognitive fluctuations were identified, with EEG changes similar to the DLB group in PD-D with fluctuations group, but not in those without. In contrast, a study assessing mismatch negativity (MMN)—a component of the auditory event-related potential (ERP) considered to represent a basic automatic change detection system—found pronounced changes with reduced MMN latency and areas in PD-D, but not in DLB or AD [53]. Another study including PD, PD-D, DLB, and controls sought evidence of posterior cortical dysfunction by rhythm reactivity to eyes opening and intermittent photic stimulation (IPS) [94]. The authors found evidence for a graded posterior cortical disconnection, with decreased reactivity to IPS in PD and DLB patients and no reaction in PD-D. However, the sample was small, with only seven PD-D patients and ten DLB patients.

Genetic studies

Exciting studies over the last few years have identified several key genes involved in the development of PD, including α-synuclein (*SNCA*), parkin (*PARK2*), *PARK7*, *LRRK2*, and *PINK1*. The potential importance of these genes and other key genetic risk factors has not yet been elucidated for DLB. A systematic review of the available literature with respect to familial occurrence of dementia with parkinsonism explored the genetic evidence pertaining to PD-D and DLB. A substantial coincidental familial occurrence of dementia and parkinsonism was evident in the 24 families described in the review [95]. In 12 families the presentation of dementia and parkinsonism fulfilled current criteria for DLB in some family members and PD-D in others, implying that the same mutation in different members of the same family caused different clinical phenotypes.

Patients with familial co-occurrence of dementia and parkinsonism displayed either mutations in *SNCA* or showed positive correlations with the *APOE* ε3/ε4 and ε4/ε4 alleles. Consistent with these observations, a three-generation Belgian family with different phenotypes involving dementia and/or parkinsonism [96] was described, with significant linkage to 2q35–q36. Further extensive sequencing within this region did not reveal a simple pathogenic mutation that co-segregated with DLB in this family [97]. A review of genetic determinants in DLB revealed that genetic variations in genes associated with AD and PD play a role in the aetiology of DLB [98]. A case–control study in patients with autopsy-proven DLB, for instance, indicated that genetic variability in all three members of the synuclein gene family affects the risk of developing DLB [99]. Together, these reports support the hypothesis of a common genetic underpinning for DLB and PD-D. The proteins encoded by genes causing genetic PD-D or DLB are related to different functions, such as mitochondria and energy metabolism, the ubiquitin–proteasome system, or synuclein, pointing to the likelihood that multiple pathways are involved in the aetiology of PD-D and DLB [100]. A recent study shows that the *5-HTTLPR* (*SLC6A4*) serotonin transporter polymorphism is associated with an increased risk for the development of delusions in DLB and PDD [101].

In addition to disease-causing mutations, other genes involved in disease susceptibility have also been uncovered. Some glucocerebrosidase (*GBA*) gene polymorphisms, in particular, are proven risk factors for PD, with different mutations occurring in different populations and increasing risk to varying degrees [102]. Most mutations cause earlier disease onset and more cognitive symptoms than found in patients with parkinsonism without these mutations [103]. The mechanisms by which *GBA* mutation operate are unknown, but misfolded glucocerebrosidase might induce lysosomal dysfunction, saturate the ubiquitin–proteasome pathway, impair clearance of α-synuclein or produce a gain-of-function mechanism to enhance aggregation of α-synuclein [102, 103].

Treatment response

Cholinesterase inhibitors

In the first placebo-controlled trial of a cholinesterase inhibitor in patients with DLB, 120 patients were treated with rivastigmine (mean dose 7 mg) or placebo for 20 weeks [104]. The primary outcome measure was 30% improvement in a four-item subscore derived from the Neuropsychiatric Inventory (NPI) (delusions, hallucinations, apathy, depression); this was attained by 63% of people treated with rivastigmine and 30% of people treated with placebo, a significant difference on the observed case analysis. On the total NPI, there was a three-point advantage for the rivastigmine-treated patients. Significant improvements were seen in attentional performance on computerized tests, with a non-significant one-point advantage for the rivastigmine-treated patients on the MMSE. More recently, a multicentre trial included 140 patients with DLB, randomized to receive placebo or 3, 5, or 10 mg of donepezil daily for 12 weeks [105]. Donepezil demonstrated significant improvement in MMSE, attention/concentration on the revised Wechsler Memory Scale, and the Wechsler Adult Intelligence Scale (third edition) symbol digit test, but not in verbal fluency or visuoperceptual tests, in a dose-dependent fashion. Neuropsychiatric symptoms assessed by the NPI were also significantly improved, as was caregiver burden and global functioning. Symptoms of parkinsonism were more frequent in the 3- and 5-mg groups than in the placebo group, although the difference did not translate to changes in the mean Unified Parkinson's Disease Rating Scale (UPDRS) part III score. Additionally, some evidence exists for cognitive benefit in DLB patients with galantamine [106].

Two large randomized, placebo-controlled, trials have examined the effect of cholinesterase inhibitors in PD-D. In one, rivastigmine conferred benefit in comparison with placebo over 24 weeks of treatment in 541 patients with PD-D (allocated 2:1 rivastigmine:placebo) [107]. Over the treatment period, the rivastigmine-treated patients had a two-point advantage on the NPI, a one-point advantage on the MMSE, an almost three-point advantage on the Alzheimer's Disease Assessment Scale—Cognition (ADAS-COG), and also superiority on more specialized assessment of attention and executive function, all differences being statistically significant. Additionally, post-hoc analyses revealed improved outcomes in basic activities of daily living (ADLs) and high-function ADLs [108]. Another trial randomized 550 PD-D patients to 5 or 10 mg of donepezil or placebo [109]: no difference was found in ADAS-COG mean changes in intention-to-treat population, but there were statistically significant differences in favour of donepezil in a post-hoc analysis removing the centre-effect. MMSE and tests of executive function and attention showed significant improvement with donepezil.

Although there are always limitations to the interpretation of comparisons of effect size across trials, the magnitude of benefit of cholinesterase inhibitor treatment in DLB and PD-D appears comparable between studies, and in DLB and PD-D [110]. There are no blinded studies that directly examine cholinesterase inhibitors in DLB and PD-D patients, but open-label trials also suggest that effect sizes and side effects are similar [111].

In both syndromes, sudden withdrawal of cholinesterase inhibitors may be detrimental, and this may be particularly pronounced in PD-D [112].

Memantine

Memantine is a N-methyl-D-aspartate (NMDA) receptor antagonist which has proven efficacy in AD and has been proposed to target the glutamatergic dysfunction described in LB disease. In case series, both cognitive improvement and worsening have been described with this treatment. Two studies have attempted to address the issue. In one double-blind, multicentre study 72 patients with LB disease (either PD-D or DLB) were randomized to memantine or placebo [113]. The main outcome variable was improvement in the Clinical Global Impression of Change scale (CGIC), while changes in MMSE, NPI, modified UPDRS, disability and cognitive speed (measured by A Quick Test of Cognitive Speed, AQT) were secondary outcome measures. High attrition was evident in both treatment arms, but a significant difference in the CGIC was demonstrated between groups at week 24. No significant differences for secondary outcome variables were found between the memantine and placebo groups between baseline and week 24. Another study randomized 199 DLB or PD-D patients to memantine or placebo [114]. In the DLB group, patients treated with memantine demonstrated significant improvement in the Alzheimer's Disease Cooperative Study (ADCS)-CGIC and NPI scales, but no changes were found in other scales or there were no statistically significant differences in any of the scales in the PD-D group [114].

Antipsychotics

Given the high frequency of psychotic symptoms in both DLB and PD-D, antipsychotic agents are frequently considered for DLB and PD-D patients. However, antipsychotic medications are often accompanied by numerous and severe adverse effects, including parkinsonism, delirium, and dystonia [115]. Only a limited number of studies have examined the effect of antipsychotic medication in patients with DLB and PD-D. One randomized controlled trial of an atypical antipsychotic in patients with dementia and PD indicated that quetiapine did not confer any greater benefit than placebo in the treatment of psychosis [116]. Another randomized trial without placebo compared the effect of citalopram and risperidone over 12 weeks in 31 DLB and 66 AD patients. Patients with DLB showed no improvement or deterioration in neuropsychiatric symptoms. In contrary, AD patients did show an improvement, and early withdrawal was significantly lower in AD patients (50%) than in DLB group (68%) [117]. Importantly, severe neuroleptic sensitivity reactions have been identified as a major clinical issue in DLB. An initial study in 1992 [118] reported that 50% of DLB patients treated with neuroleptics experienced severe drug sensitivity, with symptoms that included marked extrapyramidal features, confusion, autonomic instability, falls, and accelerated mortality. An accumulating literature of case reports and case series, as well as subsequent larger and more systematic reports, shows that severe neuroleptic sensitivity reactions occur with a wide range of typical and atypical antipsychotics, rarely including clozapine, in DLB [119, 120]. There is also evidence of similar poor tolerability in PD-D, albeit from fewer studies. A comparative study examined neurolepetic sensitivity in 94 patients (15 with DLB, 36 with PD-D, 26 with PD, and 17 with AD). Severe neuroleptic sensitivity occurred in patients with LB disease (DLB 53%, PD-D 39%, PD 27%) but not in AD. Thus, severe neuroleptic sensitivity syndrome is common in both DLB and PD-D [38]. There are other adverse effects of antipsychotic treatment in DLB and PD-D: together with the limited evidence of benefit it is recommended to prescribe antipsychotics only in patients with severe neuropsychiatric symptoms which cannot be otherwise managed.

Levodopa

Motor symptoms contribute to the disability experienced by DLB and PD-D patients and are associated with an increased risk of falls. Acute levodopa challenge in 14 DLB patients yielded some improvement in UPDRS III score, finger tapping, and walking test, but less so than in PD or PD-D [121, 122]. Of the DLB patients, 36% were classified as 'responders' on levodopa challenge, compared with 70% of the PD-D and 57% of the PD patients. Although the majority of DLB patients seemed to tolerate the drug, 15% withdrew due to confusion and gastrointestinal problems. In an extension of this study [122], acute levodopa challenge considerably improved motor function and subjective alertness in all patients, without compromising either reaction times or accuracy, but increased fluctuations were noted in both groups with dementia. Moreover, neuropsychiatric scores improved in patients with PD (both with and without dementia) on levodopa at 3 months. Sleep disturbances and VH are possible adverse effects of treatment with levodopa. Because of the common presence of these symptoms in untreated DLB there is a theoretical risk that VH and sleep disturbances may appear or be exacerbated in DLB patients with levodopa treatment. However, a study examining sleep disturbances and excessive daytime sleepiness suggest that levodopa treatment does not worsen such symptoms [123]. Conversely, in a prospective study of 19 DLB patients limited efficacy and increased risk for psychosis was observed in DLB during 3 months of levodopa treatment [124]. Overall it would therefore appear that DLB patients are less responsive to levodopa than people with PD-D, but the relative impact on neuropsychiatric symptoms and cognition remains unresolved. Treatment with dopamine receptor agonists is a feasible alternative to levodopa therapy in PD. However, dopamine receptor agonists are known to provide a higher risk for VH and sleep attacks in PD than does levodopa; therefore their use in patients with DLB is not recommended [125].

Primavanserin is a selective serotonin 5-HT2A inverse agonist without dopaminergic effects. Since VH and delusions in LB disease and some other neurodegenerative disorders have been linked to dysfunction in the serotonin system, primavanserin has been proposed as a possible treatment for these symptoms. In a recent trial, primavanserin showed improvement in psychotic symptoms in PD-D without worsening of parkinsonism. Further trials are needed to examine its effect in DLB [126].

Clinicopathological dimensions rather than categories: personal interpretation

Overall there are many similarities, but also subtle differences, between DLB and PD-D and the number of direct comparative studies is still too limited to make firm conclusions. For context, it is also important to remember that marked differences exist within the two syndromes: some DLB patients have a very characteristic clinical profile with visuospatial and executive dysfunction, VH, and parkinsonism, whereas others have a clinical profile more similar to that seen in patients with AD. Similarly, some PD patients develop dementia early in the disease course, whereas others remain without dementia or develop it late; some develop VH or severe psychosis, whereas others do not show these symptoms despite large doses of dopaminergic drugs.

Although there are no major brain differences between PD-D and DLB, subtle neurochemical and pathological differences are likely to subserve the subtle clinical differences. A more pronounced executive dysfunction in DLB may relate to the loss of the hippocampal projection to the frontal lobe in DLB but not PD, and more severe LB pathology in the inferior temporal lobe may relate to the higher frequency of VH in DLB. The differential pattern of parkinsonian features in PD and DLB is in accordance with the differential striatal changes, with changes in PD-D patients being intermediate between those found in DLB and PD patients. Similarly, within the two syndromes, the severity of AD changes is associated with a less classical DLB phenotype. In PD-D, those who develop dementia early have more pronounced cortical morphological changes. More studies are needed to address the relationship between these syndromes, by understanding the relationship between the underlying pathological and neurochemical substrates, the clinical profile, and course of PD-D and DLB. In addition, comparative studies so far conducted have been based purely upon the duration of PD prior to dementia, and no studies have yet used the new operationalized diagnostic criteria for PD-D [127] to undertake direct comparisons with DLB.

The available data strongly support a 'continuum' model, and indicate that any arbitrary clinical distinction between DLB and PD-D does not reflect the pattern of neuropathological and neurochemical changes in the cortex. As the majority of previous research has focused on the distinction between DLB and PD-D, future studies should combine DLB and PD-D patients and aim to disentangle empirically based subgroups within the continuum of LB dementia. This will enable further work to focus on the pathological and neurochemical processes underpinning the clinical phenotypes across the full spectrum, with the potential to understand prognosis and to develop and evaluate new targeted treatment approaches.

Conclusion

DLB and PD-D are characterized by similar clinical presentations with parkinsonism, VH, other psychotic symptoms, fluctuating cognition, RBD, marked sensitivity to neuroleptic drugs, and a comparable treatment response to cholinesterase inhibitors. Although there are more similarities than differences, the absence of clinically significant parkinsonism in some DLB patients, the greater asymmetry of parkinsonism in PD-D, and the reduced levodopa responsiveness in DLB are notable differences.

An arbitrary, but generally accepted, distinction has been made in current international consensus diagnostic criteria between patients presenting with parkinsonism prior to the onset of dementia (PD-D) and those who develop parkinsonism and dementia concurrently (DLB). The clinical syndromes are very similar, yet it is a priority to understand the relationship between the duration of PD prior to dementia and the distribution of the major pathological and neurochemical disease substrates in order to produce an evidence-based diagnostic conceptualization. The few studies directly comparing PD-D and DLB using the current diagnostic definitions suggested that DLB patients have significantly higher cortical LB density, greater amyloid pathology, and more pronounced atrophy than those with PD-D, and that widespread neurofibrillary tangles are rare in both disorders. Within the PD-D group there seems to be less cortical AD pathology and less cortical LB pathology in patients who have had PD for 10 years or more before the onset of dementia. Even fewer reports have directly compared neurochemical changes in DLB and PD-D, suggesting severe cholinergic deficits in both conditions but potential differences in cortical serotonergic function. The balance of evidence strongly indicates that DLB and PD-D are part of a continuum rather than distinct disorders.

Newly emerging opportunities from CSF and neuroimaging studies and an increased focus on the specific molecular impact of key risk genes will allow us to further address the relationship between DLB and PD-D. Our hypothesis is that variability is driven more by different molecular pathways than by arbitrary distinctions in the evolution of clinical symptoms.

References

1. **McKeith IG, Dickson DW, Lowe J, et al**. Diagnosis and management of dementia with Lewy bodies: third report of the DLB Consortium. Neurology 2005; **65**: 1863–72.
2. **McKeith IG, Galasko D, Kosaka K, et al**. Consensus guidelines for the clinical and pathologic diagnosis of dementia with Lewy bodies (DLB): report of the consortium on DLB international workshop. Neurology 1996; **47**: 1113–24.
3. **Cordato NJ, Halliday GM, Harding AJ, et al**. Regional brain atrophy in progressive supranuclear palsy and Lewy body disease. Ann Neurol 2000; **47**: 718–28.
4. **Aarsland D, Perry R, Brown A, et al**. Neuropathology of dementia in Parkinson's disease: a prospective, community-based study. Ann Neurol 2005; **58**: 773–6.
5. **Harding AJ, Halliday GM**. Cortical Lewy body pathology in the diagnosis of dementia. Acta Neuropathol 2001; **102**: 355–63.
6. **Tsuboi Y, Dickson DW**. Dementia with Lewy bodies and Parkinson's disease with dementia: are they different? Parkinsonism Relat Disord 2005; **11**(Suppl. 1): S47–S51.
7. **Ballard C, Ziabreva I, Perry R, et al**. Differences in neuropathologic characteristics across the Lewy body dementia spectrum. Neurology 2006; **67**: 1931–34.
8. **Harding AJ, Broe GA, Halliday GM**. Visual hallucinations in Lewy body disease relate to Lewy bodies in the temporal lobe. Brain 2002; **125**: 391–403.
9. **Samuel W, Galasko D, Masliah E, et al**. Neocortical Lewy body counts correlate with dementia in the Lewy body variant of Alzheimer's disease. J Neuropathol Exp Neurol 1996; **55**: 44–52.
10. **Ferman TJ, Arvanitakis Z, Fujishiro H, et al**. Pathology and temporal onset of visual hallucinations, misperceptions and family misidentification distinguishes dementia with Lewy bodies from Alzheimer's disease. Parkinsonism Relat Disord 2013; **19**: 227–31.
11. **Kovari E, Gold G, Herrmann FR, et al**. Lewy body densities in the entorhinal and anterior cingulate cortex predict cognitive deficits in Parkinson's disease. Acta Neuropathol 2003; **106**: 83–8.
12. **Edison P, Rowe CC, Rinne JO, et al**. Amyloid load in Parkinson's disease dementia and Lewy body dementia measured with [11C]PIB positron emission tomography. J Neurol Neurosurg Psychiatry 2008; **79**: 1331–8.
13. **Gomperts SN, Locascio JJ, Marquie M, et al**. Brain amyloid and cognition in Lewy body diseases. Mov Disord 2012; **27**: 965–73.

14. Compta Y, Parkkinen L, O'Sullivan SS, et al. Lewy- and Alzheimer-type pathologies in Parkinson's disease dementia: which is more important? Brain 2011; **134**: 1493–1505.

15. Merdes AR, Hansen LA, Jeste DV, et al. Influence of Alzheimer pathology on clinical diagnostic accuracy in dementia with Lewy bodies. Neurology 2003; **60**: 1586–90.

16. Ballard CG, Jacoby R, Del Ser T, et al. Neuropathological substrates of psychiatric symptoms in prospectively studied patients with autopsy-confirmed dementia with Lewy bodies. Am J Psychiatry 2004; **161**: 843–9.

17. Duda JE, Giasson BI, Mabon ME, et al. Novel antibodies to synuclein show abundant striatal pathology in Lewy body diseases. Ann Neurol 2002; **52**: 205–10.

18. Tsuboi Y, Uchikado H, Dickson DW. Neuropathology of Parkinson's disease dementia and dementia with Lewy bodies with reference to striatal pathology. Parkinsonism Relat Disord 2007; **13**(Suppl. 3): S221–S224.

19. Braak H, Del Tredici K, Rub U, et al. Staging of brain pathology related to sporadic Parkinson's disease. Neurobiol Aging 2003; **24**: 197–211.

20. Parkkinen L, Pirttila T, Alafuzoff I. Applicability of current staging/categorization of alpha-synuclein pathology and their clinical relevance. Acta Neuropathol 2008; **115**: 399–407.

21. Halliday G, Hely M, Reid W, et al. The progression of pathology in longitudinally followed patients with Parkinson's disease. Acta Neuropathol 2008; **115**: 409–15.

22. Gaig C, Valldeoriola F, Gelpi E, et al. Rapidly progressive diffuse Lewy body disease. Mov Disord 2011; **26**: 1316–23.

23. Beyer K, Domingo-Sabat M, Humbert J, et al. Differential expression of alpha-synuclein, parkin, and synphilin-1 isoforms in Lewy body disease. Neurogenetics 2008; **9**: 163–72.

24. Gelpi E, Navarro-Otano J, Tolosa E, et al. Multiple organ involvement by alpha-synuclein pathology in Lewy body disorders. Mov Disord 2014; **29**: 1010–18.

25. Braune S, Reinhardt M, Schnitzer R, et al. Cardiac uptake of [123I]MIBG separates Parkinson's disease from multiple system atrophy. Neurology 1999; **53**: 1020–5.

26. Siderowf A, Xie SX, Hurtig H, et al. CSF amyloid {beta} 1–42 predicts cognitive decline in Parkinson disease. Neurology 2010; **75**: 1055–61.

27. Montine TJ, Shi M, Quinn JF, et al. CSF Abeta(42) and tau in Parkinson's disease with cognitive impairment. Mov Disord 2010; **25**: 2682–5.

28. Bibl M, Mollenhauer B, Esselmann H, et al. CSF amyloid-beta-peptides in Alzheimer's disease, dementia with Lewy bodies and Parkinson's disease dementia. Brain 2006; **129**: 1177–87.

29. Mollenhauer B, Locascio JJ, Schulz-Schaeffer W, et al. Alpha-synuclein and tau concentrations in cerebrospinal fluid of patients presenting with parkinsonism: a cohort study. Lancet Neurol 2011; **10**: 230–40.

30. Parnetti L, Tiraboschi P, Lanari A, et al. Cerebrospinal fluid biomarkers in Parkinson's disease with dementia and dementia with Lewy bodies. Biol Psychiatry 2008; **64**: 850–5.

31. Andersson M, Zetterberg H, Minthon L, et al. The cognitive profile and CSF biomarkers in dementia with Lewy bodies and Parkinson's disease dementia. Int J Geriatr Psychiatry 2011; **26**: 100–5.

32. Ohrfelt A, Grognet P, Andreasen N, et al. Cerebrospinal fluid alpha-synuclein in neurodegenerative disorders-a marker of synapse loss? Neurosci Lett 2009; **450**: 332–5.

33. Paleologou KE, Kragh CL, Mann DM, et al. Detection of elevated levels of soluble alpha-synuclein oligomers in post-mortem brain extracts from patients with dementia with Lewy bodies. Brain 2009; **132**: 1093–101.

34. Tokuda T, Qureshi MM, Ardah MT, et al. Detection of elevated levels of alpha-synuclein oligomers in CSF from patients with Parkinson disease. Neurology 2010; **75**: 1766–72.

35. Ballard C, Jones EL, Londos E, et al. Alpha-synuclein antibodies recognize a protein present at lower levels in the CSF of patients with dementia with Lewy bodies. Int Psychogeriatr 2010; **22**: 321–7.

36. Maetzler W, Stapf AK, Schulte C, et al. Serum and cerebrospinal fluid uric acid levels in Lewy body disorders: associations with disease occurrence and amyloid-beta pathway. J Alzheimers Dis 2011; **27**: 119–26.

37. Piggott MA, Perry EK, Marshall EF, et al. Nigrostriatal dopaminergic activities in dementia with Lewy bodies in relation to neuroleptic sensitivity: comparisons with Parkinson's disease. Biol Psychiatry 1998; **44**: 765–74.

38. Aarsland D, Perry R, Larsen JP, et al. Neuroleptic sensitivity in Parkinson's disease and parkinsonian dementias. J Clin Psychiatry 2005; **66**: 633–7.

39. Aarsland D, Ballard CG, Halliday G. Are Parkinson's disease with dementia and dementia with Lewy bodies the same entity? J Geriatr Psychiatry Neurol 2004; **17**: 137–45.

40. Bohnen NI, Kaufer DI, Ivanco LS, et al. Cortical cholinergic function is more severely affected in parkinsonian dementia than in Alzheimer disease: an in vivo positron emission tomographic study. Arch Neurol 2003; **60**: 1745–48.

41. Bohnen NI, Kaufer DI, Hendrickson R, et al. Cognitive correlates of cortical cholinergic denervation in Parkinson's disease and parkinsonian dementia. J Neurol 2006; **253**: 242–7.

42. Ziabreva I, Ballard CG, Aarsland D, et al. Lewy body disease: thalamic cholinergic activity related to dementia and parkinsonism. Neurobiol Aging 2006; **27**: 433–8.

43. Pimlott SL, Piggott M, Owens J, et al. Nicotinic acetylcholine receptor distribution in Alzheimer's disease, dementia with Lewy bodies, Parkinson's disease, and vascular dementia: in vitro binding study using 5-[(125)I]-A-85380. Neuropsychopharmacology 2004; **29**: 108–16.

44. Ballard C, Piggott M, Johnson M, et al. Delusions associated with elevated muscarinic binding in dementia with Lewy bodies. Ann Neurology 2000; **48**: 868–76.

45. Pimlott SL, Piggott M, Ballard C, et al. Thalamic nicotinic receptors implicated in disturbed consciousness in dementia with Lewy bodies. Neurobiol Dis 2006; **21**: 50–6.

46. Perry EK, Marshall E, Kerwin J, et al. Evidence of a monoaminergic–cholinergic imbalance related to visual hallucinations in Lewy body dementia. J Neurochem 1990; **55**: 1454–6.

47. Colloby SJ, Pakrasi S, Firbank MJ, et al. In vivo SPECT imaging of muscarinic acetylcholine receptors using (R,R) 123I-QNB in dementia with Lewy bodies and Parkinson's disease dementia. NeuroImage 2006; **33**: 423–9.

48. Klein J, Eggers C, Kalbe E, et al. Neurotransmitter changes in dementia with Lewy bodies and Parkinson disease dementia in vivo. Neurology 2010; **74**: 885–92.

49. Francis PT, Perry EK. Cholinergic and other neurotransmitter mechanisms in Parkinson's disease, Parkinson's disease dementia, and dementia with Lewy bodies. Mov Disord 2007; **22**(Suppl. 17): S351–S357.

50. Aarsland D, Ballard C, Halliday G. Are Parkinson's disease with dementia and dementia with Lewy bodies the same entity? J Geriatr Psychiatry Neurol 2004; **17**: 137–45.

51. Downes JJ, Priestley NM, Doran M, et al. Intellectual, mnemonic, and frontal functions in dementia with Lewy bodies: a comparison with early and advanced Parkinson's disease. Behav Neurol 1998; **11**: 173–83.

52. Aarsland D, Litvan I, Salmon D, et al. Performance on the dementia rating scale in Parkinson's disease with dementia and dementia with Lewy bodies: comparison with progressive supranuclear palsy and Alzheimer's disease. J Neurol Neurosurg Psychiatry 2003; **74**: 1215–20.

53. Bronnick KS, Nordby H, Larsen JP, et al. Disturbance of automatic auditory change detection in dementia associated with Parkinson's disease: a mismatch negativity study. Neurobiol Aging 2010; **31**: 104–13.

54. Bonanni L, Thomas A, Tiraboschi P, et al. EEG comparisons in early Alzheimer's disease, dementia with Lewy bodies and Parkinson's disease with dementia patients with a 2-year follow-up. Brain 2008; **131**: 690–705.

55. **Perriol MP, Dujardin K, Derambure P, et al**. Disturbance of sensory filtering in dementia with Lewy bodies: comparison with Parkinson's disease dementia and Alzheimer's disease. J Neurol Neurosurg Psychiatry 2005; **76**: 106–8.

56. **Yoon JH, Lee JE, Yong SW, et al**. The mild cognitive impairment stage of dementia with Lewy bodies and Parkinson disease: a comparison of cognitive profiles. Alzheimer Dis Assoc Disord 2014; **28**: 151–5.

57. **Foltynie T, Brayne CE, Robbins TW, et al**. The cognitive ability of an incident cohort of Parkinson's patients in the UK. The CamPaIGN study. Brain 2004; **127**: 550–60.

58. **Janvin CC, Larsen JP, Aarsland D, et al**. Subtypes of mild cognitive impairment in Parkinson's disease: progression to dementia. Mov Disord 2006; **21**: 1343–9.

59. **Aarsland D, Ballard C, Larsen JP, et al**. A comparative study of psychiatric symptoms in dementia with Lewy bodies and Parkinson's disease with and without dementia. Int J Geriatr Psychiatry 2001; **16**: 528–36.

60. **Aarsland D, Brønnick K, Ehrt U, et al**. Neuropsychiatric symptoms in patients with Parkinson's disease and dementia: frequency, profile and associated caregiver stress. J Neurol Neurosurg Psychiatry 2007; **78**: 36–42.

61. **Aarsland D, Cummings JL**. Psychiatric aspects of Parkinson's disease, Parkinson's disease with dementia, and dementia with Lewy bodies. J Geriatr Psychiatry Neurol 2004; **17**: 111.

62. **Ballard C, Holmes C, McKeith I, et al**. Psychiatric morbidity in dementia with Lewy bodies: a prospective clinical and neuropathological comparative study with Alzheimer's disease. Am J Psychiatry 1999; **156**: 1039–45.

63. **Mosimann UP, Rowan EN, Partington CE, et al**. Characteristics of visual hallucinations in Parkinson disease dementia and dementia with Lewy bodies. Am J Geriatr Psychiatry 2006; **14**: 153–60.

64. **Hynninen MJ, Breitve MH, Rongve A, et al**. The frequency and correlates of anxiety in patients with first-time diagnosed mild dementia. Int Psychogeriatr 2012; **24**: 1771–8.

65. **Ballard C, O'Brien J, Swann A, et al**. One year follow-up of parkinsonism in dementia with Lewy bodies. Dement Geriatr Cogn Disord 2000; **11**: 219–22.

66. **Burn DJ, Rowan EN, Minett T, et al**. Extrapyramidal features in Parkinson's disease with and without dementia and dementia with Lewy bodies: a cross-sectional comparative study. Mov Disord 2003; **18**: 884–9.

67. **Burn DJ, McKeith IG**. Current treatment of dementia with Lewy bodies and dementia associated with Parkinson's disease. Mov Disord 2003; **18**: 72–9.

68. **Gnanalingham KK, Byrne EJ, Thornton A, et al**. Motor and cognitive function in Lewy body dementia: comparison with Alzheimer's and Parkinson's diseases. J Neurol Neurosurg Psychiatry 1997; **62**: 243–52.

69. **Alves G, Larsen JP, Emre M, et al**. Changes in motor subtype and risk for incident dementia in Parkinson's disease. Mov Disord 2006; **21**: 1123–30.

70. **McKeith IG, Rowan E, Askew K, et al**. More severe functional impairment in dementia with Lewy bodies than Alzheimer disease is related to extrapyramidal motor dysfunction. Am J Geriatr Psychiatry 2006; **14**: 582–8.

71. **Burn DJ, Rowan EN, Allan LM, et al**. Motor subtype and cognitive decline in Parkinson's disease, Parkinson's disease with dementia, and dementia with Lewy bodies. J Neurol Neurosurg Psychiatry 2006; **77**: 585–9.

72. **Hanyu H, Sato T, Hirao K, et al**. Differences in clinical course between dementia with Lewy bodies and Alzheimer's disease. Eur J Neurol 2009; **16**: 212–17.

73. **Taki J, Yoshita M, Yamada M, et al**. Significance of 123I-MIBG scintigraphy as a pathophysiological indicator in the assessment of Parkinson's disease and related disorders: it can be a specific marker for Lewy body disease. Ann Nucl Med 2004; **18**: 453–61.

74. **King AE, Mintz J, Royall DR**. Meta-analysis of 123I-MIBG cardiac scintigraphy for the diagnosis of Lewy body-related disorders. Mov Disord 2011; **26**: 1218–24.

75. **Oka H, Yoshioka M, Morita M, et al**. Reduced cardiac 123I-MIBG uptake reflects cardiac sympathetic dysfunction in Lewy body disease. Neurology 2007; **69**: 1460–5.

76. **Whitwell JL, Weigand SD, Shiung MM, et al**. Focal atrophy in dementia with Lewy bodies on MRI: a distinct pattern from Alzheimer's disease. Brain 2007; **130**: 708–19.

77. **Burton EJ, McKeith IG, Burn DJ, et al**. Cerebral atrophy in Parkinson's disease with and without dementia: a comparison with Alzheimer's disease, dementia with Lewy bodies and controls. Brain 2004; **127**: 791–800.

78. **Beyer MK, Larsen JP, Aarsland D**. Gray matter atrophy in Parkinson disease with dementia and dementia with Lewy bodies. Neurology 2007; **69**: 747–54.

79. **Lee JE, Park B, Song SK, et al**. A comparison of gray and white matter density in patients with Parkinson's disease dementia and dementia with Lewy bodies using voxel-based morphometry. Mov Disord 2010; **25**: 28–34.

80. **Kamagata K, Motoi Y, Abe O, et al**. White matter alteration of the cingulum in Parkinson disease with and without dementia: evaluation by diffusion tensor tract-specific analysis. Am J Neuroradiol 2012; **33**: 890–5.

81. **Sanchez-Castaneda C, Rene R, Ramirez-Ruiz B, et al**. Frontal and associative visual areas related to visual hallucinations in dementia with Lewy bodies and Parkinson's disease with dementia. Mov Disord 2010; **25**: 615–22.

82. **Colloby S, O'Brien J**. Functional imaging in Parkinson's disease and dementia with Lewy bodies. J Geriatr Psychiatry Neurol 2004; **17**: 158–63.

83. **Kasama S, Tachibana H, Kawabata K, et al**. Cerebral blood flow in Parkinson's disease, dementia with Lewy bodies, and Alzheimer's disease according to three-dimensional stereotactic surface projection imaging. Dement Geriatr Cogn Disord 2005; **19**: 266–75.

84. **Mito Y, Yoshida K, Yabe I, et al**. Brain 3D-SSP SPECT analysis in dementia with Lewy bodies, Parkinson's disease with and without dementia, and Alzheimer's disease. Clin Neurol Neurosurg 2005; **107**: 396–403.

85. **Firbank MJ, Molloy S, McKeith IG, et al**. Longitudinal change in ^{99m}TcHMPAO cerebral perfusion SPECT in Parkinson's disease over one year. J Neurol Neurosurg Psychiatry 2005; **76**: 1448–51.

86. **Firbank MJ, Burn DJ, McKeith IG, O'Brien JT**. Longitudinal study of cerebral blood flow SPECT in Parkinson's disease with dementia, and dementia with Lewy bodies. Int J Geriatr Psychiatry 2005; **20**: 776–82.

87. **Osaki Y, Morita Y, Fukumoto M, et al**. Cross-sectional and longitudinal studies of three-dimensional stereotactic surface projection SPECT analysis in Parkinson's disease. Mov Disord 2009; **24**: 1475–80.

88. **O'Brien JT, Firbank MJ, Mosimann UP, et al**. Change in perfusion, hallucinations and fluctuations in consciousness in dementia with Lewy bodies. Psychiatry Res 2005; **139**: 79–88.

89. **O'Brien JT, Colloby S, Fenwick J, et al**. Dopamine transporter loss visualized with FP-CIT SPECT in the differential diagnosis of dementia with Lewy bodies. Arch Neurol 2004; **61**: 919–25.

90. **Walker Z, Costa DC, Walker RW, et al**. Striatal dopamine transporter in dementia with Lewy bodies and Parkinson disease: a comparison. Neurology 2004; **62**: 1568–72.

91. **Colloby SJ, Williams ED, Burn DJ, et al**. Progression of dopaminergic degeneration in dementia with Lewy bodies and Parkinson's disease with and without dementia assessed using 123I-FP-CIT SPECT. Eur J Nucl Med Mol Imaging 2005; **32**: 1176–85.

92. **Maetzler W, Liepelt I, Reimold M, et al**. Cortical PIB binding in Lewy body disease is associated with Alzheimer-like characteristics. Neurobiol Dis 2009; **34**: 107–12.

93. **Gomperts SN, Rentz DM, Moran E, et al**. Imaging amyloid deposition in Lewy body diseases. Neurology 2008; **71**: 903–10.

94. **Pugnetti L, Baglio F, Farina E, et al**. EEG evidence of posterior cortical disconnection in PD and related dementias. Int J Neurosci 2010; **120**: 88–98.

95. **Kurz MW, Schlitter AM, Larsen JP, et al**. Familial occurrence of dementia and parkinsonism: a systematic review. Dement Geriatr Cogn Disord 2006; **22**: 288–95.

96. **Bogaerts V, Engelborghs S, Kumar-Singh S, et al**. A novel locus for dementia with Lewy bodies: a clinically and genetically heterogeneous disorder. Brain 2007; **130**: 2277–91.

97. **Meeus B, Nuytemans K, Crosiers D, et al**. Comprehensive genetic and mutation analysis of familial dementia with Lewy bodies linked to 2q35–q36. J Alzheimers Dis 2010; **20**: 197–205.

98. **Meeus B, Theuns J, Van Broeckhoven C**. The genetics of dementia with Lewy bodies: what are we missing? Arch Neurol 2012; **69**: 1113–18.

99. **Nishioka K, Wider C, Vilarino-Güell C, et al**. Association of α-, β-, and γ-synuclein with diffuse Lewy body disease. Arch Neurol 2010; **67**: 970–5.

100. **Ferrer I, López-Gonzalez I, Carmona M, et al**. Neurochemistry and the non-motor aspects of PD. Neurobiol Dis 2012; **46**: 508–26.

101. **Creese B, Ballard C, Aarsland D, et al**. Determining the association of the 5HTTLPR polymorphism with delusions and hallucinations in Lewy body dementias. Am J Geriatr Psychiatry 2014; **22**: 580–6.

102. **Guimaraes B de C, Pereira AC, Rodrigues F da C, et al**. Glucocerebrosidase N370S and L444P mutations as risk factors for Parkinson's disease in Brazilian patients. Parkinsonism Relat Disord 2012; **18**: 688–9.

103. **Sidransky E, Lopez G**. The link between the GBA gene and parkinsonism. Lancet Neurol 2012; **11**: 986–98.

104. **McKeith I, Del Ser T, Spano P, et al**. Efficacy of rivastigmine in dementia with Lewy bodies: a randomised, double-blind, placebo-controlled international study. Lancet 2000; **356**: 2031–6.

105. **Mori E, Ikeda M, Kosaka K**. Donepezil for dementia with Lewy bodies: a randomized, placebo-controlled trial. Ann Neurol 2012; **72**: 41–52.

106. **Rowan E, McKeith IG, Saxby BK, et al**. Effects of donepezil on central processing speed and attentional measures in Parkinson's disease with dementia and dementia with Lewy bodies. Dement Geriatr Cogn Disord 2007; **23**: 161–7.

107. **Emre M, Aarsland D, Albanese A, et al**. Rivastigmine for dementia associated with Parkinson's disease. N Engl J Med 2004; **351**: 2509–18.

108. **Olin JT, Aarsland D, Meng X**. Rivastigmine in the treatment of dementia associated with Parkinson's disease: effects on activities of daily living. Dement Geriatr Cogn Disord 2010; **29**: 510–15.

109. **Dubois B, Tolosa E, Katzenschlager R, et al**. Donepezil in Parkinson's disease dementia: a randomized, double-blind efficacy and safety study. Mov Disord 2012; **27**: 1230–8.

110. **Rolinski M, Fox C, Maidment I, et al**. Cholinesterase inhibitors for dementia with Lewy bodies, Parkinson's disease dementia and cognitive impairment in Parkinson's disease. Cochrane Database Syst Rev 2012; **3**: CD006504.

111. **Thomas AJ, Burn DJ, Rowan EN, et al**. A comparison of the efficacy of donepezil in Parkinson's disease with dementia and dementia with Lewy bodies. Int J Geriatr Psychiatry 2005; **20**: 938–44.

112. **Minett TS, Thomas A, Wilkinson LM, et al**. What happens when donepezil is suddenly withdrawn? An open label trial in dementia with Lewy bodies and Parkinson's disease with dementia. Int J Geriatr Psychiatry 2003; **18**: 988–93.

113. **Aarsland D, Ballard C, Walker Z, et al**. Memantine in patients with Parkinson's disease dementia or dementia with Lewy bodies: a double-blind, placebo-controlled, multicentre trial. Lancet Neurol 2009; **8**: 613–18.

114. **Emre M, Tsolaki M, Bonuccelli U, et al**. Memantine for patients with Parkinson's disease dementia or dementia with Lewy bodies: a randomised, double-blind, placebo-controlled trial. Lancet Neurol 2010; **9**: 969–77.

115. **Ballard C, Hanney ML, Theodoulou M, et al.** The dementia antipsychotic withdrawal trial (DART-AD): long-term follow-up of a randomised placebo-controlled trial. Lancet Neurol 2009; **8**: 151–7.

116. **Kurlan R, Cummings J, Raman R, et al.** Quetiapine for agitation or psychosis in patients with dementia and parkinsonism. Neurology 2007; **68**: 1356–63.

117. **Culo S, Mulsant BH, Rosen J, et al.** Treating neuropsychiatric symptoms in dementia with Lewy bodies: a randomized controlled-trial. Alzheimer Dis Assoc Disord 2010; **24**: 360–4.

118. **McKeith I, Fairbairn A, Perry R, et al.** Neuroleptic sensitivity in patients with senile dementia of Lewy body type. Br Med J 1992; **305**: 673–8.

119. **Ballard C, Grace J, McKeith I, et al.** Neuroleptic sensitivity in dementia with Lewy bodies and Alzheimer's disease. Lancet 1998; **351**: 1032–3.

120. **Sadek J, Rockwood K.** Coma with accidental single dose of an atypical neuroleptic in a patient with Lewy body dementia. Am J Geriatr Psychiatry 2003; **11**: 112–13.

121. **Molloy S, McKeith IG, O'Brien JT, et al.** The role of levodopa in the management of dementia with Lewy bodies. J Neurol Neurosurg Psychiatry 2005; **76**: 1200–3.

122. **Molloy SA, Rowan EN, O'Brien JT, et al.** Effect of levodopa on cognitive function in Parkinson's disease with and without dementia and dementia with Lewy bodies. J Neurol Neurosurg Psychiatry 2006; **77**: 1323–8.

123. **Molloy S, Minett T, O'Brien JT, et al.** Levodopa use and sleep in patients with dementia with Lewy bodies. Mov Disord 2009; **24**: 609–12.

124. **Goldman JG, Goetz CG, Brandabur M, et al.** Effects of dopaminergic medications on psychosis and motor function in dementia with Lewy bodies. Mov Disord 2008; **23**: 2248–50.

125. **Wood LD.** Clinical review and treatment of select adverse effects of dopamine receptor agonists in Parkinson's disease. Drugs Aging 2010; **27**: 295–310.

126. **Cummings J, Isaacson S, Mills R, et al.** Pimavanserin for patients with Parkinson's disease psychosis: a randomised, placebo-controlled phase 3 trial. Lancet 2014; **383**: 533–40.

127. **Emre M, Aarsland D, Brown R, et al.** Clinical diagnostic criteria for dementia associated with Parkinson's disease. Mov Disord 2007; **22**: 1689–1707; quiz 1837.

Chapter 19

Spectrum of disorders with dementia and parkinsonism

Jaime Kulisevsky and Javier Pagonabarraga

Introduction

Advances in the neuropathological basis of dementias in the past 5 to 10 years have expanded our knowledge about the different nosological entities that cause dementia associated with parkinsonism. While dementia has been clearly defined as a frequent and disabling condition associated with Parkinson's disease (PD) [1], and dementia with Lewy bodies is currently considered the second commonest cause of neurodegenerative dementia in older people [2], the actual prevalence and impact of cognitive deficits in other degenerative diseases that develop dementia and parkinsonism has not been so clearly stated.

In the 1970s, severe cognitive dysfunction leading to prototypical 'subcortical' dementia was described in patients with progressive supranuclear palsy (PSP) [3]. Patients with corticobasal degeneration (CBD) are known to suffer from profound language and visuospatial disturbances with a clinically relevant impact on global cognitive function [4]. Interestingly, some patients with PSP or CBD may present with cognitive decline instead of motor features [5], and CBD can be the underlying aetiology in patients diagnosed with frontotemporal dementia (FTD) [6]. Although dementia is an exclusion criterion for the diagnosis of multiple system atrophy (MSA), several studies have reported prominent cognitive deficits in patients with MSA when compared with control subjects [7, 8].

Frontal–subcortical circuits link the basal ganglia with regions of the frontal lobe and thalamus in functional systems that regulate motor function, cognition, emotions, and behaviour [9]. Dysfunction of frontal–subcortical circuits may account for the frequent development of cognitive and behavioural disturbances in patients with basal ganglia disorders presenting with parkinsonism. Cognitive dysfunction in diseases with parkinsonism is usually associated with a pattern of deficits characterized by impairment in cognitive domains subserved by frontal, frontostriatal, and parietal cognitive networks, namely attention and concentration, executive functions, verbal fluency, praxis, and visuospatial functioning [10, 11].

A list of major neurodegenerative disorders causing dementia and parkinsonism is given in Table 19.1.

Tauopathies and cognition

Progressive supranuclear palsy

PSP is an adult-onset neurodegenerative disorder characterized by an atypical akinetic–rigid syndrome that is usually non-responsive to levodopa, early postural instability, and vertical supra-nuclear-gaze palsy. Recent epidemiological studies have shown that the disorder is more common

Table 19.1 Spectrum of major neurodegenerative disorders causing dementia and Parkinsonism

Tauopathies:
Progressive supranuclear palsy (PSP)
Corticobasal degeneration (CBD)
Frontotemporal lobar degeneration (FTLD):
Pick's disease
Frontotemporal dementia with parkinsonism (FTDP)
Multiple system tauopathy with pre-senile dementia (MSTD)
α-Synucleinopathies:
Lewy body disease:
Parkinson's disease
Dementia with Lewy bodies
Multiple system atrophy (MSA)
Tardopathies [TAR-DNA-binding protein-43 (TDP-43) proteinopathies]:
Frontotemporal lobar degeneration with ubiquitin-positive inclusions (FTLD-U)
Frontotemporal lobar degeneration with motor-neuron disease (FTLD-MND)
Frontotemporal lobar degeneration with motor-neuron disease associated with repeat expansions in the *C9ORF72* gene [12]
Amyloidopathies:
Alzheimer's disease
Alzheimer's disease associated with mutations in the genes encoding amyloid precursor protein (*APP*), presenilin 1 (*PSEN1*), or presenilin 2 (*PSEN2*)
Miscellaneous:
Fragile X-associated tremor/ataxia syndrome (FXTAS)
Spinocerebellar ataxias (SCA type 2, 17, 21)
Fahr's syndrome (bilateral striopallidodentate calcification)
Huntington's disease

than previously recognized, with an average annual incidence for ages 50–99 years of around 5.3 cases per 100,000 population [13].

Although in their seminal paper Steele et al. [14] reported cognitive impairment in seven out of the nine patients they evaluated, and indeed the characteristic pattern of neuropsychological deficits observed in PSP gave rise to the term 'subcortical dementia' [3], traditionally more attention was paid to the motor and oculomotor abnormalities that aid in the differentiation of PSP from PD than to the cognitive and behavioural disturbances associated with it.

Behavioural and cognitive changes occur in 50 to 90% of patients with PSP, often within the first year of the disease [15, 16]. In cross-sectional studies, frequency of dementia in PSP is about 55% [17].

Cognitive changes were initially reported by Albert et al. [3] and described as a prototypical 'subcortical dementia'. The pattern of deficits could be differentiated from that seen in patients with 'cortical dementia', who usually present with aphasia, apraxia, and/or agnosia, and it was suggested that the symptoms found in PSP were similar to those which had previously been described in patients with frontal lobe lesions [11, 18]. The 'subcortical dementia' described by Albert et al. [3] was characterized by a cluster of neuropsychological deficits including forgetfulness, slowing of thought processes, emotional or personality changes (apathy, depression, irritability), and impaired ability to manipulate acquired knowledge. The neuropsychological basis for all these deficits seems to be the slowing in performance of cognitive functions rather than primary dysfunction of the cortical systems responsible for each cognitive domain, so that cognitive functions may be strikingly preserved if the patient is given sufficient time to respond. As PSP was thought to almost exclusively affect subcortical nuclei (including the pallidum and caudate nucleus, red nucleus, subthalamic nucleus, and substantia nigra), the authors proposed that cognitive impairment in PSP was due to bilateral frontal–subcortical dysfunction [3]. In keeping with this suggestion, neuroimaging studies have shown PSP to affect both the pre-synaptic and post-synaptic aspects of the dopaminergic and cholinergic neurotransmitter systems that project their efferent connections to the prefrontal cortex, and lead to early and clinically relevant cognitive dysfunction [19, 20–22].

PSP patients have a dramatically slowed speed of information processing, early and severe executive dysfunction with problems in orienting attentional resources, difficulty in planning and shifting conceptual sets, and prominent recall deficits with moderate forgetfulness [23, 24]. These cognitive deficits can also be found in PD patients and other akinetic–rigid syndromes, but patients with PSP show a greater decline in attention, processing speed, set-shifting, and categorization abilities than PD or MSA patients [25, 26]. Slowed speed of information processing and execution of responses is particularly altered in PSP. In order to disentangle whether this slowness is directly related to cognitive dysfunction or to bradykinesia, Dubois et al. [27] measured reaction times using tasks with different levels of cognitive complexity but the same motor demands. They found that central processing time in PSP is significantly increased when performing complex tasks compared with both a PD and a control group, while cognitive speed in the PD group was similar to controls. These results have been further replicated in studies using event-related potentials showing dramatically increased response latencies in complex attentional tasks in PSP that have not been observed in other dementias or parkinsonian syndromes [28].

Executive function is clearly altered in PSP, with impairment in most tests sensitive to frontal lobe dysfunction [24]. In particular, PSP patients show impairment in tasks of working memory, reasoning, problem-solving, conceptualization, planning, and social cognition [29, 30]. Characteristically, PSP patients also show perseverative errors during the performance of executive tasks, as well as deficits of response inhibition that seem not to be so frequent in other parkinsonian syndromes such as PD or MSA [29]. Similar to patients with focal prefrontal lesions, PSP patients show decreased ability to inhibit previously learned cognitive responses, while PD patients show more evident deficits in the maintenance of new cognitive programmes [31]. This cognitive dissociation has been linked to differential involvement of the medial prefrontal cortex (associated with impaired response inhibition) [32], and dysfunction of circuits connecting the striatum with the dorsolateral prefrontal cortex (associated with impairment in set maintenance) [33]. Recently, the inability to inhibit cognitive or motor responses has been claimed as a useful clinical marker that can help to discriminate PSP from PD [34]. The applause sign—the inability to stop clapping the hands after three times—was observed in 71% of PSP patients but in none of the PD patients [34]. Perseverative behaviours, due to the inability to stop an automatic activity once it has been released, have been related to dysfunction of the medial aspects of the prefrontal cortex and the caudate nucleus [35].

Thus, in PSP there seems to be a more diffuse impairment of prefrontal-based cognitive functions compared with PD. In fact, performance in a simple phonemic fluency test—which represents a reliable marker of prefrontal function—is able to separate PSP patients from those with PD. In patients with parkinsonian syndromes in the early stages (PD versus PSP versus CBD with 1–4 years of disease duration), performance on a phonemic fluency task producing seven or fewer words in a minute recently yielded high positive (81%) and negative (95%) predictive value for the diagnosis of PSP [36]. Recent data have shown direct neocortical degeneration in the prefrontal cortex beyond the well-established degeneration of subcortical nuclei [16]. It is known that clinical heterogeneity and atypical presentations result in frequent clinical misdiagnosis in the early stages of PSP [37]. In 2005, Williams et al. [38] identified two clinical phenotypes in pathologically proven PSP patients. Patients assigned to the Richardson's syndrome (RS) group (54% of all cases) developed the classical syndrome associated with PSP, with early onset of postural instability and falls, supranuclear vertical-gaze palsy, and a more severe cognitive dysfunction. By contrast, patients in the PSP-parkinsonism (PSP-P) group (32% of all cases) were characterized by asymmetric onset, tremor, and a moderate initial therapeutic response to levodopa, and were frequently confused with PD. More recently, a third type of presentation has been described [16]. In a prospective study of 152 patients with a clinical diagnosis of PSP given after a disease duration of 5 years, 20% of the subjects had predominant cognitive dysfunction and behavioural changes at disease onset associated with mild instability problems and absent or mild oculomotor disturbances. The most common initial misdiagnosis in this group was dementia, in particular FTD (35%). Volumetric magnetic resonance imaging (MRI) studies have shown that PSP patients have a greater loss of grey matter volume in both the medial and lateral aspects of the prefrontal cortex than with MSA and PD patients, which correlates with the degree of executive dysfunction but not with motor dysfunction [39]. When measuring loss of grey and white matter volume in PSP subgroups, patients with predominant cognitive versus parkinsonian symptoms have been found to have bilateral specific and higher atrophy in the prefrontal lobe [40], which reinforces the hypothesis that cognitive impairment in PSP is a direct consequence of the degeneration of the prefrontal cortex along with degeneration of subcortical nuclei.

In summary, all these findings characterize PSP as a heterogeneous clinical entity spanning a broad clinical spectrum of symptoms that may manifest as either a predominant motor disorder resembling PD, an atypical parkinsonism with postural instability, oculomotor disturbances, and cognitive impairment, or as a predominant dementing disease with prominent and early behavioural disturbances resembling FTD. Recently, clinical and pathological studies have shown that PSP can present as progressive non-fluent aphasia, with subsequent development of the parkinsonian symptoms and oculomotor disturbances of typical PSP after a delay of 3–8 years [41–43]. Such patients are more likely to progress to mutism, and to develop limb-kinetic apraxia, but progression to dementia is slower. PSP patients with progressive non-fluent aphasia have less prominent midbrain atrophy but more marked prefrontal atrophy compared with typical PSP [44].

Behavioural changes are also a frequent and characteristic feature in PSP [45]. In the first descriptive study of neuropsychiatric symptoms in PSP, almost all patients suffered from moderate to severe apathy (91%), and 36% exhibited disinhibition. Depression (18%), anxiety (18%), and irritability (9%) were infrequent, and hallucinations or delusions were not reported [46]. Apathy was significantly associated with executive dysfunction, suggesting that both cognitive dysfunction and apathy in PSP are mediated by degeneration in similar prefrontal areas or by dysfunction of similar frontal–subcortical connections [46, 47]. The impact of apathy in PSP is further stressed by the fact that PSP can be discriminated from PD and AD by more severe apathy and less depression [48, 49]. A consistent relationship of apathy with disinhibition is further evidence of the important role of the dysfunction of the orbitofrontal and medial frontal circuits in the behavioural disturbances of PSP [48], which has been replicated in recent studies showing that frontal atrophy in volumetric MRI studies correlates with behavioural changes in PSP [50]. Although hallucinations have been infrequently reported, they can be present in 9 to 16% of PSP patients [51, 52]. More detailed descriptions of behavioural disorders in PSP patients have shown the occurrence of behaviours typically ascribed to patients with FTD. In a large series of patients meeting the criteria for clinically probable PSP, disinhibition was found in 32% of the sample and eating disorders appeared in up to 40% of patients [53]. Abnormal eating behaviours, one of the core and more specific features of FTD, have been described in PSP in the form of 'greed for food', following an impulsive behaviour in which patients eat 'voraciously' and 'without biting enough before swallowing', which seems related to a need or urge to eat 'faster and faster', but without the features of hyperphagia or hyperorality [54]. In a comparative MRI study of PSP and FTD, a very similar pattern of frontal cortical atrophy was seen in the two groups, with PSP patients displaying significant atrophy in the frontal rectal gyrus, anterior temporal lobes, and thalamus [55].

Corticobasal degeneration

CBD is currently defined as a progressive neurodegenerative disease that typically presents with asymmetrical parkinsonism and cognitive dysfunction. In the initial clinical descriptions of CBD, symptoms of higher-order cortical dysfunction were restricted to ideomotor and limb-kinetic apraxia, and, in some cases, the development of alien hand syndrome, while clinically relevant cognitive and behavioural disturbances were only reported in advanced stages of the disease [56, 57].

The presence of cognitive impairment in CBD is now widely recognized. In the 1990s, detailed neuropsychological analysis of autopsy-proven cases showed not only that cognitive defects are common in CBD but that they may be present from the early stages of the disease and may help in differential diagnosis [5]. In clinico-pathological studies, a specific pattern of cognitive impairment has commonly been evident at presentation, whereas extrapyramidal motor abnormalities were present in less than half of the patients [58]. Analysing the natural history of 14 patients with autopsy-proven CBD, Wenning et al. [59] observed that 64% of them presented with ideomotor apraxia and 36% with features of 'cortical-type' dementia at the first visit. On disease evolution, the development of lateralized and focal cognitive syndromes (i.e. aphasia in 36%) and a progressive frontal syndrome led to the diagnosis of dementia in 6 out of 14 patients (43%). Moreover, 58% of patients suffered from apathy, irritability, or disinhibited behaviours. Additional data about the importance of cognitive deficits in CBD come from subsequent larger clinical series showing that 25% (36/147) of CBD patients presenting with predominant motor symptoms develop dementia during the course of the disease [60]. Further clinico-pathological studies have broadened the clinical spectrum of CBD, which can present with various clinical syndromes. Beyond the classical corticobasal syndrome (unilateral and asymmetric parkinsonism, dystonia, ideomotor apraxia, and myoclonus), CBD may also present with either progressive non-fluent aphasia, speech apraxia, PSP-like syndrome (vertical supranuclear-gaze palsy, early postural instability), or posterior cortical atrophy syndrome [61]. Conversely, classical corticobasal syndrome may be an atypical presentation of other common neurodegenerative diseases such as AD [62], PSP, or Creutzfeldt–Jakob disease [63].

Typical symptoms of FTD have also been described in CBD at disease onset, even in the absence of associated features of classical corticobasal syndrome [64, 65]. Initial reports have been confirmed in pathological studies showing a final pathological diagnosis of CBD (30% of tau-positive cases) in patients with a clinical diagnosis of FTD [6]. As in PSP, CBD patients with symptoms resembling FTD, such as altered awareness, personal and social disinhibition, and altered control of action, show a striking loss of grey matter volume and white matter integrity in medial prefrontal cortex structures [66].

The neuropsychological pattern and severity of cognitive dysfunction in CBD is highly variable between patients, but the most characteristic symptoms are asymmetric limb apraxia (usually ideomotor and limb-kinetic, with deficits in posture imitation, symbolic gesture execution, and object utilization), constructional and visuospatial difficulties, executive dysfunction, acalculia, and progressive non-fluent aphasia [4, 67] (see Table 19.2).

The most frequent cognitive symptom in CBD is apraxia, which is present in up to 70% of patients [69]. Limb apraxia in CBD is asymmetric and most often ideomotor in nature. Ideomotor apraxia impairs the ability to use tools and mimic their use, but preserves the recognition of the pattern and temporal sequence of actions when performed by others [70]. Limb-kinetic apraxia (usually coexisting with ideomotor apraxia) has been reported less often in CBD, and can be differentiated from ideomotor apraxia because it is more distal, unilateral, impairs only the production of fine finger movements and hand postures, and affects all kinds of movement, regardless of its instrumental purpose (impairment of transitive and intransitive movements) [71]. Ideational apraxia, the impairment in conceptualizing and planning the sequence of a complex motor behaviour, is infrequent in CBD, and develops in advanced stages of the disease [70]. Visuoperceptual difficulties, the difficulty in perceiving the spatial relationships of visual stimuli, are responsible for the constructional apraxia observed in CBD, especially in patients with predominant right-hemispheric frontoparietal degeneration [72]. Patients with constructional apraxia are not able to assemble into action motor behaviours that require the integration of spatial relationships [73]. In CBD, it is mainly noted by progressive impairment in drawing and writing, which is frequent in early disease or even as a presenting feature [74].

Aphasia and speech difficulties are common in CBD and represent a good clinical marker in the differential diagnosis between PD, PSP, and MSA [75, 76]. Language disturbances in CBD resemble those in FTD patients with a non-fluent progressive aphasic form of presentation [75]. Clinico-pathological studies have confirmed the development of speech and language disturbances in

Table 19.2 Pattern of cognitive and behavioural disturbances in CBD

Cognitive dysfunction [4]:
Limb apraxia (ideomotor, limb-kinetic, and ideational)
Constructional apraxia
Visuospatial difficulties (line orientation, figure rotation, motion perception)
Executive dysfunction (medial and lateral prefrontal cortex deficits)
Acalculia
Progressive non-fluent aphasia
Speech apraxia
Behavioural disturbances [68]:
75% depression
40% apathy
20% irritability
20% agitation
<10% disinhibition

CBD [5], although detailed neuropsychological investigations are needed to disclose their actual prevalence and severity in the early stages. Neuropsychological studies assessing language in CBD have shown that most patients (65%) develop progressive aphasia during the course of their illness [77]. In particular, language at baseline is more impaired in CBD patients with primarily cognitive presentation, though the evolution to aphasia in the course of the disease is similar in both primarily motor and cognitive forms of CBD [78]. Aphasia has been observed in 44% of autopsy-proven CBD cases [4].

Impairment on tests of frontal lobe function is one of the most consistent findings in CBD [79]. Measures of working memory, set-shifting, set acquisition, resistance to interference, conceptualization, mental flexibility, and social judgement [80] have been shown to be affected early and severely in the disease [67]. As is the case in PSP, these deficits highlight the extensive lateral and medial prefrontal cortex and frontal–subcortical degeneration present in tauopathies.

Visuospatial skills are usually impaired, with poor performance on tests of line orientation, mental rotation of figures, and perception of motion, reflecting a predominant dysfunction of the dorsal occipito-parietal pathway rather than a dysfunction of the ventral visual stream, which is more involved in the perception of shapes, colours, and object identification [25, 79].

Findings of memory impairment in CBD are inconsistent, with some studies reporting episodic memory impairment whereas in others memory was not altered. What seems clearer is that episodic rather than semantic memory is more preserved in CBD compared with AD, suggesting that dysfunction of semantic networks in the anterior and lateral temporal cortex, rather than hippocampal/medial temporal degeneration, may account for the memory deficits seen in CBD [81].

Frontotemporal dementia with parkinsonism

In 1996, an international consensus conference was held in order to define the cognitive, behavioural, and motor disturbances of families with FTD with parkinsonism linked to chromosome 17 (FTDP-17) [82]. The group discussed 25 families with similar symptoms of familial adult-onset behavioural disturbances, frontal lobe dementia, and parkinsonism, and identified 13 kindreds with sufficient evidence for linkage of this phenotype to chromosome 17 [82]. These families shared common, although heterogeneous, clinical features, with symptoms starting typically in the fifth decade, patients developing behavioural (disinhibition, loss of personal awareness, apathy, mental rigidity, defective judgement, stereotyped behaviours, and hyperorality with hyperphagia) and cognitive disturbances (speech disturbances with non-fluent aphasia, echolalia, palilalia, mutism, executive dysfunction, relative preservation of memory, orientation, and visuospatial functions) typical of frontotemporal lobar degeneration. Either early or during the course of the disease, patients also presented parkinsonian symptoms with early postural instability, absence of resting tremor, poor response to levodopa, and, occasionally, supranuclear ophthalmoplegia or apraxia of eyelid opening [82–85]. At that point, participants in the consensus conference decided to classify *all* these patients under the term FTDP-17, and stressed the need to identify the gene or genes responsible for this disorder [82].

In the past 5 years, advances in immunocytochemistry and molecular genetics have expanded our knowledge about the different disorders that can manifest as FTDP-17. In many kindreds with FTDP-17, mutations in the gene encoding the microtubule-associated protein tau (*MAPT*) on chromosome 17 have been found, with patients showing tau-positive inclusions on neuropathology [86]. In several other kindreds with FTDP-17, ubiquitin-positive inclusions were described, but no associated tau pathology or mutations in the *MAPT* gene were observed. In 2006, this group of patients was better defined by the identification of mutations in the gene encoding progranulin (*PGRN*), which is only 1.7 Mb centromeric to *MAPT* on chromosome 17. Symptoms of patients with *MAPT* and *PGRN* mutations are almost identical to those previously described in FTDP-17, although some clinical features may help to differentiate patients with *MAPT* or *PGRN* mutations [87]. In FTDP with *MAPT* mutations, the syndromes of mild cognitive impairment, probable AD, semantic dementia, or corticobasal syndrome have been rarely described, a few cases have been diagnosed with amyotrophic lateral sclerosis, and no cases have been reported with symptoms of posterior cortical atrophy or suggestive of dementia with Lewy bodies. In FTDP with *PRGN* mutations the syndromic diagnoses have been more variable, with patients presenting with predominant memory impairment, limb apraxia, parkinsonism, or visuospatial dysfunction; the development of a corticobasal syndrome has been frequent in the cases reported thus far [88].

In summary, the nosological entity previously called FTDP-17 is now known to include patients with different mutations and different neuropathological features. With the possible discovery of new mutations to come, current terminology for patients developing symptoms of FTDP should indicate if those patients are carrying mutations in either the *MAPT* or the *PRGN* gene.

Multiple system atrophy and cognition

Multiple system atrophy (MSA) is an adult-onset, sporadic, progressive, neurodegenerative disorder that presents clinically with autonomic failure and motor impairment, with variable combinations of poorly levodopa–responsive parkinsonism, cerebellar ataxia, and corticospinal tract dysfunction. Eighty per cent of MSA patients present with predominant parkinsonism (MSA-P) caused by nigrostriatal degeneration, while the remaining 20% present with predominant cerebellar ataxia (MSA-C) that is associated with olivopontocerebellar atrophy [89].

Neuropathologically, MSA is defined as an α-synucleinopathy and is characterized by degeneration of nigrostriatal and olivopontocerebellar structures accompanied by profuse aggregates of distinctive cytoplasmic inclusions within oligodendroglial cells (GCIs), formed by filamentous α-synuclein and a number of other proteins [90].

As is the case for CBD, the original descriptions of patients with MSA emphasized the movement disorder characteristic of the disease. To date, a minority of studies have focused on associated cognitive and behavioural disturbances. However, and although dementia still remains as an exclusion criterion for the diagnosis of MSA [89], several studies have reported prominent cognitive deficits in patients with MSA when compared with control subjects [7, 8].

The first study which assessed cognitive function in MSA using comprehensive neuropsychological testing was published in 1992 by Robbins et al. [91]. The authors used tests sensitive to frontal lobe dysfunction, memory as well as learning deficits, and compared performance with a control group. The neuropsychological deficits in MSA patients showed a prominent frontal-lobe-like syndrome, with significant deficits in all three of the frontal tests and verbal fluency, in the absence of consistent impairments in language or visual perception, and no consistent memory or learning deficits. Nevertheless, neuropsychological performance was heterogeneous, with a group of patients with high degree of intellectual competence despite severe physical disability, others with deficits restricted to tests sensitive to frontal lobe dysfunction, and others exhibiting a broader range of impairment, with clear deficits in executive tasks, memory, and language [91]. Recently, a case of MSA presenting with prominent semantic language deficits has been reported [92].

Retrospective studies have consistently reported selective impairment of executive functions in MSA. However, memory and visuospatial impairments similar to the pattern of cognitive impairment seen in PD have also been observed [93]. Several cross-sectional studies have shown MSA and PD patients to display a similar profile of cognitive dysfunction, performing poorly in visuospatial organization, construction, and visuomotor ability tests [94, 95]. Patients with MSA were found to be impaired in tests of verbal fluency, working memory, attentional set-shifting, set acquisition, planning, free recall verbal memory, and response inhibition [96, 97]. Compared with PD and PSP, executive deficits in MSA were of similar severity to those in PD, but less severe than in PSP [15]. In another cross-sectional study, executive dysfunction in MSA was even more severe and diffuse than in PD [96]. In the only comparative and longitudinal study reported to date, PD and MSA patients showed a similar overall cognitive performance and a similar pattern of cognitive impairment at baseline, except for a higher impairment of verbal fluency in MSA. After a mean follow-up of 21 months, patients with MSA deteriorated significantly more than those with PD [25]. In a recent study including motor assessment, neuropsychological examinations, MRI, and Pittsburgh compound B (PIB) PET imaging, dementia was found in 15% of MSA patients [98]. Amyloid pathology played a limited role in dementia in this sample of 152 MSA patients, and cortical thinning followed a very similar pattern to that described in dementia associated with PD [99], indicating that widespread cortical extension of oligodendroglial inclusions (involving both the prefrontal and posterior cortical areas) leads to dementia in MSA patients [98].

The first study that examined cognitive deficits in MSA-C (mean disease duration of 4.6 years) showed evidence of mild cognitive impairment, with impaired verbal memory and executive function, but none of the subjects fulfilling criteria for dementia [8]. A recent comparative study of cognitive deficits in MSA-P (mean disease duration 3.2 years) and MSA-C (mean disease duration 2.6 years), showed MSA-P patients to present with more severe and widespread cognitive dysfunction, with impairments in verbal fluency, executive function, and visuospatial and constructional tests [7]. Patients with MSA-C showed milder impairment only in visuospatial and constructional functions. Cognitive impairment in MSA-P correlated with decreased perfusion in the prefrontal cortex and posterior parietal lobes (^{99m}Tc-ethylcysteine dimer single-photon emission computed tomography), while cognitive impairment in MSA-C correlated with cerebellar hypoperfusion [7].

In accordance with these findings, a recent study identified three groups of patients with MSA with a differential degree of cognitive impairment and a different pattern of deficits in glucose metabolism as assessed by fluorodeoxyglucose PET [100]. Patients in group I had a significantly shorter disease duration, frequent memory deficits and frontal/executive dysfunction, and hypometabolism in the frontal cortex. Patients in groups II and III displayed multidomain cognitive impairment, had more severe motor deficits and showed hypometabolism not only in the frontal but also in the parieto-temporal cortex and the bilateral caudate nucleus. These findings suggest that cognitive impairment in MSA is related to cortical hypometabolism beginning in the frontal cortex and spreading to the parieto-temporal cortex [100].

Recent neuroimaging studies have demonstrated that cortical atrophy in MSA is more severe than had previously been considered. MSA is associated with volume loss in widespread cortical regions, particularly involving the lateral prefrontal cortex, but also the orbitofrontal cortex, posterior parietal cortex, hippocampus, insula, caudate nucleus, putamen, primary sensorimotor cortex, corpus callosum, and supplementary motor area [101–103].

The presence of dementia as a non-supporting feature of MSA imposes a selection bias in research studies which include patients with a clinical diagnosis. Likewise the accuracy of data regarding cognitive impairment and dementia in studies carrying out a retrospective clinical analysis of autopsy-proven cases of MSA is limited. Furthermore, it is noteworthy that most published studies comparing cognition in PD, PSP, and MSA did not include PD or PSP patients with dementia, suggesting that selection bias may question the generalization of their results.

Even though cognitive impairment seems to be of similar severity in PD and MSA, and the degree of cortical atrophy seems to be even greater in MSA, no studies have been published on the actual prevalence of dementia in MSA. A shorter disease duration, and the fact that dementia does not appear as a major complaint in patients with otherwise severe and very disabling motor symptoms, may account for the lack of data on dementia in MSA [101]. Nevertheless, data presented in this review allow us to state that cognitive impairment in MSA is common and is of similar severity to that in age and education-matched subjects with PD.

Conclusion

Disorders of the basal ganglia share a distinctive pattern of cognitive deficits, predominantly in tests of frontal lobe function. A 'frontostriatal' pattern of cognitive impairment, consisting of a frontal lobe-like syndrome without primary amnesia or genuine cortical deficits such as apraxia, aphasia, or agnosia is the classical syndrome associated with basal ganglia diseases. Recent pathological investigations, however, have revealed widespread and moderate to severe cortical atrophy in PSP, CBD, and MSA. The greater cognitive decline of PSP patients in prefrontal-based cognitive functions is probably related to the prominent frontal deafferentiation associated with direct premotor and prefrontal involvement. Likewise, progressive and significant cortical involvement in prefrontal and posterior parietal areas explain the predominant dysexecutive and visuospatial deficits found in patients with MSA. Recent advances in immunohistochemistry and molecular genetics have helped to refine the nosological entity of FTDP-17. Mutations in the *MAPT* and *PGRN* genes determine the clinical and pathological heterogeneities previously described in patients with FTDP-17. Thus, the term FTD with parkinsonism seems more adequate than FTDP-17.

References

1. **Goetz CG, Emre M, Dubois B**. Parkinson's disease dementia: definitions, guidelines, and research perspectives in diagnosis. Ann Neurol 2008; **64**(Suppl. 2): S81–S92.
2. **McKeith I, Mintzer J, Aarsland D, et al**. Dementia with Lewy bodies. Lancet Neurol 2004; **3**: 19–28.
3. **Albert ML, Feldman RG, Willis AL**. The 'subcortical dementia' of progressive supranuclear palsy. J Neurol Neurosurg Psychiatry 1974; **37**: 121–30.
4. **Graham NL, Bak TH, Hodges JR**. Corticobasal degeneration as a cognitive disorder. Mov Disord 2003; **18**: 1224–32.
5. **Bergeron C, Davis A, Lang AE**. Corticobasal ganglionic degeneration and progressive supranuclear palsy presenting with cognitive decline. Brain Pathol 1998; **8**: 355–65.
6. **Hodges JR, Davies RR, Xuereb JH, et al**. Clinicopathological correlates in frontotemporal dementia. Ann Neurol 2004; **56**: 399–406.
7. **Kawai Y, Suenaga M, Takeda A, et al**. Cognitive impairments in multiple system atrophy: MSA-C vs MSA-P. Neurology 2008; **70**: 1390–6.
8. **Burk K, Daum I, Rub U**. Cognitive function in multiple system atrophy of the cerebellar type. Mov Disord 2006; **21**: 772–6.
9. **Cummings JL**. Frontal-subcortical circuits and human behavior. Arch Neurol 1993; **50**: 873–80.
10. **Salmon DP, Filoteo JV**. Neuropsychology of cortical versus subcortical dementia syndromes. Semin Neurol 2007; **27**: 7–21.
11. **Cummings JL, Benson DF**. Subcortical dementia. Review of an emerging concept. Arch Neurol 1984; **41**: 874–9.
12. **Galimberti D, Fenoglio C, Serpente M, et al**. Autosomal dominant frontotemporal lobar degeneration due to the C9ORF72 hexanucleotide repeat expansion: late-onset psychotic clinical presentation. Biol Psychiatry 2013; **74**: 384–91.
13. **Schrag A, Ben-Shlomo Y, Quinn NP**. Prevalence of progressive supranuclear palsy and multiple system atrophy: a cross-sectional study. Lancet 1999; **354**: 1771–5.

14. **Steele JC, Richardson JC, Olszewski J.** Progressive supranuclear palsy. A heterogeneous degeneration involving the brain stem, basal ganglia and cerebellum with vertical gaze and pseudobulbar palsy, nuchal dystonia and dementia. Arch Neurol 1964; **10**: 333–59.

15. **Bak TH, Crawford LM, Hearn VC, et al.** Subcortical dementia revisited: similarities and differences in cognitive function between progressive supranuclear palsy (PSP), corticobasal degeneration (CBD) and multiple system atrophy (MSA). Neurocase 2005; **11**: 268–73.

16. **Kaat LD, Boon AJ, Kamphorst W, et al.** Frontal presentation in progressive supranuclear palsy. Neurology 2007; **69**: 723–9.

17. **Menza MA, Cocchiola J, Golbe LI.** Psychiatric symptoms in progressive supranuclear palsy. Psychosomatics 1995; **36**: 550–4.

18. **Nauta WJ.** The problem of the frontal lobe: a reinterpretation. J Psychiatr Res 1971; **8**: 167–87.

19. **Pirker W, Asenbaum S, Bencsits G, et al.** [123I]beta-CIT SPECT in multiple system atrophy, progressive supranuclear palsy, and corticobasal degeneration. Mov Disord 2000; **15**: 1158–67.

20. **Kim YJ, Ichise M, Ballinger JR, et al.** Combination of dopamine transporter and D2 receptor SPECT in the diagnostic evaluation of PD, MSA, and PSP. Mov Disord 2002; **17**: 303–12.

21. **Shinotoh H, Namba H, Yamaguchi M, et al.** Positron emission tomographic measurement of acetylcholinesterase activity reveals differential loss of ascending cholinergic systems in Parkinson's disease and progressive supranuclear palsy. Ann Neurol 1999; **46**: 62–9.

22. **Asahina M, Suhara T, Shinotoh H, et al.** Brain muscarinic receptors in progressive supranuclear palsy and Parkinson's disease: a positron emission tomographic study. J Neurol Neurosurg Psychiatry 1998; **65**: 155–63.

23. **Litvan I, Grafman J, Gomez C, et al.** Memory impairment in patients with progressive supranuclear palsy. Arch Neurol 1989; **46**: 765–7.

24. **Grafman J, Litvan I, Stark M.** Neuropsychological features of progressive supranuclear palsy. Brain Cogn 1995; **28**: 311–20.

25. **Soliveri P, Monza D, Paridi D, et al.** Neuropsychological follow up in patients with Parkinson's disease, striatonigral degeneration-type multisystem atrophy, and progressive supranuclear palsy. J Neurol Neurosurg Psychiatry 2000; **69**: 313–18.

26. **Borroni B, Turla M, Bertasi V, et al.** Cognitive and behavioral assessment in the early stages of neurodegenerative extrapyramidal syndromes. Arch Gerontol Geriat 2008; **47**: 53–61.

27. **Dubois B, Pillon B, Legault F, et al.** Slowing of cognitive processing in progressive supranuclear palsy. A comparison with Parkinson's disease. Arch Neurol 1988; **45**: 1194–9.

28. **Johnson R, Jr, Litvan I, Grafman J.** Progressive supranuclear palsy: altered sensory processing leads to degraded cognition. Neurology 1991; **41**: 1257–62.

29. **Grafman J, Litvan I, Gomez C, et al.** Frontal lobe function in progressive supranuclear palsy. Arch Neurol 1990; **47**: 553–8.

30. **Robbins TW, James M, Owen AM, et al.** Cognitive deficits in progressive supranuclear palsy, Parkinson's disease, and multiple system atrophy in tests sensitive to frontal lobe dysfunction. J Neurol Neurosurg Psychiatry 1994; **57**: 79–88.

31. **Partiot A, Verin M, Pillon B, et al.** Delayed response tasks in basal ganglia lesions in man: further evidence for a striato-frontal cooperation in behavioural adaptation. Neuropsychologia 1996; **34**: 709–21.

32. **Dillon DG, Pizzagalli DA.** Inhibition of action, thought, and emotion: a selective neurobiological review. Appl Prev Psychol 2007; **12**: 99–114.

33. **Monchi O, Petrides M, Mejia-Constain B, et al.** Cortical activity in Parkinson's disease during executive processing depends on striatal involvement. Brain 2007; **130**: 233–44.

34. **Dubois B, Slachevsky A, Pillon B, et al.** 'Applause sign' helps to discriminate PSP from FTD and PD. Neurology 2005; **64**: 2132–3.

35. **Nigg JT.** On inhibition/disinhibition in developmental psychopathology: views from cognitive and personality psychology and a working inhibition taxonomy. Psychol Bull 2000; **126**: 220–46.

36. **Rittman T, Ghosh BC, McColgan P, et al.** The Addenbrooke's Cognitive Examination for the differential diagnosis and longitudinal assessment of patients with parkinsonian disorders. J Neurol Neurosurg Psychiatry 2013; **84**: 544–51.

37. **Osaki Y, Ben-Shlomo Y, Lees AJ, et al.** Accuracy of clinical diagnosis of progressive supranuclear palsy. Mov Disord 2004; **19**: 181–9.

38. **Williams DR, de Silva R, Paviour DC, et al.** Characteristics of two distinct clinical phenotypes in pathologically proven progressive supranuclear palsy: Richardson's syndrome and PSP-parkinsonism. Brain 2005; **128**: 1247–58.

39. **Paviour DC, Price SL, Jahanshahi M, et al.** Longitudinal MRI in progressive supranuclear palsy and multiple system atrophy: rates and regions of atrophy. Brain 2006; **129**: 1040–9.

40. **Josephs KA, Whitwell JL, Dickson DW, et al.** Voxel-based morphometry in autopsy proven PSP and CBD. Neurobiol Aging 2008; **29**: 280–9.

41. **Mochizuki A, Ueda Y, Komatsuzaki Y, et al.** Progressive supranuclear palsy presenting with primary progressive aphasia—clinicopathological report of an autopsy case. Acta Neuropathol 2003; **105**: 610–14.

42. **Rohrer JD, Paviour D, Bronstein AM, et al.** Progressive supranuclear palsy syndrome presenting as progressive nonfluent aphasia: a neuropsychological and neuroimaging analysis. Mov Disord 2010; **25**: 179–88.

43. **Spagnolo F, Coppi E, Della Rosa PA, et al.** Deep magnetic stimulation in a progressive supranuclear palsy patient with speech involvement. J Neurol 2013; **260**: 670–3.

44. **Josephs KA, Duffy JR, Strand EA, et al.** Clinicopathological and imaging correlates of progressive aphasia and apraxia of speech. Brain 2006; **129**: 1385–98.

45. **Kulisevsky J, Litvan I, Berthier ML, et al.** Neuropsychiatric assessment of Gilles de la Tourette patients: comparative study with other hyperkinetic and hypokinetic movement disorders. Mov Disord 2001; **16**: 1098–104.

46. **Litvan I, Mega MS, Cummings JL, et al.** Neuropsychiatric aspects of progressive supranuclear palsy. Neurology 1996; **47**: 1184–9.

47. **Cordato NJ, Halliday GM, Caine D, et al.** Comparison of motor, cognitive, and behavioral features in progressive supranuclear palsy and Parkinson's disease. Mov Disord 2006; **21**: 632–8.

48. **Levy ML, Cummings JL, Fairbanks LA, et al.** Apathy is not depression. J Neuropsychiatry Clin Neurosci. 1998; **10**: 314–19.

49. **Aarsland D, Litvan I, Larsen JP.** Neuropsychiatric symptoms of patients with progressive supranuclear palsy and Parkinson's disease. J Neuropsychiatry Clin Neurosci 2001; **13**: 42–9.

50. **Cordato NJ, Pantelis C, Halliday GM, et al.** Frontal atrophy correlates with behavioural changes in progressive supranuclear palsy. Brain 2002; **125**: 789–800.

51. **Williams DR, Lees AJ.** Visual hallucinations in the diagnosis of idiopathic Parkinson's disease: a retrospective autopsy study. Lancet Neurol 2005; **4**: 605–10.

52. **Diederich NJ, Leurgans S, Fan W, et al.** Visual hallucinations and symptoms of REM sleep behavior disorder in Parkinsonian tauopathies. Int J Geriatr Psychiatry 2008; **23**: 598–603.

53. **Gerstenecker A, Duff K, Mast B, et al.** Behavioral abnormalities in progressive supranuclear palsy. Psychiatry Res. 2013; **210**: 1205–10.

54. **Erro R, Barone P, Moccia M, et al.** Abnormal eating behaviors in progressive supranuclear palsy. Eur J Neurol 2013; **20**: e47–e48.

55. **Lagarde J, Valabregue R, Corvol JC, et al.** Are frontal cognitive and atrophy patterns different in PSP and bvFTD? A comparative neuropsychological and VBM study. PLoS ONE 2013; **8**: e80353.

56. **Riley DE, Lang AE, Lewis A, et al.** Cortical-basal ganglionic degeneration. Neurology 1990; **40**: 1203–12.

57. **Rinne JO, Lee MS, Thompson PD, et al.** Corticobasal degeneration. A clinical study of 36 cases. Brain 1994; **117**: 1183–96.

58. **Murray R, Neumann M, Forman MS, et al.** Cognitive and motor assessment in autopsy-proven corticobasal degeneration. Neurology 2007; **68**: 1274–83.

59. **Wenning GK, Litvan I, Jankovic J, et al.** Natural history and survival of 14 patients with corticobasal degeneration confirmed at postmortem examination. J Neurol Neurosurg Psychiatry 1998; **64**: 184–9.

60. **Kompoliti K, Goetz CG, Boeve BF, et al.** Clinical presentation and pharmacological therapy in corticobasal degeneration. Arch Neurol 1998; **55**: 957–61.

61. **Wadia PM, Lang AE.** The many faces of corticobasal degeneration. Parkinsonism Relat Disord 2007; **13**(Suppl. 3): S336–S340.

62. **Alladi S, Xuereb J, Bak T, et al.** Focal cortical presentations of Alzheimer's disease. Brain 2007; **130**: 2636–45.

63. **Moreaud O, Monavon A, Brutti-Mairesse MP, et al.** Creutzfeldt–Jakob disease mimicking corticobasal degeneration clinical and MRI data of a case. J Neurol 2005; **252**: 1283–4.

64. **Boeve BF, Josephs KA, Drubach DA.** Current and future management of the corticobasal syndrome and corticobasal degeneration. Handb Clin Neurol 2008; **89**: 533–48.

65. **Boeve BF, Lang AE, Litvan I.** Corticobasal degeneration and its relationship to progressive supranuclear palsy and frontotemporal dementia. Ann Neurol 2003; **54**(Suppl. 5): S15–S19.

66. **Wolpe N, Moore JW, Rae CL, et al.** The medial frontal-prefrontal network for altered awareness and control of action in corticobasal syndrome. Brain 2014; **137**: 208–20.

67. **Pillon B, Blin J, Vidailhet M, et al.** The neuropsychological pattern of corticobasal degeneration: comparison with progressive supranuclear palsy and Alzheimer's disease. Neurology 1995; **45**: 1477–83.

68. **Litvan I, Cummings JL, Mega M.** Neuropsychiatric features of corticobasal degeneration. J Neurol Neurosurg Psychiatry 1998; **65**: 717–21.

69. **Soliveri P, Piacentini S, Girotti F.** Limb apraxia in corticobasal degeneration and progressive supranuclear palsy. Neurology 2005; **64**: 448–53.

70. **Leiguarda R, Lees AJ, Merello M, et al.** The nature of apraxia in corticobasal degeneration. J Neurol Neurosurg Psychiatry 1994; **57**: 455–9.

71. **Leiguarda RC, Merello M, Nouzeilles MI, et al.** Limb-kinetic apraxia in corticobasal degeneration: clinical and kinematic features. Mov Disord 2003; **18**: 49–59.

72. **Sawle GV, Brooks DJ, Marsden CD, et al.** Corticobasal degeneration. A unique pattern of regional cortical oxygen hypometabolism and striatal fluorodopa uptake demonstrated by positron emission tomography. Brain 1991; **114**: 541–56.

73. **Zadikoff C, Lang AE.** Apraxia in movement disorders. Brain 2005; **128**: 1480–97.

74. **Mimura M, White RF, Albert ML.** Corticobasal degeneration: neuropsychological and clinical correlates. J Neuropsychiatry Clin Neurosci 1997; **9**: 94–8.

75. **Graham NL, Bak T, Patterson K, et al.** Language function and dysfunction in corticobasal degeneration. Neurology 2003; **61**: 493–9.

76. **Frattali CM, Grafman J, Patronas N, et al.** Language disturbances in corticobasal degeneration. Neurology 2000; **54**: 990–2.

77. **Kertesz A, Martinez-Lage P, Davidson W, et al.** The corticobasal degeneration syndrome overlaps progressive aphasia and frontotemporal dementia. Neurology 2000; **55**: 1368–75.

78. **McMonagle P, Blair M, Kertesz A.** Corticobasal degeneration and progressive aphasia. Neurology 2006; **67**: 1444–51.

79. **Soliveri P, Monza D, Paridi D, et al.** Cognitive and magnetic resonance imaging aspects of corticobasal degeneration and progressive supranuclear palsy. Neurology 1999; **53**: 502–7.

80. **Dubois B, Slachevsky A, Litvan I, et al.** The FAB: a frontal assessment battery at bedside. Neurology 2000; **55**: 1621–6.

81. Massman PJ, Kreiter KT, Jankovic J, et al. Neuropsychological functioning in cortical-basal gangli-onic degeneration: differentiation from Alzheimer's disease. Neurology 1996; **46**: 720–6.

82. Foster NL, Wilhelmsen K, Sima AA, et al. Frontotemporal dementia and parkinsonism linked to chromosome 17: a consensus conference. Conference Participants. Ann Neurol 1997; **41**: 706–15.

83. Lynch T, Sano M, Marder KS, et al. Clinical characteristics of a family with chromosome 17-linked disinhibition-dementia-parkinsonism-amyotrophy complex. Neurology 1994; **44**: 1878–84.

84. van Swieten JC, Stevens M, Rosso SM, et al. Phenotypic variation in hereditary frontotemporal dementia with tau mutations. Ann Neurol 1999; **46**: 617–26.

85. van Swieten JC, Rosso SM, van Herpen E, et al. Phenotypic variation in frontotemporal dementia and parkinsonism linked to chromosome 17. Dement Geriatr Cogn Disord 2004; **17**: 261–4.

86. Hutton M, Lendon CL, Rizzu P, et al. Association of missense and 5'-splice-site mutations in tau with the inherited dementia FTDP-17. Nature 1998; **393**: 702–5.

87. Baker M, Mackenzie IR, Pickering-Brown SM, et al. Mutations in progranulin cause tau-negative frontotemporal dementia linked to chromosome 17. Nature 2006; **442**: 916–19.

88. Boeve BF, Hutton M. Refining frontotemporal dementia with parkinsonism linked to chromosome 17: introducing FTDP-17 (MAPT) and FTDP-17 (PGRN). Arch Neurol 2008; **65**: 460–4.

89. Gilman S, Wenning GK, Low PA, et al. Second consensus statement on the diagnosis of multiple system atrophy. Neurology 2008; **71**: 670–6.

90. Wenning GK, Stefanova N, Jellinger KA, et al. Multiple system atrophy: a primary oligodendrogliop-athy. Ann Neurol 2008; **64**: 239–46.

91. Robbins TW, James M, Lange KW, et al. Cognitive performance in multiple system atrophy. Brain 1992; **115**: 271–91.

92. Apostolova LG, Klement I, Bronstein Y, et al. Multiple system atrophy presenting with language impairment. Neurology 2006; **67**: 726–7.

93. Pillon B, Dubois B, Agid Y. Testing cognition may contribute to the diagnosis of movement disorders. Neurology 1996; **46**: 329–34.

94. Testa D, Fetoni V, Soliveri P, et al. Cognitive and motor performance in multiple system atrophy and Parkinson's disease compared. Neuropsychologia 1993; **31**: 207–10.

95. Pillon B, Gouider-Khouja N, Deweer B, et al. Neuropsychological pattern of striatonigral degenera-tion: comparison with Parkinson's disease and progressive supranuclear palsy. J Neurol Neurosurg Psychiatry 1995; **58**: 174–9.

96. Monza D, Soliveri P, Radice D, et al. Cognitive dysfunction and impaired organization of complex motility in degenerative parkinsonian syndromes. Arch Neurol 1998; **55**: 372–8.

97. Paviour DC, Winterburn D, Simmonds S, et al. Can the frontal assessment battery (FAB) differentiate bradykinetic rigid syndromes? Relation of the FAB to formal neuropsychological testing. Neurocase 2005; **11**: 274–82.

98. Kim HJ, Jeon BS, Kim YE, et al. Clinical and imaging characteristics of dementia in multiple system atrophy. Parkinsonism Relat Disord 2013; **19**: 617–21.

99. Pagonabarraga J, Corcuera-Solano I, Vives-Gilabert Y, et al. Pattern of regional cortical thinning associated with cognitive deterioration in Parkinson's disease. PLoS ONE 2013; **8**: e54980.

100. Lyoo CH, Jeong Y, Ryu YH, et al. Effects of disease duration on the clinical features and brain glucose metabolism in patients with mixed type multiple system atrophy. Brain 2008; **131**: 438–46.

101. Watanabe H, Saito Y, Terao S, et al. Progression and prognosis in multiple system atrophy: an analy-sis of 230 Japanese patients. Brain 2002; **125**: 1070–83.

102. Konagaya M, Konagaya Y, Sakai M, et al. Progressive cerebral atrophy in multiple system atrophy. J Neurol Sci 2002; **195**: 123–7.

103. Brenneis C, Seppi K, Schocke MF, et al. Voxel-based morphometry detects cortical atrophy in the Parkinson variant of multiple system atrophy. Mov Disord 2003; **18**: 1132–8.

Chapter 20

Diagnosis of dementia in Parkinson's disease

Murat Emre

Introduction

In essence, diagnosis of dementia in a patient with Parkinson's disease (PD) is no different from diagnosing dementia in any other patient. The diagnostic approach can be conceptualized as a two-step process: diagnosis of dementia and differential diagnosis with regard to its aetiology. The first step involves excluding other conditions which can mimic dementia, as well as evaluating whether mental impairment is severe enough to affect normal functioning by itself in order to fulfil the current definition of dementia. The second step includes the assessment of the aetiology, i.e. whether dementia is due to PD, by excluding other potential causes. Although rather straightforward in a patient with a typical history and symptoms of PD, this step involves considering other conditions which can present with dementia and parkinsonism, particularly in patients for whom the history is not reliable or when atypical features are present.

Compared with other patients with suspected dementia, diagnosis of dementia in patients with PD can be more difficult. There are several confounding factors related to the disease itself, its treatment, and co-morbid conditions which are more frequent in this patient population. These include adverse effects of medication, acute or prolonged confusion due to systemic abnormalities or diseases, and the presence of depression, all of which can mimic symptoms of dementia. At times, severe motor impairment renders it difficult to judge whether impairment in function, a prerequisite for the diagnosis of dementia, is due to mental or motor dysfunction. Conditions that can mimic dementia in patients with PD are listed in Table 20.1 and the general approach to diagnosis is summarized in the rest of this chapter.

Diagnosis of dementia

Diagnosing dementia in patients with PD (PD-D) is principally a clinical undertaking, with little help from auxiliary methods. The diagnostic process involves several components, including a careful history from patients and their family members with emphasis on typical features of PD-D [1], assessment of cognitive functions, behavioural symptoms, and activities of daily living (ADL). In typical cases auxiliary examinations are of least help—they usually serve the purpose of excluding alternative aetiologies in suspected patients.

Taking the history

Along with cognitive testing, a detailed history is the most powerful tool for the diagnosis of dementia. Of particular interest are the mode of onset of mental dysfunction, the profile and time course of cognitive and behavioural symptoms, the presence of typical features for PD-D,

Table 20.1 Conditions which may mimic dementia in patients with Parkinson's disease (PD)

Worried patients or their families
Mild cognitive impairment of PD
Depression
Acute or prolonged confusion (delirium)
Adverse effects of drugs

presence/absence of depressive symptoms, and symptoms and signs of acute confusion. Typically, cognitive impairment due to PD-D has an insidious onset and slow progression. Current medication and recent changes in treatment should be reviewed, in particular administration of drugs known to cause mental dysfunction, such as anticholinergics, along with recently initiated treatments and changes in doses.

PD patients who are destined to develop dementia frequently present typical early symptoms. It is useful to specifically ask for the presence of such features when taking the history from patients and their family members. Changes in the sleep–wake cycle are frequent, including excessive daytime sleepiness, disturbance of night sleep, and brief confusion or transient hallucinations on awakening. Rapid eye movement (REM) sleep behaviour disorder (RBD; dream-enacting behaviour such as speaking, screaming, or movements in sleep) may be seen also in patients without dementia; however, it is more common in patients with dementia, it presents a risk factor for dementia, and it may precede the development of dementia by many years. Prior to overt psychosis, 'phantom boarder' phenomenon or a 'feeling of presence' may develop, where patients believe that somebody is standing behind them, a shadow has just passed-by, or there is somebody else in the house, although they do not see this person. The development of hallucinations or psychosis shortly after initiating dopaminergic medication may be another early sign of incipient dementia. The presence of visual hallucinations, usually well-formed, coloured objects, insects, animals, or humans should also be specifically asked for. Patients and their families may not volunteer this information because of fear that patients are going 'mad', but may admit it when asked. Other early signs include loss of interest, apathy, social withdrawal, forgetfulness, inattentiveness, and difficulties with concentration when reading a book, watching a movie, or following a conversation. Early signs of functional impairment include difficulties in handling personal or family finances and navigating or finding directions especially in unfamiliar, but sometimes also in familiar, environments.

Assessment of cognitive functions

Cognitive functions can be examined either by using formal, validated scales or by administering several tests for each cognitive domain. For each purpose one can use either simple scales or a limited number of easy to administer bedside tests for screening purposes, or more elaborate scales and more complex neuropsychological tests for a detailed and quantitative evaluation. A two-level approach, simpler screening scales and tests for routine clinical practice, versus a more detailed assessment for complex cases or for research purposes, was also proposed in the recommendations for the diagnosis of PD-D published by a Task Force of the Movement Disorder Society [2]. A validation study revealed that the proposed screening checklist showed 100% specificity but only 46.7% sensitivity, the most problematic items for lack of sensitivity were absence of depression and a Mini-Mental State Examination (MMSE) score of less than 26 [3]. Another validation study also found a high specificity but low sensitivity and suggested that replacing MMSE by a more specific screening scale such as Mini-Mental Parkinson with a cut-off value of 27 points may increase the sensitivity [4].

Composite cognitive scales

Simple, easy to administer, and less time-consuming scales include those which are not specific for PD as well as those developed specifically for screening patients with PD (Table 20.2). General-purpose scales, such as the most widely known MMSE, can be used for brief screening. The Montreal Cognitive Assessment (MoCA) is probably more sensitive for detecting cognitive deficits in PD as it includes a more detailed assessment of executive functions [5]. It has a high test–retest and inter-rater reliability and a cut-off score of 21/30, yielding a sensitivity of 90% in PD-D patients [6]. Addenbrooke's Cognitive Examination (ACE) scale takes longer to complete than the other screening batteries [7]. However, it offers the advantages that a more complete and extensive cognitive evaluation can be achieved, and a MMSE score can be extracted from this scale. In a validation study in which the Mattis Dementia Rating Scale (DRS) was used as a reference it was found to be a valid tool for assessing dementia in PD, displaying good correlation with both the PD-specific Scales for Outcomes in Parkinson's Disease–Cognition (SCOPA-COG) scale (see later in this section), as well as with the less specific MMSE; a cut-off score of 83 points was proposed for the PD population [8].

Screening batteries specifically developed for PD include the Parkinson Neuropsychometric Dementia Assessment (PANDA) [9] and the Mini-Mental Parkinson [10]. These scales specifically include tests assessing common deficits seen in patients with PD. Another screening instrument which focuses on impairment in frontal-executive functions, one of the core deficits in PD-D, and also including assessment of some behavioural symptoms, is the Frontal Assessment Battery (FAB) [11].

More elaborate scales are reserved for a more detailed and quantitative assessment, and these are usually administered in the context of research studies or in early stage patients with a high level of education who can show a normal performance on simple screening scales. These also include two categories: those not specific for PD, and those specifically developed to assess typical deficits in PD. Among the established and validated scales in the former group are the most widely used composite cognitive scale, the Alzheimer Disease Assessment Scale–Cognitive Section (ADAS-COG) [12] and the Mattis DRS [13], which is more sensitive for PD as it includes an extensive executive functions component. In a study performed in a Hungarian PD population in which ACE, FAB, Mattis DRS, and MMSE were compared, the Mattis DRS was proposed to have the best clinicometric profile to detect PD-D, with a cut-off core of 125 points [14]. In a clinical trial to assess the long-term outcome of treatment with the cholinesterase inhibitor rivastigmine, the Mattis DRS was found to be sensitive to change induced by treatment as well detecting changes occurring in the course of the disease [15]. SCOPA-COG [16] and Parkinson Disease–Cognitive Rating Scale (PD-CRS) [17] were both specifically developed to assess cognitive functions in patients with PD, and can also be used for follow-up purposes to assess change over time.

When using composite scales and trying to interpret their scores it is important that one should consider not only the total score but also the profile of deficits. For example a score of 27 on the MMSE is nominally a normal score. This score, however, may be abnormal in a well-educated patient when the errors include difficulties copying the intersecting pentagons, failing to remember one out of three words, and one mistake on subtracting serial sevens. These show typical deficits in attention, visuospatial function, and free recall and may indicate an abnormal performance in this particular patient despite a nominally normal MMSE score.

Table 20.2 Composite scales which can be used to evaluate cognitive functions in Parkinson's disease (PD)

A: Screening scales

General-purpose scales:

- Mini-Mental State Examination (MMSE)
- Montreal Cognitive Assessment (MoCA)
- Addenbrooke's Cognitive Assessment (ACE)
- Frontal Assessment Battery (FAB)

PD-specific scales:

- Mini-Mental Parkinson
- Parkinson Neuropsychometric Dementia Assessment (PANDA)

B: More quantitative scales

General-purpose scales:

- Alzheimer Disease Assessment Scale–Cognitive Section (ADAS-COG)
- Mattis Dementia Rating Scale (DRS)

PD-specific scales:

- Scales for Outcomes in Parkinson's Disease–Cognition (SCOPA-COG)
- Parkinson Disease–Cognitive Rating Scale (PD-CRS)

Neuropsychological tests

A full neuropsychological evaluation, with several tests for each cognitive domain including attention, memory, language, praxis, visuospatial and executive functions, tailored for the age, education, and general mental status of the patient, is the most appropriate way to assess cognitive functions. However, this is time-consuming and needs special expertise to choose the tests, perform them, and interpret their results. For routine clinical practice, easy-to-administer bedside tests may be sufficient to rapidly assess the cognitive status of the patient. In accordance with the profile of cognitive impairment in PD-D, several simple tests for the most affected cognitive domains can be administered (Table 20.3). These include serial sevens (subtracting 7 from 100 backwards) or months/days recited backwards to assess attention; verbal fluency (both lexical and semantic) and clock-drawing tests for executive functions; copying a three-dimensional cube or intersecting pentagons, mimicking complex hand figures (such as intercalating fingers) to assess visuospatial functions; and simple memory tests such as learning a three- to five-word list or a five-item address, assessing both free recall and recognition (after cueing and after providing alternatives) following sufficient learning trials. The most yielding are probably verbal fluency and clock-drawing tests, which are described below.

The lexical fluency task consists of naming as many words as possible within a minute which start with a certain letter. The letters used in the English language are F, A, and S, names of humans (such as Peter) or geographical places (such as New York) are not allowed. The semantic fluency test requires the naming of as many objects as possible within a minute which belong to a certain semantic category, such as animals or vegetables. In PD patients both tests are sensitive to detect impairment, basically in internally cued search strategies, lexical fluency tapping more frontal functions and semantic fluency more temporal ones. The cut-off scores vary depending on age,

Table 20.3 Neuropsychological tests to evaluate individual cognitive domains

A: Bedside tests

- Attention: serial sevens, months or days backwards
- Memory: learning a three- to five-word list, or a five-item address, with delayed free recall, recall after cueing and recognition
- Executive functions: verbal (lexical and category) fluency, clock-drawing test
- Visual–spatial functions: copying intersecting pentagons or a three-dimensional cube; imitating hand figures such as intercalating fingers
- Language: spontaneous speech (word-finding difficulties, pauses), naming common and rarer objects, understanding complex sentences

B: More comprehensive tests

- Attention: forward and backward Digit Span, continuous performance tests
- Memory: Rey Auditory Learning, California Verbal Learning, Buschke Selective Reminding Tests
- Executive functions: Wisconsin Card Sorting, Stroop test, Tower of London test, Trails A and B
- Visual–spatial functions: Rey–Osterreich Complex Figure, Picture Completion, Recognizing Embedded Figures, Line Orientation and Benton Facial Recognition tests
- Language: Boston Naming Test

culture, and education; usually 12–14 words for each letter or items in each category are regarded as normal. The clock-drawing test is a simple but very sensitive test, it taps executive functions such as planning as well as visuospatial functions. The patient is given an empty circle about 5 cm in diameter on a blank sheet, with the centre and the top marked, and asked to place all the numbers of a clock in the appropriate location and then to draw the arms of the clock to indicate 11:10. The following are evaluated: whether the patient starts with adequate planning by placing 12, 3, 6, and 9 first; whether all the numbers are located in the right place; whether the whole circle is used; and whether 11:10 is correctly indicated.

Examples of more elaborate neuropsychological tests are listed in Table 20.3. These include: forward and backward digit span and computerized continuous performance tests for attention; Wisconsin Card Sorting, Tower of London, or Stroop tests for assessing planning, mental set-building and set-shifting, Trails A and B for psychomotor speed, and set-shifting for the assessment of various components of executive functions; California Verbal Learning, Rey's 15 words and 15 shapes, or Bushke's Selective Reminding Test for memory; copying Rey–Osterreich complex figure, picture completion test, recognizing embedded figures, line orientation, and face recognition tests to assess visuospatial functions; and the Boston Naming Test for confrontational naming. The extent of testing and types of tests should be tailored according to the age, intellectual capacity, and general condition of the patient.

Assessment of behavioural symptoms

At the bedside or in the office setting, the most efficient and practical way to assess behavioural symptoms is through a semi-structured interview with the patient and a well-informed family member. As patients and caregivers may not voluntarily report psychotic symptoms, these should be specifically asked for, in particular the existence of typical symptoms such as infidelity, phantom boarder or 'feeling of presence' delusions, and visual hallucinations, typically of insects, animals, or people. A tactful way of asking may be: 'Patients with this disease may sometimes have dreams when they are awake, does this happen to you?'. Likewise loss of interest and motivation, apathy, social withdrawal, depressive symptoms such as sadness and anhedonia, excessive daytime sleepiness, transient confusion and disorientation on awakening, and symptoms of RBD must be explored.

The most widely used formal scale to assess behavioural and neuropsychiatric symptoms is the Neuropsychiatric Inventory [18]. There are 10- and 12-item versions, and also the possibility to capture caregiver burden. The scale is easy to use with screening questions for each symptom answered by an informed caregiver. When the occurrence of a particular symptom is confirmed the severity is measured semi-quantitatively by assessing the frequency of its occurrence and the grade of discomfort caused by it.

Assessment of functional impairment

This is probably the most difficult part of the assessment, yet the most critical one to ascertain the diagnosis of dementia as per current definitions. It is generally less difficult to decide if a patient has functional impairment. The more difficult part is to judge whether and how much of the functional impairment is due to motor versus mental dysfunction. This can be especially difficult in patients who have severe motor impairment, in particular axial involvement such as postural imbalance and speech disorder, symptoms which are more frequent in PD-D patients. Elderly patients may have stopped taking care of themselves for many years, simply because it is more convenient to rely on their caregivers for ADL. In such cases it may be difficult to judge whether they have any functional impairment as they do not attempt to do much by themselves.

Given all these limitations the most direct and useful way to assess functional impairment is to ask family members what the patient was able to do before cognitive symptoms become apparent that she/he is not able to do anymore. Instrumental (such as handling finances and money, shopping, travelling alone) and basic (such as choosing clothes, dressing, bathing, personal hygiene) ADL, as well as occupational and social activities should be assessed by asking lead-questions. Once newly developed functional impairment is acknowledged, one should attempt to qualify if the impairment is more due to mental or motor dysfunction. Questions for various daily activities should be asked, based on the age, sex, social, and occupational status of the patient. It was proposed that the ability of a patient to organize and remember his/her own medication schedule can be used to assess functional impairment, as all PD patients receive medication [2]. This proposal was validated in a large number of PD patients; although the Pill Questionnaire demonstrated acceptable basic properties as a screening tool for dementia, its positive predictive value was low [19].

Although there is none specifically developed for PD, ADL scales such as the Alzheimer Disease Consortium Study–Activities of Daily Living (ADCS-ADL) scale [20] or the Disability Assessment in Dementia (DAD) [21] scale can be used to quantitatively assess functional impairment.

Auxillary methods

These include laboratory examinations and neuroimaging; occasionally electrophysiological investigations such as electroencephalography may be needed. Laboratory examinations may help to differentiate acute confusion (delirium) from dementia, and also to exclude or reveal other causes of dementia such as metabolic, endocrine, or toxic disorders. One should not forget that PD patients with mental dysfunction are usually elderly people—they are also prone to other causes of dementia which can affect the elderly population at large. Therefore, a basic laboratory screening should be performed in PD patients who develop mental dysfunction, including haematological, biochemical, and urine tests. The array of laboratory examinations can be limited or expanded based on the clinical presentation. In typical cases with an insidious onset and slow progression, laboratory examinations may still be helpful to exclude concomitant diseases such as diabetes.

In a patient with established, long-standing PD who then develops symptoms of dementia with a clinical presentation typical for PD-D, renewed structural imaging may not be necessary. There is no single pattern of atrophy in computed tomography or magnetic resonance imaging (MRI) scans that would help to diagnose dementia in individual patients; nevertheless imaging may help to exclude an alternative diagnosis. Findings in structural and functional imaging are described in detail in Chapter 10, whereas those relevant for diagnosis are summarized here.

In structural imaging with MRI there is a four-fold increased rate of whole-brain atrophy and also more cortical atrophy in PD-D compared with PD without dementia and controls [22]. In general, medial temporal lobe atrophy including the hippocampus and parahippocampal gyrus is more severe in AD patients, with more severe atrophy of the thalamus and parieto-occipital lobes in patients with PD-D [23].

Functional imaging will rarely be required for routine diagnosis. Cerebral blood flow studies as assessed using single photon emission computed tomography (SPECT), often demonstrate frontal hypoperfusion or bilateral temporo-parietal deficits in PD-D patients [24]. Perfusion deficits in the precuneus and inferior lateral parietal regions, areas associated with visual processing, have also been described in PD-D compared with AD, where perfusion deficits are found in a more anterior and inferior location [25]. Reduced metabolism in temporo-parietal regions of patients with PD-D compared with PD is also observed in ^{18}F-fluorodeoxyglucose positron emission tomography (^{18}F-FDG-PET) studies [26], both PD-D and DLB patients demonstrating similar patterns of decreased metabolism in bilateral inferior and medial frontal lobes and the right parietal lobe [27].

2β-Carbomethoxy-3β-(4-iodophenyl)-N-(3-fluoropropyl)-N-nortropane (FP-CIT) SPECT demonstrates the integrity of nigrostriatal dopaminergic pre-synaptic terminals and can help to differentiate Lewy body-related dementias from AD with extrapyramidal features, for example due to neuroleptic use. Significant reductions were found in [^{123}I]-FP-CIT binding in the caudate, anterior, and posterior putamen in subjects with DLB and PD-D compared with those with AD and controls, the greatest loss in all three areas being seen in patients with PD-D [28].

Another imaging method which can differentiate Lewy body-related dementias from other disorders such as AD is metaiodobenzylguanidine (MIBG)-SPECT. [^{123}I]-MIBG is an analogue of noradrenaline, and its imaging with SPECT can be used to quantify post-ganglionic sympathetic cardiac innervation. The heart to mediastinum (H:M) ratio is lower in PD and DLB, but normal in patients with AD [29, 30].

Finally, another method, still in its infancy with regard to routine diagnosis, is imaging of specific protein depositions in the brain. Imaging of α-synuclein has not yet been achieved in humans, but amyloid burden can be quantified using substances binding to amyloid-beta. In PET studies with the Pittsburgh compound B (PIB), mean cortical levels of amyloid were increased two-fold in AD [31] and by 60% in DLB [32]. In PD-D the mean cortical amyloid load was not significantly elevated, although 20% of individuals showed an AD pattern of increased PIB uptake [33]. Once established with reliable cut-off values, quantitative assessment of amyloid versus α-synuclein burden may help in differential diagnosis.

There are as yet no blood or cerebrospinal fluid (CSF) biomarkers to diagnose PD-D. CSF levels of α-synuclein may help to diagnose PD, with no further value to diagnose PD-D [34]. CSF levels of amyloid-beta and tau proteins, which are helpful for diagnosing AD, have been suggested to predict dementia in PD [35, 36]; they may also help to differentiate PD from DLB and AD [37], but this assertion needs further confirmation (see Chapter 11).

Diagnostic criteria for PD-D

Historically, diagnosis of PD-D in clinical practice was made empirically, while diagnosis in research studies was mainly based on the Diagnostic and Statistical Manual (DSM)-IV criteria, which group 'dementia due to PD' along with 'other causes of dementia' without providing specifics. This gap was recognized by the Movement Disorder Society (MDS), and a Task Force of international experts was called together to develop specific clinical diagnostic criteria for PD-D [38].

According to these criteria, the first step in the diagnostic process is the diagnosis of PD in accordance with the Queen Square (UK) Brain Bank criteria for the diagnosis of PD. The second step involves identification of a dementia syndrome diagnosed on the basis of history and clinical and mental examination, with insidious onset, slow progression, and typical clinical features (Table 20.4). The later steps involve screening for other conditions, in the presence of which diagnosis of dementia would be uncertain or impossible. Diagnostic certainty relies on the presence of typical or atypical cognitive and behavioural features as well as the presence or absence of other conditions. Based on these features, diagnostic criteria are described for 'probable' and 'possible' PD-D (Table 20.5). Probable PD-D is diagnosed when dementia with typical features develops on the background of established PD, in the absence of any other conditions which may contribute to, or cause, dementia. A diagnosis of possible PD-D is justified when either there is one or more atypical clinical feature, or in the presence of one or more conditions which would make the diagnosis of PD-D uncertain. In a validation study including 299 PD patients, agreement between MDS Task Force and DSM-IV criteria was substantial; MDS Task Force criteria were, however, more sensitive than DSM-IV for the diagnosis of PD-D. Old age, absence of psychiatric symptoms, and severe motor impairment were the likely factors hindering the diagnosis of PD-D [39].

Differential diagnosis

As mentioned above, diagnosis of dementia in patients with PD can be difficult because of several confounders, notably the presence of severe motor and speech impairment as well as co-morbid conditions such as depression, systemic disorders, and adverse drug events. The onset, the course, and the pattern of neuropsychological and behavioural symptoms and the presence or absence of systemic and laboratory findings are important factors in deciding whether the patient is suffering from dementia associated with PD or from conditions which can mimic dementia. Once these are excluded and a dementia syndrome is diagnosed, other disorders with combined motor and mental dysfunction should be excluded before diagnosing PD-D. As for PD-D, a Task Force of the MDS developed diagnostic criteria for mild cognitive impairment of PD (PD-MCI) [40]. These criteria are structured similarly to those for PD-D; applying both sets of criteria together would help to differentiate PD patients with cognitive impairment but no dementia from those with dementia. This may be particularly useful for research purposes as well as for treatment decisions.

The main prerequisite for the diagnosis of PD-D is that dementia develops in the background of established PD. Yet, this may not always be easy to ascertain, especially in those patients who develop dementia relatively soon after developing motor symptoms or when this temporal relationship cannot be determined. In such patients, other disorders that present with parkinsonism and dementia should be considered in the differential diagnosis, including other neurodegenerative diseases and symptomatic forms. Applying the Queen Square (UK) Brain Bank diagnostic criteria for PD as well as the diagnostic criteria for PD-D would easily exclude an alternative diagnosis in the majority of patients. There remains, however, a group of patients in whom a careful differential diagnosis becomes necessary. Other disorders which present with a combination of parkinsonism and cognitive dysfunction are listed in Table 20.6 and are briefly summarized below.

Table 20.4 Clinical features of dementia associated with Parkinson's disease (PD-D)

I. Core features

1. Diagnosis of PD according to Queen Square Brain Bank criteria

2. A dementia syndrome with insidious onset and slow progression, developing within the context of established PD and diagnosed by history, clinical, and mental examination, defined as:

- Impairment in more than one cognitive domain

- Representing a decline from pre-morbid level

- Deficits severe enough to impair daily life (social, occupational, or personal care), independent of the impairment ascribable to motor or autonomic symptoms

II. Associated clinical features

1. Cognitive features:

- Attention: impaired. Impairment in spontaneous and focused attention, poor performance in attentional tasks; performance may fluctuate during the day and from day to day

- Executive functions: impaired. Impairment in tasks requiring initiation, planning, concept formation, rule-finding, set-shifting or set maintenance; impaired mental speed (bradyphrenia)

- Visuospatial functions: impaired. Impairment in tasks requiring visual–spatial orientation, perception, or construction

- Memory: impaired. Impairment in free recall of recent events or in tasks requiring learning new material, memory usually improves with cueing, recognition is usually better than free recall

- Language: core functions largely preserved. Word-finding difficulties and impaired comprehension of complex sentences may be present

2. Behavioural features:

- Apathy: decreased spontaneity; loss of motivation, interest, and effortful behaviour

- Changes in personality and mood including depressive features and anxiety

- Hallucinations: mostly visual, usually complex, formed visions of people, animals or objects

- Delusions: usually paranoid, such as infidelity, or phantom boarder (unwelcome guests living in the home) delusions

- excessive daytime sleepiness

III. Features which do not exclude PD-D, but make the diagnosis uncertain

- Coexistence of any other abnormality which may by itself cause cognitive impairment, but judged not to be the cause of dementia, e.g. the presence of relevant vascular disease in imaging

- Time interval between the development of motor and cognitive symptoms not known

IV. Features suggesting other conditions or diseases as the cause of mental impairment, which, when present, make it impossible to reliably diagnose PD-D

- Cognitive and behavioural symptoms appearing solely in the context of other conditions such as: (1) acute confusion due to (a) systemic diseases or abnormalities or (b) drug intoxication; or (2) major depression according to DSM-IV

- Features compatible with 'probable vascular dementia' criteria according to NINDS-AIREN (dementia in the context of cerebrovascular disease as indicated by focal signs in neurological examination such as hemiparesis, sensory deficits, and evidence of relevant cerebrovascular disease by brain imaging *and* a relationship between the two as indicated by the presence of one or more of the following: onset of dementia within 3 months after a recognized stroke, abrupt deterioration in cognitive functions, and fluctuating, stepwise progression of cognitive deficits)

Emre M, Aarsland D, Brown R, et al, Mov Disord, Clinical diagnostic criteria for dementia associated with Parkinson's disease, 22, 1689–1707 ©2007

Table 20.5 Diagnostic criteria for probable and possible PD-D

Probable PD-D

A. Core features: both must be present

B. Associated clinical features:

- Typical profile of cognitive deficits including impairment in at least two of the four core cognitive domains (impaired attention which may fluctuate, impaired executive functions, impairment in visuospatial functions, and impaired free recall memory which usually improves with cueing)

- The presence of at least one behavioural symptom (apathy, depressed or anxious mood, hallucinations, delusions, excessive daytime sleepiness) supports the diagnosis of 'probable' PD-D; however, lack of behavioural symptoms does not exclude the diagnosis

C. None of the group III features [Table 20.4] present

D. None of the group IV features [Table 20.4] present

Possible PD-D

A. Core features: both must be present

B. Associated clinical features:

- Atypical profile of cognitive impairment in one or more domains, such as prominent or receptive-type (fluent) aphasia, or pure storage-failure type amnesia (memory does not improve with cueing or in recognition tasks) with preserved attention

- Behavioural symptoms may or may not be present

OR:

C. One or more of the group III features present

D. None of the group IV features present

Emre M, Aarsland D, Brown R, et al, Mov Disord, Clinical diagnostic criteria for dementia associated with Parkinson's disease, 22, 1689–1707 ©2007

Table 20.6 Disorders which may present with parkinsonism and dementia

Degenerative disorders:

- Dementia with Lewy bodies

- Progressive supranuclear palsy

- Corticobasal ganglionic degeneration

- Frontotemporal dementia–parkinsonism complex

- (Multiple system atrophy)

Symptomatic forms:

- Cerebrovascular disease (subcortical vascular encephalopathy, lacunar state)

- Normal-pressure hydrocephalus

- Drug intoxications such as with neuroleptics, anticonvulsants

The main degenerative disorder which overlaps with PD-D is dementia with Lewy bodies (DLB). The clinical and pathological features of DLB and PD-D grossly overlap; clinically it is the time course of the symptoms and presenting features that differentiate these two disorders. The clinical and pathological overlap between these two conditions led to the suggestion that they represent two clinical entities on the spectrum of Lewy body-related dementias, with different temporal and spatial sequences of events [41, 42]. The original Consortium Criteria for DLB stipulated that mental dysfunction should precede motor symptoms by at least 1 year or that they should occur within 1 year of each other [43]. There is, however, no clinical or pathological basis to suggest a fixed time interval between the development of motor versus mental symptoms in differentiating PD-D from DLB. In fact, it is often difficult to determine retrospectively when cognitive or behavioural changes emerged in relation to motor symptoms. These aspects were acknowledged in the subsequent revision of the DLB criteria, and accordingly it was proposed that the '1-year rule' between the onset of dementia and parkinsonism should be maintained in research studies in which distinction is made between DLB and PD-D [44]. In practice, however, it is suggested that a diagnosis of PD-D should be entertained when dementia develops following the diagnosis of idiopathic PD, whereas a diagnosis of DLB is warranted when the symptoms of dementia precede or coincide with the development of motor symptoms. The diagnostic difficulty mostly arises when the temporal relationship between the occurrence of motor versus mental dysfunction is unknown or uncertain. In cases where this temporal relationship cannot be determined, it may be easier to use a more generic term such as 'Lewy body disease'.

Other degenerative disorders that can present with a combination of parkinsonism and mental dysfunction include progressive supranuclear palsy, corticobasal ganglionic degeneration, frontotemporal dementia–parkinsonism complex, and occasional cases of multiple system atrophy. Symptomatic forms of dementia associated with extrapyramidal features include cerebrovascular disease (in particular subcortical vascular encephalopathy and lacunar state), normal-pressure hydrocephalus, and drug intoxications, such as with neuroleptics or anticonvulsants, for example valproate.

A detailed history, including a review of current treatment, deliberate questioning for features known to be associated with PD-D, and use of appropriate neuropsychological tests, are the essential tools in differential diagnosis. Laboratory investigations and neuroimaging may reveal the presence of alternative aetiologies or may help to exclude them. The pattern of atrophy or the presence of vascular pathology in structural imaging, and the selective distribution of hypometabolism in functional imaging, may be helpful. FP-CIT SPECT may help to differentiate patients with PD-D from AD patients with extrapyramidal symptoms. Auxiliary investigations may be particularly helpful in the differential diagnosis of atypical or complex cases.

Conclusion

The diagnosis of dementia associated with PD is a two-step process. The first step involves exclusion of other causes of mental dysfunction and an evaluation of how much ADL are impaired due to cognitive deficits. A detailed history, an adequate evaluation of cognitive functions, behavioural symptoms, and ADL are the main diagnostic tools, whereas auxiliary examinations are of less importance in standard cases. The application of clinical diagnostic criteria for PD-D facilitates the diagnostic process. Although not necessary when dementia with typical features for PD-D develops in the context of established PD, differential diagnosis with regard to other causes of parkinsonism associated with dementia may be required in complex cases.

References

1. Emre M. Dementia associated with Parkinson's disease. Lancet Neurol 2003; **2**: 229–37.

2. Dubois B, Burn D, Goetz C, et al. Diagnostic procedures for Parkinson's disease dementia: recommendations from the Movement Disorder Society task force. Mov Disord 2007; **22**: 2314–24.

3. Barton B, Grabli D, Bernard B, et al. Clinical validation of Movement Disorder Society-recommended diagnostic criteria for Parkinson's disease with dementia. Mov Disord 2012; **27**: 248–53.

4. Isella V, Mapelli C, Siri C, et al. Validation and attempts of revision of the MDS-recommended tests for the screening of Parkinson's disease dementia. Parkinsonism Relat Disord 2014; **20**: 32–6.

5. Nasreddine ZS, Phillips NA, Bedirian V, et al. The Montreal Cognitive Assessment, MoCA: a brief screening tool for mild cognitive impairment. J Am Geriatr Soc 2005; **53**: 695–9.

6. Dalrymple-Alford JC, MacAskill MR, Nakas CT, et al. The MoCA: well-suited screen for cognitive impairment in Parkinson disease. Neurology 2010; **75**: 1717–25.

7. Mioshi E, Dawson K, Mitchell J, et al. The Addenbrooke's Cognitive Examination Revised (ACE-R): a brief cognitive test battery for dementia screening. Int J Geriatr Psychiatry 2006; **21**: 1078–5.

8. Reyes MA, Perez-Lloret S, Roldan Gerschcovich E, et al. Addenbrooke's Cognitive Examination validation in Parkinson's disease. Eur J Neurol 2009; **16**: 142–7.

9. Kalbe E, Calabrese P, Kohn N, et al. Screening for cognitive deficits in Parkinson's disease with the Parkinson neuropsychometric dementia assessment (PANDA) instrument. Parkinsonism Relat Disord 2008; **14**: 93–101.

10. Mahieux F, Fénelon G, Flahault A, et al. Neuropsychological prediction of dementia in Parkinson's disease. J Neurol Neurosurg Psychiatry 1998; **64**: 178–83.

11. Dubois B, Slachevsky A, Litvan I, et al. The FAB: a frontal assessment battery at bedside. Neurology 2000; **55**: 1621–6.

12. Rosen WG, Mohs RC, Davis KL. A new rating scale for Alzheimer's disease. Am J Psychiatry 1984; **141**: 1356–64.

13. Mattis S. *Dementia rating scale*. Odessa, FL: Psychological Assessment Resources Inc., 1988.

14. Kaszás B, Kovács N, Balás I, et al. Sensitivity and specificity of Addenbrooke's Cognitive Examination, Mattis Dementia Rating Scale, Frontal Assessment Battery and Mini Mental State Examination for diagnosing dementia in Parkinson's disease. Parkinsonism Relat Disord 2012; **18**: 553–6.

15. Emre M, Poewe W, De Deyn P et al. Long-term safety of rivastigmine in Parkinson disease dementia: an open-label, randomized study. Clin Neuropharmacol 2014; **37**: 9–16.

16. Marinus J, Visser M, Verwey NA, et al. Assessment of cognition in Parkinson's disease. Neurology 2003; **61**: 1222–8.

17. Pagonabarraga J, Kulisevsky J, Llebaria G, et al. Parkinson's disease-cognitive rating scale: a new cognitive scale specific for Parkinson's disease. Mov Disord 2008; **23**: 998–1005.

18. Cummings JL, Mega M, Gray K, et al. The Neuropsychiatric Inventory: comprehensive assessment of psychopathology in dementia. Neurology 1994; **44**: 2308–14.

19. Martinez-Martin P. Dementia in Parkinson's disease: usefulness of the pill questionnaire. Mov Disord 2013; **28**: 1832–7.

20. Galasko D, Bennett D, Sano M, et al. An inventory to assess activities of daily living for clinical trials in Alzheimer's disease. The Alzheimer's Disease Cooperative Study. Alzheimer Dis Assoc Disord 1997; **11**(Suppl. 2): S33–S39.

21. Gélinas I, Gauthier L, McIntyre M, et al. Development of a functional measure for persons with Alzheimer's disease: the disability assessment for dementia. Am J Occup Ther 1999; **53**: 471–81.

22. Burton EJ, McKeith IG, Burn DJ, et al. Brain atrophy rates in Parkinson's disease with and without dementia using serial magnetic resonance imaging. Mov Disord 2005; **20**: 1571–6.

23. Burton EJ, McKeith IG, Burn DJ, et al. Cerebral atrophy in Parkinson's disease with and without dementia: a comparison with Alzheimer's disease, dementia with Lewy bodies amnd controls. Brain 2004; **127**: 791–800.

24. **Bissessur S, Tissingh G, Wolters EC, et al.** rCBF SPECT in Parkinson's disease patients with mental dysfunction. J Neural Transm Suppl 1997; **50**: 25–30.

25. **Firbank MJ, Colloby SJ, Burn DJ, et al.** Regional cerebral blood flow in Parkinson's disease with and without dementia. NeuroImage 2003; **20**: 1309–19.

26. **Peppard RF, Martin WR, Carr GD, et al.** Cerebral glucose metabolism in Parkinson's disease with and without dementia. Arch Neurol 1992; **49**: 1262–8.

27. **Yong SW, Yoon JK, An YS, Lee PH.** A comparison of cerebral glucose metabolism in Parkinson's disease, Parkinson's disease dementia and dementia with Lewy bodies. Eur J Neurol 2007; **14**: 1357–62.

28. **O'Brien JT, Colloby S, Fenwick J, et al.** Dopamine transporter loss visualized with FP-CIT SPECT in the differential diagnosis of dementia with Lewy bodies. Arch Neurol 2004; **61**: 919–25.

29. **Yoshita M.** Differentiation of idiopathic Parkinson's disease from striatonigral degeneration and progressive supranuclear palsy using iodine-123 meta-iodobenzylguanidine myocardial scintigraphy. J Neurol Sci 1998; **155**: 60–7.

30. **Yoshita M, Taki J, Yamada M.** A clinical role for [(123)I]MIBG myocardial scintigraphy in the distinction between dementia of the Alzheimer's type and dementia with Lewy bodies. J Neurol Neurosurg Psychiatry 2001; **71**: 583–8.

31. **Edison P, Archer HA, Hinz R, et al.** Amyloid, hypometabolism, and cognition in Alzheimer disease. An [11C]PIB and [18F]FDG PET study. Neurology 2007; **68**: 501–8.

32. **Rowe CC, Ng S, Ackermann U, et al.** Imaging β-amyloid burden in aging and dementia. Neurology 2007; **68**: 1718–25.

33. **Edison P, Rowe CC, Rinne JO, et al.** Amyloid load in Parkinson's disease dementia and Lewy body dementia measured with [11C]PIB-PET. J Neurol Neurosurg Psychiatry 2008; **79**: 1331–8.

34. **Mollenhauer B.** Quantification of α-synuclein in cerebrospinal fluid: how ideal is this biomarker for Parkinson's disease? Parkinsonism Relat Disord 2014; **20**(Suppl. 1): S76–S79.

35. **Leverenz JB, Watson GS, Shofer J, et al.** Cerebrospinal fluid biomarkers and cognitive performance in non-demented patients with Parkinson's disease. Parkinsonism Relat Disord 2011; **17**: 61–4.

36. **Beyer MK, Alves G, Hwang KS, et al.** Cerebrospinal fluid Aβ levels correlate with structural brain changes in Parkinson's disease. Mov Disord 2013; **28**: 302–10.

37. **Kaerst L, Kuhlmann A, Wedekind D, et al.** Using cerebrospinal fluid marker profiles in clinical diagnosis of dementia with Lewy bodies, Parkinson's disease, and Alzheimer's disease. J Alzheimers Dis 2014; **38**: 63–73.

38. **Emre M, Aarsland D, Brown R, et al.** Clinical diagnostic criteria for dementia associated with Parkinson's disease. Mov Disord 2007; **22**: 1689–707.

39. **Martinez-Martin P, Falup-Pecurariu C, Rodriguez-Blazquez C, et al.** Dementia associated with Parkinson's disease: applying the Movement Disorder Society Task Force criteria. Parkinsonism Relat Disord 2011; **17**: 621–4.

40. **Litvan I, Goldman JG, Tröster AI, et al.** Diagnostic criteria for mild cognitive impairment in Parkinson's disease: Movement Disorder Society Task Force guidelines. Mov Disord 2012; **27**: 349–56.

41. **Lippa CF, Duda JE, Grossman M, et al.** DLB and PDD boundary issues: diagnosis, treatment, molecular pathology and biomarkers. Neurology 2007; **68**: 812–19.

42. **Lippa CF, Emre M.** Characterizing clinical phenotypes: the Lewys in their life or the life of their Lewys?. Neurology 2006; **67**: 1910–11.

43. **McKeith IG, Galasko D, Kosaka K, et al.** Consensus guidelines for the clinical and pathologic diagnosis of dementia with Lewy bodies (DLB): report of the consortium on DLB international workshop. Neurology 1996; **47**: 1113–24.

44. **McKeith IG, Dickson DW, Lowe J, et al.** Diagnosis and management of dementia with Lewy bodies: third report of the DLB Consortium. Neurology 2005; **65**: 1863–72.

Chapter 21

Management of Parkinson's disease dementia and dementia with Lewy bodies

Ian McKeith and Murat Emre

Introduction

The management of the Lewy body dementias, namely Parkinson's disease dementia (PD-D) and dementia with Lewy bodies (DLB), can be one of the most complex tasks facing neurologists, psychiatrists, geriatricians, primary-care physicians, or others caring for such patients [1]. On the one hand there is the risk of provoking severe neuroleptic sensitivity reactions, which can sometimes be fatal [2], on the other are the potentially gratifying beneficial effects of cholinesterase inhibitors (ChE-Is) [3]. Polypharmacy is the norm, with multiple treatment targets including motor impairment, cognitive deficits, sleep disorders, psychiatric symptoms, and autonomic dysfunction. Non-pharmacological treatments similarly need to be directed towards a variety of symptom complexes. Depending on the availability of resources it is apparent that the best delivery of care to a person with PD-D or DLB and his or her carers will be devised and reviewed by a multidisciplinary team of experienced specialists and delivered, when possible, in the patient's home, minimizing the need for multiple hospital attendances. The general principles described in this chapter are applicable to most patients with a Lewy body-related dementia [4], the details of administration, dosing, and response varying more according to the individual person's symptom mix rather than any particular diagnostic label (PD-D or DLB) which they might carry [5].

Making and disclosing the diagnosis

The clinical diagnostic approach and criteria have been described in Chapter 20. Although operationalized criteria [5, 6] can help clinicians to make confident and reliable diagnoses, common problems which remain in diagnosing PD-D are deciding whether cognitive impairment is severe enough to warrant a diagnosis of dementia [7] and the extent to which impairment of activities of daily living (ADL) is due to motor and autonomic symptoms alone. The distinction between PD-D and DLB also causes difficulties for some, but for the purposes of clinical management this may not be particularly important. The key is that the clinician is able to give a confident diagnostic label to the patient and family and follow this up with explanations for common questions, for example has the person with PD developed another disorder, such as Alzheimer's disease (AD), to explain the dementia or whether the onset of confusion and hallucinations is due to side effects of medication or a consequence of disease progression. For lay people who do not have a grounding in neuroanatomy and physiology it can be difficult to understand how a single disorder can produce such widely variable symptoms as tremor, instability, constipation, hallucinations, sleep disturbance, and cognitive impairment. Time spent at this early stage in explaining the diagnosis and the mechanisms underlying symptoms, and checking out how well the patient and family understand what they have been told, is an essential part of forming the therapeutic alliance which will be required for the next stages of management. This is a particularly important step in developing non-pharmacological management strategies which need to address the manifestations of dementia in general plus the additional unique features of PD-D and DLB. The latter include fluctuating levels of cognitive and communicative ability, which are particularly perplexing and stressful for carers [8]. Useful materials to aid in this process can be found on a variety of websites produced by carer support organizations, statutory care providers, or specialist clinics, the latter often tailored to regional or local needs.

Making a problem list, managing antiparkinsonian medications, and non-pharmacological approaches

Having negotiated a common framework and terminology for diagnosis and understanding, the next step is to produce a problem list, working systematically through the domains of motor, cognitive, neuropsychiatric, and autonomic functions, and sleep. Having established this list, the next step is to ask the patient and carer to identify the symptoms that they find most disabling or distressing and which carry the highest priority for treatment. There may be discrepant views about this which have to be resolved, for example a carer may complain that his/her sleep is being disrupted by the patient's nocturnal restlessness, whereas the patient is more preoccupied with motor slowness through the day. Patients with a long-established history of PD will usually be familiar with the concept of trading benefits of treatment in one domain against potential adverse events in another, for example dyskinesias, worsening of nightmares, or emergence of hallucinations, as the cost of improved mobility with increased dopaminergic drug dose. What must also be stated is that some wearing off of dopaminergic drug responsiveness may occur as a consequence of disease progression at that same time as the emergence of side effects starts to become disproportionate to dose elevation. In other words chasing maintenance of motor function by continuing to increase antiparkinsonian drugs may not only become less effective than in the earlier stages of PD, but the risk of precipitating or exacerbating cognitive and psychiatric symptoms in particular is increased. The therapeutic ratio of these agents therefore begins to fall and the potential for unwanted symptoms to persist becomes greater, even after the medication which clearly precipitated their onset is withdrawn. This phenomenon of confusional states and visual hallucinations following closely on the heels of changes in antiparkinsonian treatments is generally interpreted as the symptoms having been 'caused' by medications. The reality is, however, that dementia and related symptoms in PD typically occur because of diffuse spread of the disease process, cortical involvement in particular producing a vulnerable cerebral substrate. Substances which affect neurotransmitter systems can under such circumstances 'bring forward in time' symptoms which were destined to emerge eventually, independent of such treatment. There is unlikely ever to be a randomized controlled trial of this proposition, but there is substantial corroborating clinical experience and circumstantial evidence.

In addition to providing adequate information to the patient and the family about the disease, non-pharmacological measures should be taken, including sufficient mental and physical activation and avoidance of aggravating factors such as undue sensory stimuli and inappropriate environmental factors. Other than these general measures cognitive-stimulation techniques can be employed in appropriate patients, although a systematic review of non-pharmacological and non-invasive therapies in PD revealed no studies in PD-D patients [9]. All together there were nine controlled trials, including six randomized controlled ones. Although five trials showed positive results, only one study of cognitive training achieved satisfactory grading for evidence of efficacy, demonstrating a significant benefit for cognitive training in the domains of attention, executive function, memory, and visuospatial function [10].

Before initiating a pharmacological treatment, other conditions which can trigger or aggravate mental dysfunction should be excluded. These include systemic abnormalities and diseases, depression, and adverse events of antiparkinsonian medication and treatment for concomitant diseases. Drugs which can aggravate mental dysfunction, such as anticholinergics, tricyclic antidepressants, and benzodiazepines, should be discontinued. Before reverting to medication the need for treatment, especially of behavioural symptoms, should be determined, based on the frequency, severity, and burden of symptoms. Whenever possible, one drug should be introduced at a time at a low dose and titrated up as needed. Non-specific treatment for behavioural symptoms should be tapered and discontinued once sufficient symptom control is attained.

Specific treatments for cognitive impairment

Cholinesterase inhibitors

Evidence suggests that cholinergic deficit is a major biochemical substrate of cognitive dysfunction in PD-D and DLB [11]. ChE-Is inhibit the enzyme acetylcholinesterase, which breaks down acetylcholine in the synaptic cleft, terminating its post-synaptic effects. The synaptic half-life of acetylcholine is prolonged through this inhibition and cholinergic transmission is enhanced. The first report of a ChE-I in PD-D was of a small, open-label study with tacrine, the first ChE-I which became available for clinical use [12]; this suggested favourable effects on mental symptoms without worsening of motor functions. All available ChE-Is, including donepezil, rivastigmine, and galantamine, have subsequently been tested in PD-D and DLB. Despite open-label designs and small sample sizes in most of these studies, a consistent pattern was seen, with improvements in cognitive and behavioural symptoms [3]. Worsening of motor symptoms, usually a dose-related increase in tremor, was seen in only a few cases. These preliminary findings prompted the initiation of one large-scale, placebo-controlled randomized trial with rivastigmine in DLB, and two studies in PD-D, one with rivastigmine and the other with donepezil. The first [13] to be conducted assessed the effect of rivastigmine in DLB patients over a period of 20 weeks, followed by a 3-week withdrawal period. A total of 120 patients with a clinical diagnosis of probable DLB and a Mini-Mental State Examination (MMSE) score between 10 and 23 were treated with up to 12 mg per day of rivastigmine (mean dose 9.4 mg/day) or placebo. A four-item subscore of the Neuropsychiatric Inventory (NPI), comprising delusions, hallucinations, apathy, and depression, was used as the primary efficacy criterion [14]. Approximately twice as many patients on rivastigmine (63.4%) as on placebo (30.0%) showed at least a 30% improvement from baseline on their NPI-4 scores ($p = 0.001$), these symptoms re-emerged during a 3-week washout period. Statistically non-significant improvements were also seen at 20 weeks in MMSE score and Clinical Global Impression of Change (CGIC)-plus rating in favour of the rivastigmine-treated group. Parkinsonian signs did not worsen on treatment, although emergent tremor was noted in four rivastigmine-treated patients. Predominant adverse effects were cholinergic in nature and the frequency of nausea (37%), vomiting (25%), anorexia (19%), and somnolence (9%) was significantly higher in the rivastigmine-treated patients. Most adverse events were rated as either mild or moderate, but 7 of 59 patients receiving rivastigmine withdrew for this reason. Long-term follow-up of some of the study participants [15] found MMSE and NPI scores to be stable over the first 12 months of treatment, then to gradually worsen, although not significantly so, even 2 years after baseline.

Unified Parkinson's Disease Rating Scale (UPDRS) motor scores tended to improve, probably because some antiparkinsonian treatment was initiated during this time.

In the EXPRESS study 541 patients with mild to moderate PD-D were assigned to rivastigmine or placebo over 24 weeks [16r]. Rivastigmine was slowly titrated in monthly increments of 3 mg/day over the first 16 weeks up to 12 mg/day and then maintained at the highest tolerated dose for another 8 weeks; the mean dose at the end of the study was 8.6 mg/day. Primary efficacy parameters included the Alzheimer's Disease Assessment Scale—Cognition subscale (ADAS-COG) for the assessment of cognitive functions and a CGIC scale for the assessment of changes in the overall state from baseline. Both primary end points showed statistically significant improvements on rivastigmine treatment compared with placebo. Patients on rivastigmine showed an improvement of 2.1 points in ADAS-COG score at week 24, whereas patients on placebo deteriorated by 0.7 points ($p < 0.001$). The mean score for the CGIC at week 24 was 3.8 in the rivastigmine group and 4.3 in the placebo group (a score of 4 indicating no change, lower scores indicating improvement, and higher scores indicating worsening from baseline). More patients on rivastigmine showed any degree of improvement (40.8% on rivastigmine versus 29.7% on placebo) and more patients on placebo had any degree of deterioration (42.5% on placebo versus 33.7% on rivastigmine) ($p = 0.007$). Similarly, all secondary efficacy measures revealed statistically significant differences in favour of rivastigmine, including neuropsychiatric symptoms (NPI), the clock-drawing test, verbal fluency, computer-based attention tests, and MMSE score. ADL scores showed a minimal worsening from baseline in patients on rivastigmine, whereas those on placebo worsened significantly more. Adverse events were significantly more frequent with rivastigmine, mainly nausea (29.0% on rivastigmine versus 11.2% on placebo) and vomiting (16.6.% on rivastigmine versus 1.7% on placebo). Worsening of parkinsonian symptoms was more frequently reported on rivastigmine (27.3% versus 15.6% on placebo); this was principally driven by worsening of tremor (10.2% on rivastigmine versus 3.9% on placebo). UPDRS motor scores did not, however, reveal any significant differences between the groups.

In order to assess the long-term effects of rivastigmine, the EXPRESS study had a further 6-month extension during which all patients received active treatment [17]. The results demonstrated that the beneficial effects seen during the first 6 months were largely maintained, although treatment effects started to decline. Patients who initially received placebo and then switched to rivastigmine showed similar benefits to those who had been on rivastigmine for the entire duration of the study, but not in all parameters, suggesting that there may be potential benefits to starting treatment earlier. Importantly, there was no evidence of worsening motor function over the course of 1 year of treatment [18].

The second large randomized, double-blind, placebo-controlled study in PD-D used donepezil [19]. In this study 550 patients with mild to moderate PD-D were randomized into three groups to receive either placebo, donepezil 5 mg, or donepezil 10 mg for 24 weeks. The primary efficacy parameters were ADAS-COG and a global measure of change from baseline (CIBIC-plus). At week 24, there was a 0.3-point improvement in ADAS-COG on placebo, a 2.45-point improvement on 5 mg, and a 3.72-point improvement on 10 mg. These differences did not reach statistical significance in the primary analysis because of a country interaction, but did so when this was controlled for ($p < 0.001$). In the latter analysis the CIBIC-plus showed statistically significant superiority for the 10 mg dose but not for 5 mg. Statistically significant differences in favour of donepezil were also found on some secondary measures including MMSE, Brief Test of Attention, and the Verbal Fluency Test, whereas there were no statistically significant differences from placebo on the ADL scale Disability Assessment in Dementia and the behavioural scale NPI. UPDRS motor scores did not reveal any significant worsening of motor functions on donepezil.

In a later trial of donepezil in DLB [20], 140 patients recruited from 48 specialty centres in Japan were randomly assigned to receive placebo, 3, 5, or 10 mg of donepezil daily for 12 weeks. Effects on cognitive function were assessed using the MMSE and several domain-specific neuropsychological tests. Changes in behaviour were evaluated using the NPI, caregiver burden using the Zarit Caregiver Burden Interview, and global function using the Clinician's Interview-Based Impression of Change-plus Caregiver Input (CIBIC-plus). Safety measures included the UPDRS part III. Donepezil at 5 and 10 mg/day was significantly superior to placebo on both the MMSE (5 mg, mean difference 3.8; 10 mg, mean difference 2.4) and on CIBIC-plus ($p < 0.001$ for each); 3 mg/day was significantly superior to placebo on CIBIC-plus but not on the MMSE. Significant improvements were also found in behavioural measures at 5 and 10 mg/day and caregiver burden at 10 mg/day. The safety results were consistent with the known profile of donepezil and similar among groups. A subsequent open-label follow-up study suggested that benefits lasted at 52 weeks. [21].

Using ChE-Is in practice: predictors of outcome, side effects, and discontinuation

Visual hallucinations are known from post-mortem studies to be associated with more severe cholinergic deficits in the Lewy body dementias [22], and patients with hallucinations might therefore be expected to benefit more from cholinergic enhancement. This was demonstrated to be the case in both the DLB [23] and the PD-D studies with rivastigmine [24]. The presence of visual hallucinations in Lewy body disease is also associated with a greater degree of impairment in attentional performance and a faster rate of cognitive decline, the common factor probably being greater cholinergic deficit—the activity of enzyme butyryl-cholinesterase may play a role [25] which may increase in functional importance as acetylcholinesterase levels diminish with disease progression. Other clinical indicators suggestive of central cholinergic failure, and therefore potentially predictive of a good ChE-I response, include apathy and daytime drowsiness. In practice the majority of PD-D and DLB patients will have such symptoms, visual hallucinations, or both. Given the lack of any demonstrable alternatives, a trial of a ChE-I seems to be the preferred action for any PD-D or DLB patient with significant cognitive impairments.

The side-effect profile of ChE-Is in Lewy body dementias is broadly similar to that reported in the AD population, but there are additional effects to be considered which probably reflect the pre-existing impact of the disease on cholinergic autonomic activity. The drugs are generally well tolerated at doses in the usual AD range, with dropout rates from 10 to 31% being reported. In addition to the well-recognized gastrointestinal side effects, troublesome hypersalivation, rhinorrhoea, and lachrymation occurred in about 15% of DLB and PD-D patients treated with donepezil, and postural hypotension, falls, and syncope in up to 10% [26]. The same open-label study found no difference in treatment responsiveness or side-effect profile when PD-D and DLB patients were compared. Worsening parkinsonism occurred in 9% of patients on 10 mg of donepezil, but this was rarely clinically significant and it could usually be improved by dose reduction. Abrupt withdrawal of ChE-Is may be associated with rapid return of neuropsychiatric symptoms and cognitive decline in DLB and PD-D [27]. Although reinstatement of treatment may reverse such deterioration, it is recommended that patients with Lewy body-related dementias who are assessed as responding to ChE-Is are maintained on treatment for the long term. Since attempts at switching from one ChE-I to another may be associated with clinically significant withdrawal effects [28], this treatment strategy should be considered carefully and patients who are switched should be closely monitored. A preliminary comparison of datasets from treatment studies in DLB using different ChE-Is suggests that there are no major differences between the available agents [29].

Rivastigmine has a marketing approval for treatment of patients with mild to moderate PD-D, both in the European Union and the Unites States. Licensing approval has not been obtained for any of the other ChE-Is in PD-D, nor for the use of any of them in DLB. Much prescribing is therefore 'off label', creating difficulties for those drafting good practice guidelines and dealing with reimbursement issues. Given the scale of the clinical problem and the lack of safe alternatives, this is an unsatisfactory situation and there is a good case for investment in more clinical trials, particularly those measuring longer-term outcomes, cost-effectiveness, and practical aspects of drug administration.

N-methyl-D-aspartate (NMDA) antagonists and dopaminergic drugs

The NMDA antagonist memantine is approved for the treatment of moderate to severe AD. Conflicting results have been described in the few case reports or case series in patients with DLB, reporting both worsening or improvement in equal measure [30, 31]. Three double-blind, randomized controlled studies comparing memantine with placebo have been reported. The first, a study of 22 weeks' duration, included 25 patients with PD-D [32]. At the end of the study there were no significant differences between the two groups on any efficacy parameters; however, 6 weeks after withdrawal more patients who had been treated with memantine deteriorated on a global scale ($p = 0.04$), suggesting that they had had some beneficial effects while being treated. The second study lasted 24 weeks and included 72 patients with either PD-D or DLB of mild to moderate severity randomized either to memantine 20 mg daily or placebo. [33]. The primary end point, the CGIC score was significantly in favour of memantine ($p = 0.03$) and the effect was stronger in the PD-D group. Except for the improved speed in an attentional task in the memantine group, there were no other significant differences in secondary outcome measures between the two groups. The treatment was well tolerated with similar withdrawals in both groups.

In another study of similar design, 199 patients with mild to moderate PD-D or DLB were randomized either to memantine 20 mg once daily given in the morning or placebo. The mean CGIC score was lower (better) in the total population on memantine treatment, but this difference was not statistically significant except in the DLB group who also showed a statistically significant improvement in total NPI score at 24 weeks compared with patients treated with placebo. There were no consistent effects of memantine on cognitive tests, nor on ADL scores in either PD-D or DLB [34].

Taken together these latter two trials suggest a possible benefit of memantine in patients with Lewy body dementias but there is no consistent message as to which patients might benefit (DLB or PD-D) or which symptoms might improve. There were minor differences in the trial populations, most notably the use of ChE-Is in the former but not the latter study, but these are likely insufficient to explain the variable results. A more plausible explanation is that there is considerable heterogeneity within both DLB and PD-D groups, with different patterns of response in different individuals which are not adequately captured by a pooled-group design. The same response heterogeneity is also seen with antipsychotics and ChE-Is and argues that individual case studies or responder analysis might prove better ways of determining treatment effects in the Lewy body dementias.

The effects of dopaminergic treatment on mental functions have barely been studied in patients with PD-D, most formal studies having been performed in patients without dementia. The results have been equivocal, describing either no effects or improvement in some and worsening in other functions. In one of the few studies which specifically included patients with dementia, subjects with PD, PD-D, or DLB were tested for cognitive functions and behavioural symptoms after acute levodopa challenge and following 3 months of treatment. After acute challenge, patients reported improvement in subjective alertness, but fluctuations increased; reaction time and accuracy remained unchanged in those with PD-D. After 3 months of treatment neuropsychiatric scores improved in both PD and PD-D, mean global cognitive score was better, but attention and memory scores were worse in PD patients without dementia. Reaction time became slower in those with PD-D, but no patients showed a marked deterioration [35].

Drug treatment of psychiatric and behavioural symptoms

In common with other types of dementia, it is the psychiatric and behavioural symptoms which cause the greatest distress to patients and carers, and which eventually lead to requests for treatment and institutional care [36]. In Lewy body dementias such symptoms are frequent and contribute to greater impairment in quality of life and costs of care than for AD patients with equivalent cognitive impairments [37, 38]. In addition to the cognitive effects of ChE-Is described earlier, the same agents have also been reported to improve a range of neuropsychiatric symptoms in PD-D and DLB, particularly apathy, visual hallucinations, anxiety, sleep disturbances, and delusions [3]. It is possible that these behavioural effects are largely mediated via improvements in attention and cognitive processing. Since cognitive and neuropsychiatric symptoms often go hand in hand, the choice of a ChE-I as the first-line drug treatment is often directed at both domains.

Agitation and related behaviours are less likely to improve with ChE-Is and occasionally may even be aggravated. The mainstay of treatment for agitation, aggression, and psychotic symptoms in dementia has generally been with D2 receptor antagonists, but these drugs, particularly traditional neuroleptic agents, can provoke severe neuroleptic sensitivity reactions in up to 50% of DLB patients and 25% of PD-D patients, with a two- to three-fold increased mortality [2, 39–41], therefore they are contraindicated in this patient population. These reactions are generally acute or subacute, becoming evident within the first few doses or after increase from a previously tolerated dose. When acute deterioration occurs in a confused elderly patient following neuroleptic administration, Lewy body disease should always be considered as part of the differential diagnosis. Following initial positive case reports of the use of newer atypical antipsychotics in DLB, further case studies indicate that neuroleptic sensitivity does occur with both risperidone and olanzapine, especially as the dose is increased [42, 43]. Quetiapine did not appear to significantly worsen motor symptoms in a recent, small placebo-controlled trial of 36 patients with DLB [44], but was not associated with significant improvement in psychiatric or cognitive outcome measures. Clozapine may also be useful in treating PD psychosis, but its antimuscarinic properties may increase confusion in patients with dementia [45]. The frequent occurrence of electroencephalogram abnormalities with transient temporal slow waves has prompted the use of carbamazepine and sodium valproate as agents to treat behavioural disturbance, but no systematic reports of efficacy or side effects are available. The 5-HT3 antagonist ondansetron was reported as having antipsychotic effects in PD patients with hallucinations, but this has not been independently replicated and the high doses required make the cost prohibitive for routine practice [46]. There are sporadic reports of the traditional Japanese medicine yokukansan being effective and well-tolerated in the treatment of ChE-I-resistant visual hallucinations and neuropsychiatric symptoms in patients with DLB, but this needs confirmation [47].

Although disorders of affect and depressive features are among the most frequent behavioural symptoms in PD and PD-D, surprisingly there have been no randomized, controlled studies of antidepressants in the PD-D population. A meta-analysis of all studies in PD patients with depression revealed large effect sizes, both under active treatment and placebo. There were, however, no statistically significant differences between them; increasing age and major depression predicted better response [48]. In another systematic review, amitriptyline was reported to be the only compound with evidence of efficacy in PD depression [49]. In the past few years there have been several placebo-controlled randomized trials in PD patients with depression, although none were specifically in PD-D patients. In one study desipramine and citalopram were both significantly better than placebo [50], in another nortriptyline was significantly better than placebo whereas paroxetine was not [51]. In contrast, both paroxetine and venlafaxine were significantly better than placebo in a larger randomized trial [52]. The dopamine agonist pramipexole was shown to be significantly better than placebo in a large randomized placebo-controlled trial in patients without dementia but with depressive symptoms [53]; agonists, however, can worsen psychosis and cognition in PD-D patients. It should be remembered that all randomized controlled trials were conducted in patients without dementia. There is a hint that tricyclics such as amitriptyline and nortriptyline may have larger effect sizes, but they should be avoided in PD-D patients because of their anticholinergic effects and hence the potential to worsen cognition. Although an evidence base is lacking, empirically selective serotonin reuptake inhibitors (SSRIs) or selective serotonin and noradrenaline reuptake inhibitors (SNRIs) should be preferred in these patients. Elevated 5-HT1A receptor density has been reported in the temporal cortex of PD-D and DLB patients with a history of depression, suggesting that a 5-HT1A receptor antagonist adjuvant may improve treatment of depression in this group [54].

Disturbances of the sleep–wake cycle, including excessive daytime sleepiness and rapid eye movement (REM) sleep behaviour disorder (RBD), frequently occur in patients with PD-D or DLB [55]. Disturbed sleep with thrashing limb movements, vocalizations, and vivid dreams may precede Lewy body disease as an early manifestation, and may persist, sometimes in attenuated form. Treatment of RBD lacks a double-blind, placebo-controlled, evidence base. Clonazepam has been reported as effective and well tolerated [56] in suppressing the motor features, but does not restore REM sleep atonia [57]. Melatonin has been reported to be beneficial, with control of symptoms or significant improvement being noted in 10 of 14 patients who had failed to respond to clonazepam or were unable to tolerate therapeutic doses [58]. Memantine has also been reported to reduce physical activity in DLB and PD-D during sleep, but no significant change was observed in the severity of excessive daytime sleepiness which is also a frequent problem [59]. In studies performed in PD patients without dementia, modafinil, an agent that promotes wakefulness through undetermined mechanisms, was found to be significantly better than placebo in two small randomized, placebo-controlled studies [60, 61], but its use in DLB may be associated with agitation and psychosis [62]. Armodafinil, the racemic form of modafinil, was reported as showing mild to marked clinical improvement in 90% of participants in a small open-label trial, with moderate to marked improvement seen in half of these. Significant improvement over baseline was reported in the ability to maintain wakefulness and also in apathy, with some improvement in visual hallucinations, delusions, and anxiety. Treatment was well tolerated, and this appears to be a promising avenue for further evaluation [63].

Conclusion

The management of patients with Lewy body-related dementias involves both pharmacological and non-pharmacological measures. The management plan should be developed considering the whole symptom complex and the impact of symptoms on the family and the patient. Patients with PD-D or DLB should be offered treatment with a ChE-I, taking into account expected benefits and potential risks. It is not yet known whether early intervention with ChE-Is confers an advantage compared with later administration. Some behavioural symptoms such as apathy may benefit from a ChE-I, but treatment with antipsychotics may become necessary in some patients with psychotic behaviour. In such instances classical neuroleptics, as well as risperidone and olanzapine, should be avoided. Quetiapine might be considered; however the strongest evidence for efficacy exists for clozapine. The clinician must remain vigilant whichever agent is selected. Although evidence from randomized controlled studies is lacking, SSRIs or SNRIs should be given priority in the treatment of depressive features. Clonazepam, melatonin, and memantine can be tried to treat RBD, and armodafinil may emerge as useful for the treatment of excessive daytime sleepiness.

There are so far no disease-modifying agents available to treat Lewy body diseases; until our understanding of the basic neurobiology of the dementing process improves it is probably premature to expect their development. If successful disease-modifying treatments for AD are demonstrated, for example directed against amyloid neurotoxicity, it is likely that these could also be extended to the Lewy body dementias. For the present time symptomatic treatments are likely to remain the only clinically available options, and given the multiple targets and multiple underlying neurotransmitter abnormalities it seems logical to expect that patient treatment regimens will usually be multiagent and individually tailored.

References

1. **McKeith IG, Galasko D, Wilcock GK, et al**. Lewy body dementia–diagnosis and treatment. Br J Psychiatry 1995; **167**: 709–17.

2. **McKeith I, Fairbairn A, Perry R, et al**. Neuroleptic sensitivity in patients with senile dementia of Lewy body type. Br Med J 1992; **305**: 673–8.

3. **Aarsland D, Mosimann UP, McKeith IG**. Role of cholinesterase inhibitors in Parkinson's disease and dementia with Lewy bodies. J Geriatr Psychiatry Neurol 2004; **17**: 164–71.

4. **Barber R, Newby J, McKeith IG**. Lewy body disease. In: Richter RW, Zoeller Richter B (ed.), *Current clinical neurology. Alzheimer's disease: a physician's guide to practical management*. Totowa, NJ: Humana Press, 2003; pp. 127–35.

5. **McKeith I, Dickson D, Emre M, et al**. Dementia with Lewy bodies: diagnosis and management: Third Report of the DLB Consortium. Neurology 2005; **65**: 1863–72.

6. **Emre M, Aarsland D, Brown R, et al**. Clinical diagnostic criteria for dementia associated with Parkinson disease. Mov Disord 2007; **22**: 1689–707.

7. **Dubois B, Feldman HH, Jacova C, et al**. Research criteria for the diagnosis of Alzheimer's disease: revising the NINCDS-ADRDA criteria. Lancet Neurol 2007; **6**: 734–46.

8. **Cohen-Mansfield J**. Non-pharmacological management of DLB. In O'Brien J, McKeith I, Ames D, et al. (ed.), *Dementia with Lewy bodies*. Taylor and Francis London, 2005; pp. 103–206.

9. **Hindle JV, Petrelli A, Clare L, et al**. Nonpharmacological enhancement of cognitive function in Parkinson's disease: a systematic review. Mov Disord 2013; **28**: 1034–49.

10. **París AP, Saleta HG, de la Cruz Crespo Maraver M, et al**. Blind randomized controlled study of the efficacy of cognitive training in Parkinson's disease. Mov Disord 2011; **26**: 1251–8.

11. **Tiroboschi P, Hansen LA, Alford M, et al**. Cholinergic dysfunction in diseases with Lewy bodies. Neurology 2000; **54**: 407–11.

12. **Hutchinson M, Fazzini E**. Cholinesterase inhibitors in Parkinson's disease. J Neurol Neurosurg Psychiatry 1996; **61**: 324–5.

13. **McKeith I, Del Ser T, Spano PF, et al**. Efficacy of rivastigmine in dementia with Lewy bodies: a randomised, double-blind, placebo-controlled international study. Lancet 2000; **356**: 2031–6.

14. **Del-Ser T, McKeith I, Anand R, et al**. Dementia with Lewy bodies: findings from an international multicentre study. Int J Geriatr Psychiatry 2000; **15**: 1034–45.

15. **Grace J, Daniel S, Stevens T, et al.** Long-term use of rivastigmine in patients with dementia with Lewy bodies: an open-label trial. Int Psychogeriatr 2001; **13**: 199–205.

16. **Emre M, Aarsland D, Albanese A, et al.** Rivastigmine for dementia associated with Parkinson's disease. N Engl J Med 2004; **351**: 2509–18.

17. **Poewe W, Wolters E, Emre M, et al.** Long-term benefits of rivastigmine in dementia associated with Parkinson's disease: an active treatment extension study. Mov Disord 2006; **21**: 456–61.

18. **Oertel W, Poewe W, Wolters E, et al.** Effects of rivastigmine on tremor and other motor symptoms in patients with Parkinson's disease dementia–a retrospective analysis of a double-blind trial and an open-label extension. Drug Safety 2008; **31**: 79–94.

19. **Dubois B, Tolosa E, Katzenschlager R et al.** Donepezil in Parkinson's disease dementia: a randomized, double-blind efficacy and safety study Mov Disord 2012; **27**: 1230–8.

20. **Mori E, Ikeda M, Kosaka K** on behalf of Donepezil-DLB Study Investigators. Donepezil for dementia with Lewy bodies: a randomized, placebo-controlled trial. Ann Neurol 2012; **72**: 41–52.

21. **Ikeda M, Mori E, Kosaka K. et al** on behalf of Donepezil-DLB Study Investigators. Long-term safety and efficacy of donepezil in patients with dementia with Lewy bodies: results from a 52-week, open-label, multicenter extension study. Dem Ger Cog Disord 2013; **36**: 229–41.

22. **Perry EK, McKeith I, Thompson P, et al.** Topography, extent, and clinical relevance of neurochemical deficits in dementia of Lewy body type, Parkinson's disease and Alzheimer's disease. Ann NY Acad Sci 1991; **640**: 197–202.

23. **Wesnes KA, McKeith IG, Ferrara R, et al.** Effects of rivastigmine on cognitive function in dementia with Lewy bodies: a randomised placebo-controlled international study using the Cognitive Drug Research computerised assessment system. Dementia Geriatr Cogn Dis 2002; **13**: 183–92.

24. **Wesnes KA, McKeith I, Edgar C, et al.** Benefits of rivastigmine on attention in dementia associated with Parkinson disease. Neurology 2005; **65**: 1654–6.

25. **O'Brien KK, Saxby BK, Ballard CG, et al.** Regulation of attention and response to therapy in dementia by butyrylcholinesterase. Pharmacogenetics 2003; **13**: 231–9.

26. **Thomas AJ, Burn DJ, Rowan EN, et al.** A comparison of the efficacy of donepezil in Parkinson's disease with dementia and dementia with Lewy bodies. Int J Geriatr Psychiatry 2005; **20**: 938–44.

27. **Minett TSC, Thomas A, Wilkinson LM, et al.** What happens when donepezil is suddenly withdrawn? An open label trial in dementia with Lewy bodies and Parkinson's disease with dementia. Int J Geriatr Psychiatry 2003; **18**: 988–93.

28. **Bhanji NH, Gauthier S.** Dementia with Lewy bodies: preliminary observations on cholinesterase inhibitor switching. Int Psychogeriatrics 2003; **15**: 179.

29. **Bhasin M, Rowan E, Edwards K, et al.** Cholinesterase inhibitors in dementia with Lewy bodies–a comparative analysis. Int J Geriatr Psychiatry 2007; **22**: 890–5.

30. **Ridha BH, Josephs KA, Rossor MN.** Delusions and hallucinations in dementia with Lewy bodies: worsening with memantine. Neurology 2005; **65**: 481–2.

31. **Sabbagh M, Hake A, Ahmed S, et al.** The use of memantine in dementia with Lewy bodies. J Alzheimers Dis 2005; **7**: 285–9.

32. **Leroi I, Overshott R, Byrne EJ, et al.** Randomized, controlled trial of memantine in dementia associated with Parkinson's disease. Mov Disord 2009; **24**: 1217–21.

33. **Aarsland D, Ballard C, Walker Z, et al.** Memantine in patients with Parkinson's disease dementia or dementia with Lewy bodies: a double-blind, placebo controlled, multicentre trial. Lancet Neurol 2009; **8**: 613–18.

34. **Emre M, Tsolaki M, Bonuccelli U, et al.** Memantine for patients with Parkinson's disease dementia or dementia with Lewy bodies: a randomised, double-blind, placebo-controlled trial. Lancet Neurol 2010; **9**: 969–77.

35. **Molloy S, McKeith I, O'Brien JT, et al.** The role of levodopa in the management of dementia with Lewy bodies. J Neurol Neurosurg Psychiatry 2005; **76**: 1200–3.

36. **Aarsland D, Larsen JP, Karlsen K, et al.** Mental symptoms in Parkinson's disease are important contributors to caregiver stress. Int J Geriatr Psychiatry 1999; **14**: 866–74.

37. **Bostrom F, Jonsson L, Minthon L, et al.** Patients with dementia with Lewy bodies have more impaired quality of life than patients with Alzheimer disease. Alzheimers Dis Assoc Disord 2007; **21**: 150–4.

38. **Bostrom F, Jonsson L, Minthon L, et al.** Patients with Lewy body dementia use more resources than those with Alzheimer's disease. Int J Geriatr Psychiatry 2007; **22**: 713–19.

39. **McKeith IG, Fairbairn AF, Perry RH, et al.** Neuroleptic sensitivity in patients with senile dementia of Lewy body type Br Med J 1992; **305**: 673–8.

40. **Ballard C, Grace J, McKeith I, et al.** Neuroleptic sensitivity in dementia with Lewy bodies and Alzheimer's disease Lancet 1998; **35**: 1032–3.

41. **Aarsland D, Ballard C, Larsen JP, et al.** Marked neuroleptic sensitivity in dementia with Lewy bodies and Parkinson's disease. J Clin Psychiatry 2005; **66**: 633–7.

42. **McKeith IG, Ballard CG, Harrison RWS.** Neuroleptic sensitivity to risperidone in Lewy body dementia. Lancet 1995; **346**: 699.

43. **Walker Z, Grace J, Overshot R, et al.** Olanzapine in dementia with Lewy bodies: a clinical study. Int J Geriatr Psychiatry 1999; **14**: 459–66.

44. **Kurlan R, Cummings J, Raman R, et al.** Quetiapine for agitation or psychosis in patients with dementia and parkinsonism. Neurology 2007; **68**: 1356–63.

45. **Burke WJ, Pfeiffer RF, McComb RD.** Neuroleptic sensitivity to clozapine in dementia with Lewy bodies. J Neuropsychiatry Clin Neurosci 1998; **10**: 227–9.

46. **Harrison RH, McKeith IG.** Senile dementia of Lewy body type—a review of clinical and pathological features: implications for treatment. Int J Geriatr Psychiatry 1995; **10**: 919–26.

47. **Iwasaki K, Kosaka K, Mori H, et al.** Improvement in delusions and hallucinations in patients with dementia with Lewy bodies upon administration of a traditional Japanese medicine. Psychogeriatrics 2012; **12**: 235–41.

48. **Weintraub D, Morales KH, Moberg PJ, et al.** Antidepressant studies in Parkinson's disease: a review and meta-analysis. Mov Disord 2005; **20**: 1161–9.

49. **Miyasaki JM, Shannon K, Voon V, et al.** Practice parameter: evaluation and treatment of depression, psychosis, and dementia in Parkinson disease (an evidence-based review). Report of the Quality Standards Subcommittee of the American Academy of Neurology. Neurology 2006; **66**: 996–1002.

50. **Devos D, Dujardin K, Poirot I, et al.** Comparison of desipramine and citalopram treatments for depression in Parkinson's disease: a double-blind, randomized, placebo-controlled study. Mov Disord 2008; **23**: 850–7.

51. **Menza M, Dobkin RD, Marin H, et al.** A controlled trial of antidepressants in patients with Parkinson disease and depression. Neurology 2009; **72**: 886–92.

52. **Richard IH, McDermott MP, Kurlan R, et al.** A randomized, double-blind, placebo-controlled trial of antidepressants in Parkinson disease. Neurology 2012; **78**: 1229–36.

53. **Barone P, Poewe W, Albrecht S, et al.** Pramipexole for the treatment of depressive symptoms in patients with Parkinson's disease: a randomised, double-blind, placebo-controlled trial. Lancet Neurol 2010; **9**: 573–80.

54. **Sharp SI, Ballard CG, Ziabreva I, et al.** Cortical serotonin 1a receptor levels are associated with depression in patients with dementia with Lewy bodies and Parkinson's disease dementia. Dementia Geriatr Cogn Disord 2008; **26**: 330–8.

55. **Boeve B, Silber M, Ferman T, et al.** Association of REM sleep behavior disorder and neuro-degenerative disease may reflect an underlying synucleinopathy. Mov Disord 2001; **16**: 622–30.

56. **Olson EJ, Boeve BF, Silber MH.** Rapid eye movement sleep behaviour disorder: demographic, clinical and laboratory findings in 93 cases. Brain 2000; **123**: 331–9.

57. **Lapierre O, Montplaisir J.** Polysomnographic features of REM-sleep behavior disorder–development of a scoring method. Neurology 1992; **42**: 1371–4.

58. **Boeve BF, Silber MH, Ferman TJ.** Melatonin for treatment of REM sleep behavior disorder in neurologic disorders: results in 14 patients. Sleep Med 2003; **4**: 281–4.

59. **Larsson V, Aarsland D, Ballard C, et al.** The effect of memantine on sleep behaviour in dementia with Lewy bodies and Parkinson's disease dementia. Int J Psychogeriatr 2010; **25**: 1030–8.

60. **Adler CH, Caviness JN, Hentz JG, et al.** Randomized trial of modafinil for treating subjective daytime sleepiness in patients with Parkinson's disease. Mov Disord 2003; **18**: 287–93.

61. **Hogl B, Saletu M, Brandauer E, et al.** Modafinil for the treatment of daytime sleepiness in Parkinson's disease: a double-blind, randomized, crossover, placebo-controlled polygraphic trial. Sleep 2002; **25**: 905–9.

62. **Prado E, Paholpak P, Ngo M, et al.** Agitation and psychosis associated with dementia with Lewy bodies exacerbated by modafinil use. Am J Alzheimers Dis Other Demen 2012; **27**; 468–73.

63. **Boeve B, Kuntz K, Drubach D, et al.** Safety, tolerability, and efficacy of armodafinil therapy for hypersomnia associated with dementia with Lewy bodies. Mov Disord 2012; **27**(Suppl. 1): 62.

Chapter 22

Parkinson's disease: what will the future bring?

John Hardy

Introduction

Predicting the future is a notorious a way to ensure that you appear foolish in 20 years' time. However, it is now more than 50 years since the discovery of the effects of levodopa in reserpinized (dopamine-depleted) animals and nearly 50 years since the first human levodopa treatment trials [1]. Hence it is perhaps worth taking stock of progress and thinking about how things might progress from here.

Since the miracle of dopamine replacement therapy, there has been incremental improvement in the pharmacological treatment of Parkinson's disease (PD), first with peripheral decarboxylase inhibition and then dopamine agonists [2]. Surgical therapies, too, had initially startling clinical effects, and have subsequently shown steady progress [3]. Neither current medical nor surgical interventions are believed to have any effects on the progression of the neurodegenerative process. In early disease, initial therapy leads to remarkable benefits. Indeed, dopaminergic therapy has more than doubled the life expectancy of patients after their diagnosis [4].

Despite this I am sure that the current situation leads to great frustration among patients and caregivers. In nearly all other neurodegenerative diseases, patients get the diagnosis, for example Alzheimer's disease (AD), motor neuron disease, or Huntington's disease, and are told, at diagnosis, that there is no effective treatment to halt disease progression. While this is a cruel outcome, there is no arguing with it. Currently, there are no effective treatments for these diseases and patients and their families cope with that outcome as best they can. With PD, early treatment really is miraculous and, for a period of a few years, it allows patients and their families to return to a near-normal life. Yet the effectiveness of this treatment gradually and frustratingly lessens and the disease gains the upper hand, finally leading to disability and death in a manner no less unpleasant than that caused by the less-teasing diseases which have no treatment at all. It must seem to patients and caregivers that we are close to 'curing' the disease, and yet, of course, we are not.

Since it seems likely that only incremental improvements are going to be made through either further advances in dopaminergic drugs or surgical treatment, clearly we need to make substantive progress towards either preventing the disease or in mechanistic therapy. It is in this area that we have to hope we can make progress.

Progress towards understanding disease mechanisms

Over the past 10 years we have made enormous advances in understanding some of the genetic causes of PD [5] (Table 22.1). A large number of genes have been discovered which, when mutated, lead either to clinically defined PD or to Lewy body disease. Together, mutations in these

Table 22.1 Loci for parkinsonism and Lewy body disease

Locus (OMIM)	Gene	Mode of inheritance	Pathology	Comments
PARK1 (168601)	*SNCA*	Dominant	Lewy bodies	Point mutations and gene duplications
PARK2 (600116)	*PARK2*	Recessive	Usually no Lewy bodies	Loss of function variants
PARK6 (605909)	*PINK1*	Recessive	Not known	Loss of function variants
PARK7 (606324)	*DJ1*	Recessive	Not known	Loss of function variants
PARK8 (607060)	*LRRK2*	Dominant	Usually, but not always Lewy bodies	Variable pathology is a real puzzle
PARK9 (610513)	*ATP13A2*	Recessive	Not known	
	VPS35	Dominant	Not known	Not known
Parkinson—pyramidal syndrome	*FBXO7*	Recessive	Not known	
Gaucher's disease	*GBA*	Recessive for Gaucher's, risk locus (OR ~ 5) for PD	Lewy bodies	PD has Lewy bodies, Gaucher's disease cases also have Lewy bodies
NBIA1 (234200)	*PANK2*	Recessive	Tangle pathology	Variable phenotype: later-onset cases have levodopa-responsive parkinsonian dystonia
INAD1/NBIA2 (256600)	*PLA2G6*	Recessive	Lewy bodies: often brain iron	Identical to above: parkinsonian disorder
Neimann–Pick C type 1 (607623)	*NPC1*	Recessive	Lewy bodies and tangles	Neuropathology includes both Lewy bodies and tangles
MAPT (260540)	*MAPT*	Autosomal dominant and complex	Tangles, but contributes to risk of Lewy body disease	Autosomal dominant disease has tangle-like inclusions: haplotype predisposes to PSP and Lewy body PD

PD, Parkinson's disease; OR, odds ratio; PSP, progressive supranuclear palsy.

The numbers in the brackets refer to the OMIM number for the syndrome.

Reprinted from Curr Opin Genet Dev, 19, Hardy J, Lewis P, Revesz, T, Lees, AJ, Paisan Ruiz C, The genetics of Parkinson's syndromes: a critical review, 254–65, Copyright (2009), with permission from Elsevier.

genes explain a small but significant proportion of the risk of getting PD. This proportion is perhaps 5% in general European populations, but as much as 30% in Ashkenazi Jews or the North African Berber population [6, 7].

The general belief is that these genes should map out one or more pathways to disease—based on an analogy with AD where the three autosomal dominant genes map onto a pathway of amyloid precursor protein (APP) metabolism [8] (see Table 22.2).

Over the last few years we have come to see that some, at least, of these genes map to defined pathways. The best evidence relating to at least one pathway to disease is for *PINK1*, *PARK2* (*parkin*), and *FBXO7* [9–11]. It is clear from cell biology and from work in *Drosophila* that these genes are involved in a mitochondrial pathway to disease, and that *PARK2* is downstream in this pathway. However, *PARK2* cases do not have Lewy bodies and it has been argued that we should use a pathological, rather than a clinical, definition of disease [5]. On this basis, I would contend that whereas this work clearly sketched a pathway to parkinsonism, it is unlikely to be the pathway which is operating in that vast majority of people with disease who have Lewy body pathology [13].

Most of the other genes for PD affect more neuronal regions than *PINK1* and *PARK2* mutations, which are very selective for the substantia nigra. *SNCA*, *LRRK2*, *GBA*, and the other genes from Table 22.1 affect a much wider range of neurons, and are usually, though not always, associated with Lewy body pathology. It is not yet entirely clear which pathway(s) these genes map to, but it is certain that many (e.g. *GBA*, *ATP13A2*) are lysosomal; an increasing amount of evidence suggests that autophagy is the process to which they all contribute [13]. Since mitophagy is the process in which *PINK1* and *PARK2* are involved, the notion that the broader disease is associated with a defect in the general process of autophagy rather than the specific process of mitophagy has appeal. This is currently an active area of research and we can expect considerable process from both cell biological investigations and the identification of more genes involved in the disorder from genome-wide association studies.

From mechanism to treatment

Let us suppose that very soon we will have developed a reasonably clear understanding of the biochemical pathways which appear to be dysregulated in typical PD with Lewy bodies. Then our task will be to try to interfere in this pathway and to design clinical trials to test these potential therapies. At that stage we will want to design small molecules to intervene in those pathways and to start to think about designing clinical trials to slow disease progression. Both of these are formidable undertakings. A comparison of AD research and PD research (Table 22.2) really shows the magnitude of this task. Mechanistic PD research started 13 years later than mechanistic AD research, and we are, optimistically, still several years away from the first mechanistic therapies for AD.

Our current problems are clearly both practical (so far we have no good animal model of the disease) and philosophical (there is no generally agreed pathway to disease). Furthermore, we should not forget that AD research has not yet led to disease-modifying treatments, and currently AD researchers are worrying that trials of mechanistic therapies will need to be long and will therefore be extremely expensive to run. Additionally therapies need to be tested in individuals who are at a very early stage in the disease, possibly even completely asymptomatic. I think, therefore, that we are facing a rather distressing paradox. It would seem likely that we are more than a decade away from mechanistic therapies. From a practical perspective this means that we have nothing to offer anyone who currently has the disease except the hope that future generations will not suffer as they are suffering. While to the patient and the caregiver it seems as if we need just one more push to cure the disease, the truth is that this goal is still beyond the horizon.

Table 22.2 Progress and problems on the road to Alzheimer disease (AD) therapies: comparison with Parkinson's disease (PD)

Year	Progress	Comment	Lesson
1984	Aβ identified	α-Synuclein identified in 1997	PD started 13 years behind
1991	APP mutations identified	α-Synuclein mutations identified in 1993	
1992	Amyloid hypothesis	As yet no PD equivalent	
1995	Presenilin genes discovered	Many other PD genes discovered	Note that AD was defined by pathology
1995	Animal model with some pathology made	AD model was incomplete, but it did at least have plaques	As yet no generally accepted pathological model of PD has been developed
1998	Presenilins shown to be involved in APP metabolism as γ-secretase	Connection between any two parkinsonism genes has yet been found	
1998	Delineation of other elements of APP metabolism such as BACE as other targets for intervention		No parkinsonism equivalent as yet
1998	*MAPT* mutations found in FTD	Led to mice with other pathological elements being developed and eventually to heavily engineered mice with full pathology	
1999	Aβ immunization works in mice	Probably an accidental finding, but depended on having mice with pathology	
2003	First active human vaccination trial halted because of immunogenic side effects		
2008	Ambivalent phase 2 results reported on passive Aβ antibody trial. Phase 3 trials of this and other agents begin		
2009	Planning stages of next-generation compounds. Drug companies start to plan other approaches such as anti-tau therapies using mice with tangles	The following are the present concerns: Are the AD trials beginning early enough in the disease? Does the amyloid hypothesis relate only to the autosomal dominant form of the disease? How long should a trial be to show disease modification?	We need to be ready with cohorts of high-risk genetically defined individuals so that we can organize trials in defined and characterized individuals

Table 22.2 (continued) Progress and problems on the road to Alzheimer disease (AD) therapies: comparison with Parkinson's disease (PD)

Year	Progress	Comment	Lesson
2012	Planned reporting of passive immunization trial: phase 3 trials at least 3 years behind this	28 years from amyloid identification	

Aβ, amyloid-beta; APP, amyloid precursor protein; BACE, β-secretase; FTD, frontotemporal dementia.

Reprinted from Neuron, 52, Hardy J, A hundred years of Alzheimer's disease research, 3–13, Copyright (2006), with permission from Elsevier.

References

1. **Honykiewicz O.** Dopamine miracle, from brain homogenate to dopamine replacement. Mov Disord 2002; **17**: 501–8.

2. **Schapira AH, Olanow CW.** Drug selection and timing of initiation of treatment in early Parkinson's disease. Ann Neurol 2008; **64**(Suppl. 2): S47–S55.

3. **Benabid AL, Chabardès S, Seigneuret E, et al.** Surgical therapy for Parkinson's disease. J Neural Transm 2006; **70**(Suppl.): 383–92.

4. **Gwinn-Hardy K, Evidente VG, et al.** L-dopa slows the progression of familial parkinsonism. Lancet 1999; **353**: 1850–1.

5. **Hardy J, Lewis P, Revesz, T, et al.** The genetics of Parkinson's syndromes: a critical review. Curr Opin Genet Dev 2009; **19**: 254–65.

6. **Clark LN, Wang Y, Karlins E, et al.** Frequency of LRRK2 mutations in early- and late-onset Parkinson disease. Neurology 2006; **67**: 1786–91.

7. **Clark LN, Ross BM, Wang Y, et al.** Mutations in the glucocerebrosidase gene are associated with early-onset Parkinson disease. Neurology 2007; **69**: 1270–7.

8. **Hardy J.** A hundred years of Alzheimer's disease research. Neuron 2006; **52**: 3–13.

9. **Park J, Lee SB, Lee S, et al.** Mitochondrial dysfunction in Drosophila PINK1 mutants is complemented by parkin. Nature 2006; **441**: 1157–61.

10. **Clark IE, Dodson MW, Jiang C, et al.** Drosophila pink1 is required for mitochondrial function and interacts genetically with parkin. Nature 2006; **441**: 1162–6.

11. **Burchell VS, Nelson DE, Sanchez-Martinez A, et al.** The Parkinson's disease-linked proteins Fbxo7 and Parkin interact to mediate mitophagy. Nat Neurosci 2013; **16**: 1257–65.

12. **Hughes AJ, Daniel SE, Ben-Shlomo Y, et al.** The accuracy of diagnosis of parkinsonian syndromes in a specialist movement disorder service. Brain 2002; **125**: 861–70.

13. **Manzoni C, Lewis PA.** Dysfunction of the autophagy/lysosomal degradation pathway is a shared feature of the genetic synucleinopathies. FASEB J 2013; **27**: 3424–9.

Index